# EEG Primer

# EEG Primer


**R. SPEHLMANN**

*Professor of Neurology*
*Northwestern University Medical School*
*Director of EEG Laboratories*
*VA Lakeside Medical Center, Chicago*
*and Evanston Hospital, Evanston, Illinois, U.S.A.*



ELSEVIER BIOMEDICAL PRESS — AMSTERDAM • NEW YORK • OXFORD

ISBN – hardbound: 0-444-80260-6
– paperback: 0-444-80299-1

First edition: 1981
Second printing: 1982
Third printing: 1985
Fourth printing: 1987
Fifth printing: 1987

Published by:
Elsevier Biomedical Press
P.O. Box 211
1000 AE Amsterdam, The Netherlands

Sole distributors for the U.S.A. and Canada:
Elsevier Science Publishing Company, Inc.
52 Vanderbilt Avenue
New York, N.Y. 10017

**Library of Congress Cataloging in Publication Data**

Main entry under title:

EEG primer.

Includes bibliographies and index.
1. Electroencephalography. I. Spehlmann, Rainer, 1931- [DNLM: 1. Electroencephalography. WL 150 E104]
RC386.6.E43E15 616.8'047547 80-26037
ISBN 0-444-80260-6 (Elsevier North-Holland)

PRINTED IN THE NETHERLANDS

# Preface

This book is written mainly for beginners in EEG. It may help several groups: Resident physicians who are in neurology training and need to learn EEG interpretation as part of this training; residents in other fields, interns and medical students who have become interested in EEG; neuroscientists who wish to understand the methods and clinical applications of EEG; EEG technicians who want to gain more insight into the test they perform; and anyone who wants to find out how clinical EEG is done and what it can do. On the other hand, even persons with some experience in EEG may find the book useful because it leads to fairly advanced levels. To make learning easier for the beginner, several methods have been adopted:

(1) Explanations start with simple concepts and build up in steps following an order which generally corresponds with the steps of recording and reading an EEG.

(2) The reader can choose the depth at which he wishes to master a topic. Each chapter is preceded by a summary. Reading all summaries takes from one to two hours and gives a rough overview of clinical EEG. Each part of the summary refers to numbered sections of the text which expand on the summarized material. Each section presents the most important material at the start and then gives the details, allowing the reader to go as far as desired.

(3) The book adopts widely accepted standards wherever they are available. The text is written in the terminology recommended by the International Federation of Societies for EEG and Clinical Neurophysiology. It incorporates the guidelines of the American EEG Society for proper EEG recording. The sections on epileptiform patterns conform with the international classification of epileptic seizures recently endorsed by federations of several societies.

(4) The clinical correlation of the EEG reverses the conventional order of listing diseases and describing the attendant EEG abnormalities. In this text, abnormal EEG patterns are described first and then correlated with clinical abnormalities. This method is chosen because it corresponds with the situation of the EEG reader who faces an EEG pattern and searches for its clinical correlates. Although this approach leads to repetition of some diseases under the heading of several EEG patterns, it causes much less repetition than the conventional method which repeats a few EEG abnormalities under the headings of many different diseases. The various EEG manifestations of a disease can be found through cross-references in the text and through the index.

(5) The main goal of this text is a didactic presentation of clinical EEG and its role in the diagnosis of cerebral disorders. Therefore, I have favored the established over the controversial and preferred modern insights to historical details. References for suggested reading are listed at the end of each chapter. They emphasize the more recent publications through which the reader may find the older ones.

It is a pleasure to acknowledge the many sources of help I have had in writing this book. I thank the residents, students and technicans who I taught EEG reading; they asked many of the questions which I tried to answer in this text. Dr. Donald W. Klass reviewed the manuscript and gave me his critical advice. Special thanks are due to Dr. Karyl Norcross who thoroughly revised several drafts of the text. Mr. Clifford C. Smathers helped me to design the technical illustrations. Mrs. Thelma Howell typed the manuscript without ever tiring.

# Contents

*Preface* *v*

## *Part A: Technical background*

*Introduction* *3*

1 *The source of the EEG* *7*

1.1 The generator of the EEG 7
1.2 Rhythmical EEG activity 13
1.3 Recording of electrical potentials with scalp electrodes 15

2 *Recording electrodes* *21*

2.1 Electrode shapes and application methods 21
2.2 Electrical properties of recording electrodes 26
2.3 Electrode placement 30

3 *The EEG machine: Parts and functions* *37*

3.1 The input board 38
3.2 Input selector switches 39
3.3 Calibration 40
3.4 The amplifiers 41
3.5 Filters 49
3.6 Writing units 57

4 *Recording strategy* *63*

4.1 Multichannel recordings 63
4.2 Specific montages 72
4.3 Electrode combinations for monitoring of extracerebral activity 75

5 *The product of the recording: The clinical EEG record* *83*

5.1 General technical standards 85
5.2 Standards for recordings from infants and small children 92
5.3 Standards for all-night sleep recordings 95
5.4 Standards for recordings in cases of suspected cerebral death 96
5.5 Telephone transmission 101

6 *Artifacts* *105*

6.1 Artifacts from the patient 105
6.2 Interference 113
6.3 Artifacts from recording electrodes and equipment 115

7 *Other methods of recording and analysis* *119*

7.1 Oscilloscope displays 119
7.2 Telemetry and portable magnetic tape recordings 120
7.3 Magnetic tape recording 121
7.4 Computer analysis 122
7.5 Computer analysis of spontaneous EEG 123
7.6 Computer averaging of evoked potentials: General techniques 128

*Part B: The normal EEG*

8 *Definition of the normal EEG, relation to brain function* *143*

8.1 Definition of the normal EEG 143
8.2 A normal EEG does not always mean normal brain function 145

8.3 An abnormal EEG does not necessarily mean abnormal brain function 145

9 *Descriptors of EEG activity* *147*

9.1 Wave form 147
9.2 Repetition 150
9.3 Frequency 150
9.4 Amplitude 152
9.5 Distribution 153
9.6 Phase 154
9.7 Timing 155
9.8 Persistence 156
9.9 Reactivity 156

10 *The normal EEG from premature age to the age of 19 years* *159*

10.1 Premature infants of 24 to 27 weeks of conceptional age 159
10.2 Premature infants of 28 to 31 weeks of conceptional age 161
10.3 Premature infants of 32 to 35 weeks of conceptional age 161
10.4 Premature infants of 36 to 40 weeks of conceptional age 163
10.5 Infants from full term to 3 months of age 165
10.6 Infants of 3 to 12 months of age 170
10.7 Infants, children and adolescents from 1 to 19 years of age 177
10.8 Major abnormalities 179

11 *The normal EEG of wakeful resting adults of 20 to 60 years of age* *183*

11.1 Alpha rhythm 183
11.2 Beta rhythms 189
11.3 Mu rhythm 191
11.4 Lambda waves 193
11.5 Vertex sharp transients (V waves) 193
11.6 Kappa rhythm 194
11.7 Normal posterior theta rhythms 194
11.8 The low voltage EEG 195
11.9 Major abnormalities 195

12 *The normal sleep EEG of adults over 20 years* 201

12.1 Elements of normal sleep activity 201
12.2 Sleep stages 203
12.3 Sleep cycles 207
12.4 Major abnormalities 208

13 *The normal EEG of adults over 60 years of age* 213

13.1 Alpha rhythm 213
13.2 Beta rhythm 214
13.3 Sporadic generalized slow waves 214
13.4 Intermittent temporal slow waves 215
13.5 Sleep stages 217
13.6 Major abnormalities 217

14 *Activation procedures* 219

14.1 Hyperventilation 219
14.2 Sleep 222
14.3 Photic stimulation 223
14.4 Other stimuli 227
14.5 Pentylene tetrazol, bemegride and other convulsant drugs 228

*Part C: The abnormal EEG*

*15 Abnormal EEG patterns, correlation with underlying cerebral lesions and neurological diseases* 235

15.1 Definition of the abnormal EEG 235
15.2 Correlation between abnormal EEG patterns, general cerebral pathology and specific neurological diseases 236
15.3 The diagnostic value of the EEG 240

## 16 *Classification of seizures* *245*

16.1 Definitions 245
16.2a Classification of seizures—General 247
16.2b Classification of seizures—Specific 250

## 17 *Localized epileptiform patterns* *261*

17.1 Description of patterns 262
17.2 Clinical significance of focal epileptiform activity 268
17.3 Other EEG abnormalities associated with focal epileptiform activity 272
17.4 Grading of focal epileptiform activity 275
17.5 Mechanisms underlying focal epileptiform activity 275
17.6 Specific disorders causing focal epileptiform activity 277

## 18 *Generalized epileptiform patterns* *285*

18.1 Description of patterns 286
18.2 Clinical significance of generalized epileptiform activity 298
18.3 Other EEG abnormalities associated with generalized epileptiform activity 301
18.4 Grading of generalized epileptiform activity 302
18.5 Mechanisms underlying generalized epileptiform activity 302
18.6 Specific disorders causing generalized epileptiform activity 304

## 19 *Special epileptiform patterns* *309*

19.1 The infantile and juvenile patterns of hypsarrhythmia, slow spike-and-wave discharges and multifocal independent spikes 309
19.2 Periodic complexes 317
19.3 Ictal patterns without spikes and sharp waves 327
19.4 Epileptiform patterns without proven relation to seizures ('pseudo-epileptogenic patterns') 331

## 20 *Local slow waves* *341*

20.1 Description of pattern 341

20.2 Clinical significance of local slow waves 344
20.3 Other EEG abnormalities associated with focal slow waves 347
20.4 Grading of focal slow waves 351
20.5 Mechanisms causing focal slow waves 351
20.6 Specific disorders causing local slow waves 352

21 *Generalized asynchronous slow waves* *359*

21.1 Description of pattern 359
21.2 General clinical significance of generalized asynchronous slow waves 364
21.3 Other EEG abnormalities associated with generalized asynchronous slow waves 365
21.4 Grading of generalized asynchronous slow waves 365
21.5 Mechanisms causing generalized asynchronous slow waves 366
21.6 Specific disorders causing generalized asynchronous slow waves 366

22 *Bilaterally synchronous slow waves* *379*

22.1 Description of pattern 381
22.2 Clinical significance of bisynchronous slow waves 386
22.3 Other EEG abnormalities associated with bisynchronous slow waves 387
22.4 Grading of bisynchronous slow waves 388
22.5 Mechanisms causing bisynchronous slow waves 388
22.6 Specific disorders causing bilaterally synchronous slow waves 389

23 *Localized and lateralized changes of amplitude: Asymmetries* *397*

23.1 Description of pattern 397
23.2 Clinical significance of asymmetries 401
23.3 Other abnormalities associated with asymmetries 402
23.4 Grading of asymmetries 403
23.5 Mechanisms causing local changes of amplitude 403
23.6 Specific disorders causing asymmetries of amplitude 404
23.7 Asymmetries of alpha, beta, mu and other rhythms 410

24 *Generalized changes of amplitude: Symmetrically high and low amplitude* *415*

24.1 Description of patterns 418
24.2 Clinical significance of high and low amplitude 419
24.3 Other EEG abnormalities associated with high and low amplitude 420
24.4 Grading of amplitude changes 420
24.5 Mechanisms causing generalized changes of amplitude 420
24.6 Specific disorders causing a generalized decrease of amplitude of all types of activity 422
24.7 Generalized decrease or absence of alpha rhythm 427
24.8 Generalized increase of beta rhythm 428
24.9 Changes of amplitude of sleep patterns 429

25 *Deviations from normal patterns* *431*

25.1 Abnormal frequency of alpha rhythm 431
25.2 Abnormal reactivity of alpha rhythm 437
25.3 Activity of alpha frequency in coma and seizures 438
25.4 Abnormal timing and incidence of sleep patterns 441
25.5 Abnormal photic responses 445
25.6 Immature patterns 449

26 *The EEG report* *451*

26.1 Description of the record 452
26.2 EEG diagnosis 456
26.3 Clinical interpretation 457

*Appendix* *461*

*Subject index* *463*

# Part A
# Technical background

# Introduction

The steps involved in recording an EEG are illustrated in Figure 0.1 and described in Chapters 1 to 7 comprising Part A of this text.

(1) *The Source* of the EEG are electrical potentials generated by nerve cells in the cerebral cortex in response to various kinds of input, including that from pacemakers of rhythmical activity in the depth of the brain. These fluctuating potentials summate and penetrate to the scalp where they can be recorded as the scalp EEG.

(2) *Recording electrodes* usually consist of small metal cups or discs which are attached to the scalp so that they make good mechanical and electrical contact. They cover the surface of the head at regular intervals.

(3) *The EEG machine* receives electrical input from the scalp electrodes which are connected to an input board. The cable of the input board terminates at the input selector switches which are used to select a pair of electrodes, or a calibration voltage, as the input of each recording channel. The input is connected to differential amplifiers which increase the size of the electrical potential differences between the two electrodes and reject interference simultaneously affecting both electrodes. High and low frequency filters are used to reduce the size of very slow and very fast potential changes and to emphasize clinically important electrical activity in the medium frequency range. A 60 Hz filter can eliminate the most common electrical interference in EEG recordings, namely that from power lines, if it cannot be eliminated by other means. The amplified electrical potentials are used to drive an ink pen, or other writing devices, up and down on chart paper which is pulled along at a constant speed.

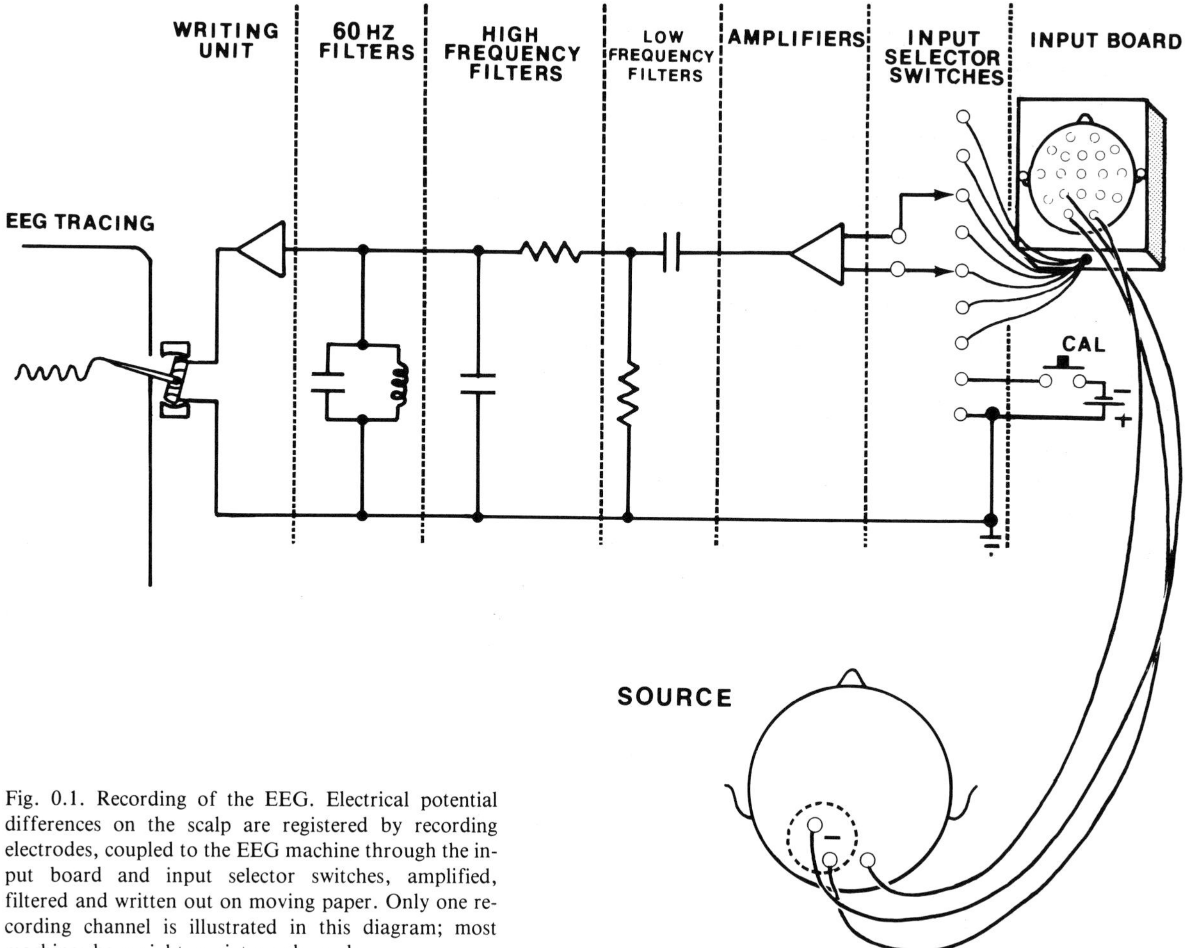


Fig. 0.1. Recording of the EEG. Electrical potential differences on the scalp are registered by recording electrodes, coupled to the EEG machine through the input board and input selector switches, amplified, filtered and written out on moving paper. Only one recording channel is illustrated in this diagram; most machines have eight or sixteen channels.

(4) *Recording strategy* uses several different combinations of electrodes, or montages, to display the potential changes from all parts of the head and to localize the origin of abnormal potential changes.

(5) *The product* of the recording, namely the clinical EEG record, must satisfy a number of technical requirements to be acceptable. Requirements for routine clinical recordings differ from those for recordings from infants and small children, for all-night sleep recordings, for recordings in cases of suspected cerebral death and for recordings transmitted by telephone.

(6) *Artifacts* are pen deflections that are not due to cerebral activity and may come from such extracerebral activity as eye movements, heart beat and muscle contraction or from electrical interference, malfunctioning recording electrodes, or defects of the EEG machine. They must be eliminated or clearly explained to avoid confusion with cerebral activity.

(7) *Other methods of recording and analyzing the EEG* use magnetic tape recorders, computers and other instruments to answer questions which cannot be answered by the conventional method of examining the pages of a paper record.

# The source of the EEG

# 1

SUMMARY

(1.1) *The EEG* is generated by the nerve cells of the cerebral cortex which line the surface of the hemispheres. The fluctuations of electrical potential recorded in the scalp EEG reflect changes of a steady electrical charge on the cell membrane induced by impulses arriving from other cells. These electrical changes summate in the cortex and extend through the coverings of the brain to the scalp. Although the incoming impulses may cause some cortical neurons to give off action potentials to other neurons, these events are extremely brief and contribute little or nothing to the surface EEG.

(1.2) *Rhythmical EEG activity* is probably due to the projection of periodic impulses from a subcortical pacemaker which causes cortical neurons to respond with rhythmical activity. Desynchronization of rhythmical activity may be due to the interaction of other centers with the pacemaking center, the cortex, or both.

(1.3) *Scalp electrodes* record mainly the summated potential changes of neurons in the underlying cortex, favoring slow potential changes generated in large areas near the recording electrode. Scalp electrodes rarely record potentials produced in distant parts of the brain. However, subcortical structures may send synchronizing impulses to the cortex and induce synchronous potential changes in cortical neurons in large parts of the brain. Scalp electrode recordings may also show extracerebral potential changes produced either by biological activity such as eye movements, heart beat and scalp muscle activity, or by interference or defects of the recording equipment.

## 1.1 THE GENERATOR OF THE EEG

The EEG is generated by changes in the electrical charge of the membrane of cortical nerve cells (Fig. 1.1). These neurons, like other nerve cells, have a *resting potential* which is a difference in electrical potential between the interior of the cell and the extracellular space. The resting potential fluctuates as a result of impulses arriving from other neurons at contact points, or synapses, located on the cell body

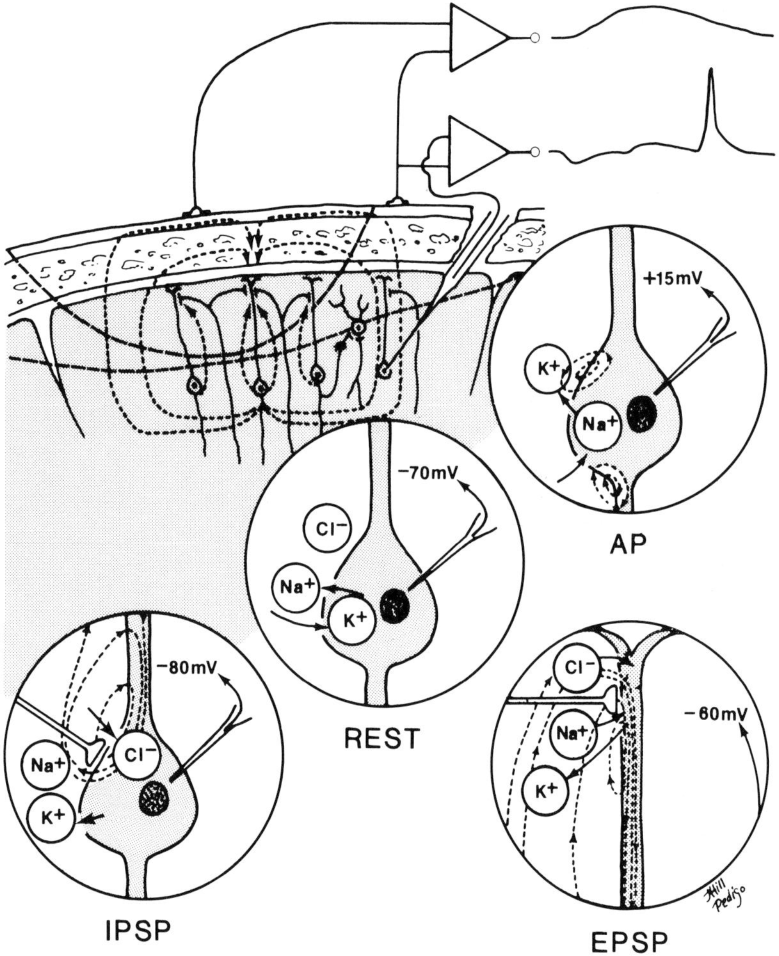


Fig. 1.1. The generation of the EEG by the cerebral cortex. Scalp electrodes record potential differences which are caused by postsynaptic potentials in the membrane of cortical neurons. The closed loops of the lighter dashed lines represent the summation of extracellular currents produced by the postsynaptic potentials; the open segments of heavier dashed lines connect all points having the same voltage level. The two scalp electrodes are at different voltage levels and record this difference, as it changes with time, in the form of a wave which is indicated by the first of the two tracings at the upper right. A simultaneous recording made with a microelectrode from a single cortical neuron is indicated by the second tracing and bears no close relation to the scalp EEG. The round insets show the major ionic and electrical events at single neurons. *REST*: The uneven distribution of ions across the cell membrane, partly maintained by the semipermeable membrane, partly by the active extrusion of sodium ions and intrusion of potassium ions, causes a steady potential difference of 70 mV recordable with an intracellular microelectrode. *IPSP*: An inhibitory postsynaptic potential is caused by activation of an inhibitory synpase on the cell body which transiently increases the permeability of the postsynaptic membrane to potassium and chloride ions and thereby increases the membrane potential, generating electrical current flow of decreasing intensity along the cell membrane. *EPSP*: An excitatory postsynaptic potential, caused by activation of an excitatory synapse on a dendritic process of the neuron, causes a nonselective increase of permeability to ions including sodium ions and thereby transiently decreases the membrane potential locally, generating current flow which tends to depolarize the membrane of the cell body. *AP*: An action potential is initiated at the axon hillock of the cell body by the summation of excitatory postsynaptic potentials which reduce the membrane potential to a level at which the membrane suddenly becomes freely permeable to all ions so that the membrane potential momentarily collapses and reverses; local current flow depolarizes neighboring membrane parts and results in the propagation of an action potential along the membrane of the cell body and axon.

and its processes. Such impulses generate relatively sustained local *postsynaptic potentials* which cause electrical current flow along the membrane of the cell body and dendrites. These changes may reduce the membrane potential to a critical level at which the membrane loses its charge completely, generating an *action potential* of brief duration which is propagated along the axon. The fluctuations in the surface EEG are produced mainly by the temporal and spatial summation of electrical currents caused by the relatively slow postsynaptic potentials with little or no contribution by the brief action potentials.

**1.1.1** *The resting potential* of a neuron measures 50–100 mV and is negative on the inside of the cell membrane with respect to the outside. It is the result of (a) passive and (b) active properties of the cell membrane. (a) *The passive properties* are those which do not require metabolic energy. They result from unequal permeability of the membrane to sodium, potassium, chloride and other ions (Fig. 1). Diffusion and electrical charge tend to drive ions in or out of the cell so that they distribute unevenly on both sides of the membrane, sodium and chloride being more concentrated on the outside and potassium being more concentrated on the inside; this uneven distribution causes a steady difference of electrical potential at rest. (b) *Active properties* require metabolic energy to counteract some leakage of ions across the membrane; leaking ions are continuously transported against diffusional and electrical gradients back to concentrations appropriate for resting conditions. Most important is the active transport of sodium out of the cell, coupled with the transport of potassium into the cell. Conditions which disrupt cerebral metabolism, such as anoxia or ischemia, may reduce or abolish this pumping action of the membrane, causing reduction of the membrane potential which can result in increased excitability or complete collapse of neuronal function.

**1.1.2** *Postsynaptic potentials* in a neuron are caused by impulses arriving from other neurons via axons which terminate in a specialized contact zone, or synapse, located on the cell body or its processes. The impulse in the afferent neuron causes release of a neurotransmitter substance from its nerve terminal which diffuses across the synaptic cleft to the postsynaptic neuronal membrane patch where it interacts with a specialized receptor. The interaction produces a transient change in permeability to some ion species in the membrane portion near the synapse; this causes a local change in the resting potential or a postsynaptic potential (PSP). An *excitatory post*-synaptic potential (EPSP, Fig. 1.1) is a transient partial reduction in membrane potential which is usually due to an increased local permeability to sodium and other ions, whereas an *inhibitory postsynaptic potential* (IPSP, Fig. 1.1) is a transient increase in membrane potential which is usually the result of a local increase of permeability to potassium or chloride ions. The potential difference between the postsynaptic membrane portion and the other parts of the neuronal membrane causes an electrical current to flow along the neuronal membrane and to change the membrane potential of the cell body. Postsynaptic potentials alter the neuronal membrane potential by several millivolts and last for up to over 100 msec. The potentials generated at synapses on different parts of the cell are thus summated in the membrane potential of the cell body. EPSPs decrease the membrane potential or depolarize the cell and make it more likely to fire an action potential; IPSPs increase the membrane potential or hyperpolarize the cell and make it less likely to fire.

**1.1.3** *Action potentials* occur when the neuronal membrane is depolarized beyond a critical level or threshold (Fig. 1.1). This threshold is lowest at the junction of the cell body and the axon, or the axon hillock. A depolarization of the resting potential by about 30 mV at this point triggers a self-limited sequence of events consisting of a brief increase of the membrane permeability to sodium and potassium ions which leads to a sudden collapse, brief reversal and quick restitution of the membrane potential. This electrical change is the action potential; it has an amplitude up to over 100 mV and lasts only about 1 msec. By depolarizing and inducing the same sequence of events in neighboring membrane parts, the action potential spreads as a wave of excitation over the cell membrane; it travels from the axon hillock down to the terminal where the depolarization releases neurotransmitter and causes an EPSP or IPSP in other neurons. The action potential itself causes only a very brief local current which does not penetrate far into the extracellular space.

**1.1.4** *Summation of electrical potential changes in the cortex* occurs mainly at the vertically oriented large pyramidal cells of the cortex. These neurons are especially suited for this role for several reasons. (a) The dendrites of the pyramidal cells extend through nearly all layers of the cortex, guiding the flow of currents generated by postsynaptic potentials at either the cell body in the deep layers of the cortex or at dendrites in the more superficial layers through the entire thickness of the cortex. (b) These neurons are closely packed and oriented parallel to each other, facilitating spatial summation of the currents generated by each neuron. (c) Groups of these neurons receive similar input and respond to it with potential changes of similar direction and timing; the currents generated by these neurons summate in the extracellular space as indicated in Fig. 1.1. Most of the current is limited to the cortex. However, a small fraction penetrates through the meningeal coverings, spinal fluid and skull to the scalp where it causes different parts of the scalp to be at different potential levels. These potential differences, having amplitudes of usually only 10–100 $\mu$V, can be recorded between two electrodes and constitute the EEG.

Although the EEG is a result of neuronal potential changes, it is far too complex to be deciphered in terms of the underlying neuronal events. For instance, a potential change recorded at the scalp may be caused by a potential change of the same polarity produced at dendrites near the surface of the cortex, but it may also be caused by a potential change of the opposite polarity occurring at the cell bodies

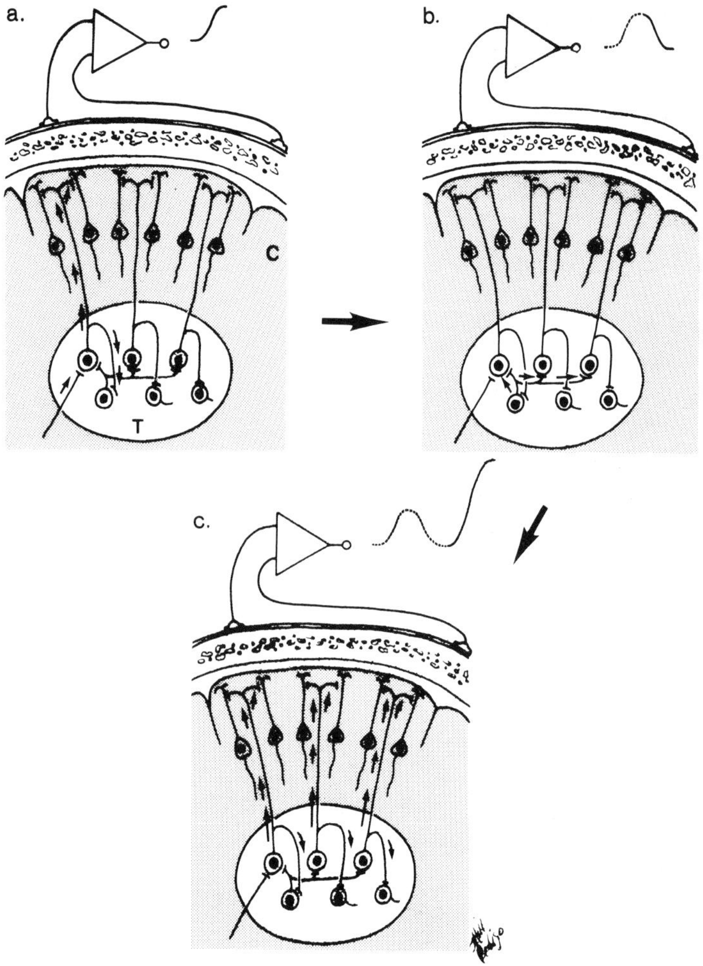


Fig. 1.2. Steps in the production of rhythmical EEG activity in the cortex (C) by impulses from a hypothetical pacemaker in the thalamus (T). – a. A thalamic projection neuron is excited by an afferent and sends an impulse simultaneously to cortical neurons and to an inhibitory thalamic interneuron. Postsynaptic potentials of cortical neurons generate the first deflection in the cortical EEG. – b. The output of the inhibitory thalamic interneuron suppresses the activity of several thalamic projection neurons. The resultant disappearance of postsynaptic potentials at cortical neurons causes the end of the first deflection of the cortical EEG. – c. Several thalamic projection neurons, simultaneously released from inhibition by interneurons, send synchronous impulses to cortical neurons, causing another, larger, deflection of the cortical EEG. Simultaneous impulses to larger numbers of inhibitory thalamic interneurons initiate the next cycle of rhythmical activity.

in the depth of the cortex. Excitation in one place can therefore not be distinguished from inhibition in another place, and the activity of single neurons or specific groups of neurons can only be speculated about. Thus, although the cellular mechanisms which generate the EEG are now rather clearly known, this knowledge cannot be applied directly to the clinical interpretation of EEGs.

## 1.2 RHYTHMICAL EEG ACTIVITY

Although one might expect that the complex neuronal activities of the brain would result in rather irregular EEG waves, the EEG of human subjects, awake and at rest, commonly contains rhythmical potential changes, for instance alpha, beta and mu rhythm (11.1–11.3). Attempts to explain the production of rhythmical activity are based mainly on animal experiments; it is not known whether rhythmical activity in humans is produced in the same manner. The animal experiments indicate that rhythmical activity in the cortex depends on synchronizing impulses from a central pacemaker which generates rhythmical impulses through a network consisting of thalamic projection neurons and thalamic interneurons (Fig. 1.2). Thalamic projection neurons send fibers to most parts of the cerebral cortex; these fibers give off branches which turn back and end on thalamic interneurons. Fibers of thalamic interneurons terminate on several of the projection neurons. The firing of one or a few thalamic projection neurons, in addition to affecting a few cortical neurons, excites thalamic interneurons via recurrent collateral fibers (Fig. 1.2a). The output of the interneurons inhibits a large number of projection neurons (Fig. 1.2b). At the end of the period of inhibition, the pool of projection neurons overshoots into excitation, giving off a volley which is again distributed both to cortical neurons and to inhibitory interneurons (Fig. 1.2c). The interneurons inhibit an even larger number of projection neurons, thus generating another cycle of rhythmical dis-

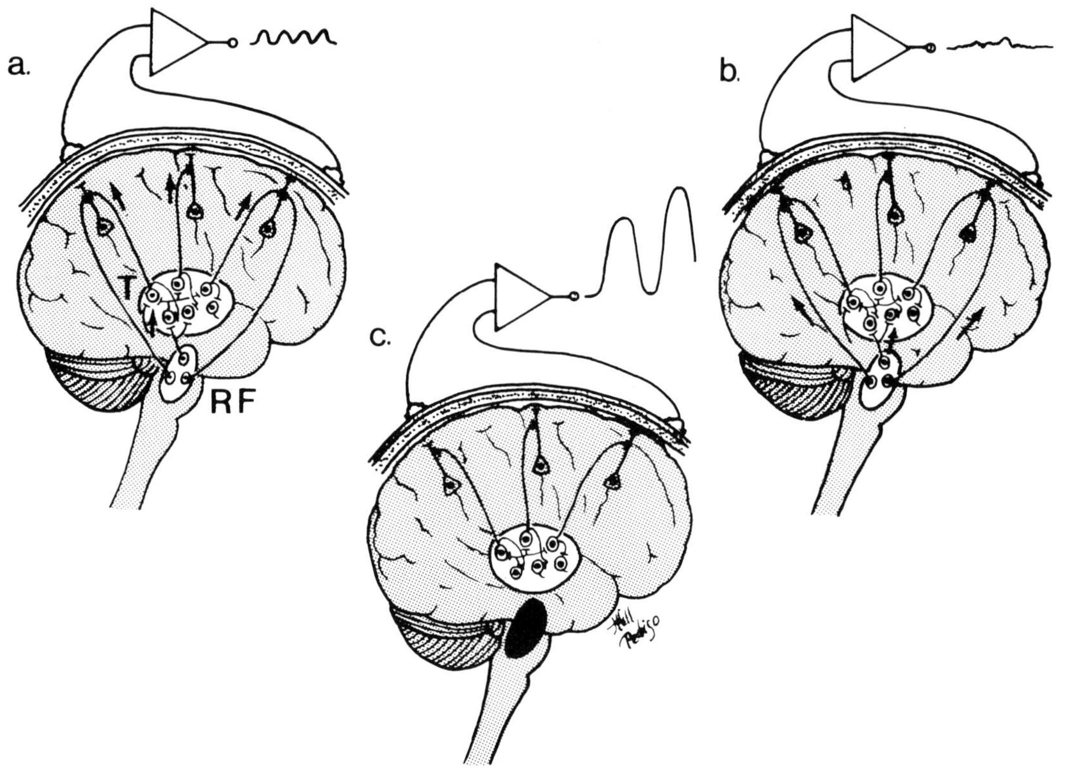


Fig. 1.3. Postulated effect of the mesencephalic reticular formation (RF) on rhythmical cortical activity induced by a thalamic pacemaker (T). – a. Rhythmical activity is generated by the pacemaker system in the absence of strong activating impulses from the reticular formation. – b. Activating impulses from the reticular formation to the cortex and the thalamus abolish rhythmical cortical activity. – c. Lesions destroying or inactivating the reticular formation or its rostral connections result in the appearance of rhythmical slow waves, presumably caused by release of synchronizing centers from a tonic desynchronizing input by the reticular formation.

charges. Interneurons which have an inhibitory action lasting a tenth of a second would thus cause periodic and synchronous inhibition and rebound excitation of thalamo-cortical projection neurons ten times a second. The projection of these impulses to the cortex induces postsynaptic potentials at that rate which are recorded as EEG waves of 10 Hz with scalp electrodes.

The rhythmical activity in the thalamus may stop for various reasons. It may cease when slight differences of conduction speed in the thalamic networks desynchronize the steps in the cycle. The cycle may be actively interrupted by changes in the activity of the midbrain reticular activating system. This system receives input from practically all sensory systems and cortical areas and sends its output to the entire cortex both through direct connections and through relays in the diencephalon (Fig. 1.3a). It can thus interrupt the production of rhythmical cortical activity both by directly interfering with the activity of cortical neurons generating this activity and by influencing the thalamic interneurons producing pacemaker impulses (Fig. 1.3b). Either an increase or a decrease of the tonic activity of the ascending reticular activating system causes rhythmical cortical activity to disappear: Cortical rhythms in humans may be abolished by arousal and heightened attention or by drowsiness and sleep. However, rhythmical activity may be facilitated by structures in the lower brain stem which inhibit the desynchronizing effect of the ascending reticular activating system. Abnormal rhythmical activity may thus appear as the result of brain stem damage which reduces the desynchronizing action of the reticular formation and increases the synchronizing action of other centers (Fig. 1.3.c).

## 1.3 RECORDING OF ELECTRICAL POTENTIALS WITH SCALP ELECTRODES

Electrodes on the scalp record mainly the summated electrical changes of the underlying cortex; they may also record some potential changes generated in distant parts of the brain and potential changes produced outside the brain. The amplitude of the recorded potentials depends on the intensity of the electrical source, on its distance and spatial orientation, and on the electrical resistance and capacitance of the structures between the source and the recording electrodes. These factors favor the recording of potential changes which (a) occur near the recording electrodes, (b) are generated in a large area of tissue and (c) rise and fall at slow speed.

**1.3.1** *Potentials generated in the underlying cortex* are the major source of the scalp EEG. However, the EEG recorded with scalp electrodes differs from that recorded simultaneously with electrodes placed directly on the underlying cortex ('electrocorticogram', 'ECoG'). The scalp EEG is of lower amplitude and may be distorted in shape. Generally, faster frequencies are attenuated more than slower ones. Very fast and brief potential changes may be lost completely in scalp recordings or may be picked up only over their production site whereas slower potentials may be conducted farther and thus be recorded over greater distances. These distortions depend in part on the electrical properties of structures between cortex and scalp electrodes. The amplitude of the scalp EEG may decrease as a result of either (a) an increase of electrical impedance between the source and the recording electrodes, for instance an increase in the thickness of the skull, which reduces the flow of currents between the source and the recording electrodes, or (b) a decrease in the impedance across the path of these currents, for instance a collection of subdural blood or of cerebrospinal fluid which shunts the currents before they reach the recording electrodes.

Even though the scalp EEG directly reflects mainly local potential changes, it may indirectly reveal abnormalities at distant sites which can give rise to cortical potentials of very similar shape and timing over wide parts of the brain. This mechanism has been called 'projection' or 'bilateral synchrony' and the resulting rhythms have been called 'projected rhythms' or 'rhythmes à distance'. Because the pacemaker for bilaterally synchronous discharges is presumed to be located at the center of the brain, the term 'centrencephalic' has also been used. Although these rhythms may be induced by the action of distant centers, they are generated by the cortex under the recording electrodes, not by distant sites.

**1.3.2** *Potentials generated at distant sites* are only rarely recorded by scalp electrodes. This is illustrated by the observation that scalp electrodes over an area of cortex with completely abolished function will generally show complete absence of electrical activity. However, some types of activity of high amplitude, such as slow waves deep in the frontal pole or spikes in the mesial and basal parts of the brain are occasionally conducted electrically through the volume of the interposed tissue and appear in scalp electrodes at considerable distance, superimposed on the EEG representing local cortical activity. Electrical conduction probably also accounts for the appearance of EEG potentials at scalp electrodes over partially or completely removed hemispheres and for the recording of a depth EEG ('DEEG') by electrodes which have been inserted surgically into the brain but may be located at some distance from nerve cells generating EEG potentials.

**1.3.3** *Potentials generated by sources other than the brain* are often picked up by scalp electrodes and recorded together with the EEG; such extracerebral potentials are usually called 'artifacts' (6). For instance, muscle fiber activity may be recorded by a scalp electrode located over muscle. Movements of the eyes, tongue and other large and electrically charged structures can generate changing electrical fields, which are recorded by scalp electrodes. Heart muscle contraction can induce potential changes at scalp electrodes similar to the potential changes recorded in the electrocardiogram. Strong sources of alternating current near the recording site may interfere with the recording.

## REFERENCES


Abraham, K. and Ajmone Marsan, C. (1958) Patterns of cortical discharges and their relation to routine scalp electroencephalography. Electroenceph. clin. Neurophysiol. 10: 447–461.

Andersen, P. and Andersson, S.A. (1968) Physiological Basis of the Alpha Rhythm. Appleton, New York.

Andersen, P. and Andersson, S.A. (1974) Section IV. Thalamic origin of cortical rhythmical activity. In: Rémond, A. (Ed.), Handbook of Electroenceph. clin. Neurophysiol., Vol. 2C, Elsevier, Amsterdam, pp. 90–118.

Ball, G.J., Gloor, P. and Thompson, C.J. (1977) Computed unit-EEG correlations and laminar profiles of spindle waves in the electroencephalogram of cats. Electroenceph. clin. Neurophysiol. 43: 330–345.

Brookhart, J.M. and Mountcastle, V.B. (1977) Section 1: The nervous system. American Physiological Society, Bethesda.

Cooper, R., Winter, A.L., Crow, H.J. and Walter, W.G. (1965) Comparison of subcortical, cortical and scalp activity using chronically indwelling electrodes in man. Electroenceph. clin. Neurophysiol. 18: 217–228.

Creutzfeldt, O. and Houchin, J. (1974) Section I. Neuronal basis of EEG-waves. In: Rémond, A. (Ed.), Handbook of Electroenceph. clin. Neurophysiol., Vol. 2C, Elsevier, Amsterdam, pp. 5–55.

DeLucchi, M.R., Garoutte, B. and Aird, R.B. (1962) The scalp as an electroencephalographic averager. Electroenceph. clin. Neurophysiol. 14: 191–196.

Elul, R. (1972) The genesis of the EEG. Int. Rev. Neurobiol. 15: 227–272.

Leissner, P., Lindholm, L.-E. and Petersén, I. (1970) Alpha amplitude dependence on skull thickness as measured by ultrasound technique. Electroenceph. clin. Neurophysiol. 29: 392–399.

Lopes da Silva, F.H., Lierop, T.H.M.T. van, Schrijer, C.F. and Storm van Leeuwen, W. (1973) Essential differences between alpha rhythms and barbiturate spindles: Spectra and thalamo-cortical coherences. Electroenceph. clin. Neurophysiol. 35: 641–645.

Lopes da Silva, F.H., Lierop, T.H.M.T. van, Schrijer, C.F. and Storm van Leeuwen, W. (1973) Organization of the thalamic and cortical alpha rhythms: Spectra and coherences. Electroenceph. clin. Neurophysiol. 35: 627–639.

Lopes da Silva, F.H. and Storm van Leeuwen, W. (1978) The cortical alpha rhythm in dog: The depth and surface profile of phase. In: Brazier, M.A.B., Petsche, H. (Eds.), Architectonics of the Cerebral Cortex. Internat. Brain Res. Organization Monograph Series, Vol. 3, Raven Press, New York, pp. 319–333.

Mountcastle, V.B. (1974) Medical Physiology. Vol. 1, 13th Ed., Mosby, St. Louis.

Pfurtscheller, G. and Cooper, R. (1975) Frequency dependence of the transmission of the EEG from cortex to scalp. Electroenceph. clin. Neurophysiol. 38: 93–96.

Rayport, M., Sandler, B. and Katzman, R. (1966) Observations on the passive electrical properties of the envelopes of cat brain. Electroenceph. clin. Neurophysiol. 20: 513–519.

Ruch, T.C. and Patton, H.D. (1973–1979) Physiology and Biophysics, 20th Ed., Saunders, Philadelphia.

Schlag, J. (1974) Section V. Reticular influences on thalamo-cortical activity. In: Rémond, A. (Ed.), Handbook of Electroenceph. clin. Neurophysiol., Vol. 2C, Elsevier, Amsterdam, pp. 119–134.

# Recording electrodes

# 2

SUMMARY

Recording electrodes couple differences of electrical potential at the recording site to the input of the recording machine.

(2.1) *Electrode types* most commonly used in clinical EEG are metal discs or cups attached to the scalp and other recording sites. Needle electrodes which are inserted into the scalp are rarely used. Nasopharyngeal and sphenoidal electrodes require special insertion procedures and are used in some laboratories in addition to scalp electrodes to record the EEG from the undersurface of the temporal lobe.

(2.2) *Electrical properties* should enable recording electrodes to couple potential changes from the head to the input of the EEG machine without distortion. Electrodes should have a surface made of gold, chlorided silver or other materials which do not interact chemically with the scalp. Electrodes must be applied so as to make electrical contact having impedances between 100 and 5000 Ω. Electrodes with much higher impedances can attenuate the recording and cause 60 Hz artifact; impedances of less than 100 Ω are usually the result of accidental short-circuits between electrodes. Polarization and bias potentials develop at the interface between electrode and tissue and can be minimized by careful technique.

(2.3) *Placement of electrodes* should cover the entire head evenly and be reproducible between subjects and laboratories. This is accomplished with the International 10–20 System. This system uses measurements between bony landmarks on the skull to determine the coordinates for 21 recording electrodes with provisions for additional electrodes as needed. Fewer electrodes may be used in infants.

## 2.1 ELECTRODE SHAPES AND APPLICATION METHODS

In general, electrodes consist of a conductor connected by a lead wire and plug to the input of the recording machine. Scalp electrodes are applied after determining the precise location and after preparing the scalp to reduce electrical impedance. Metal surface electrodes should be cleansed with a solution of an antiseptic soap

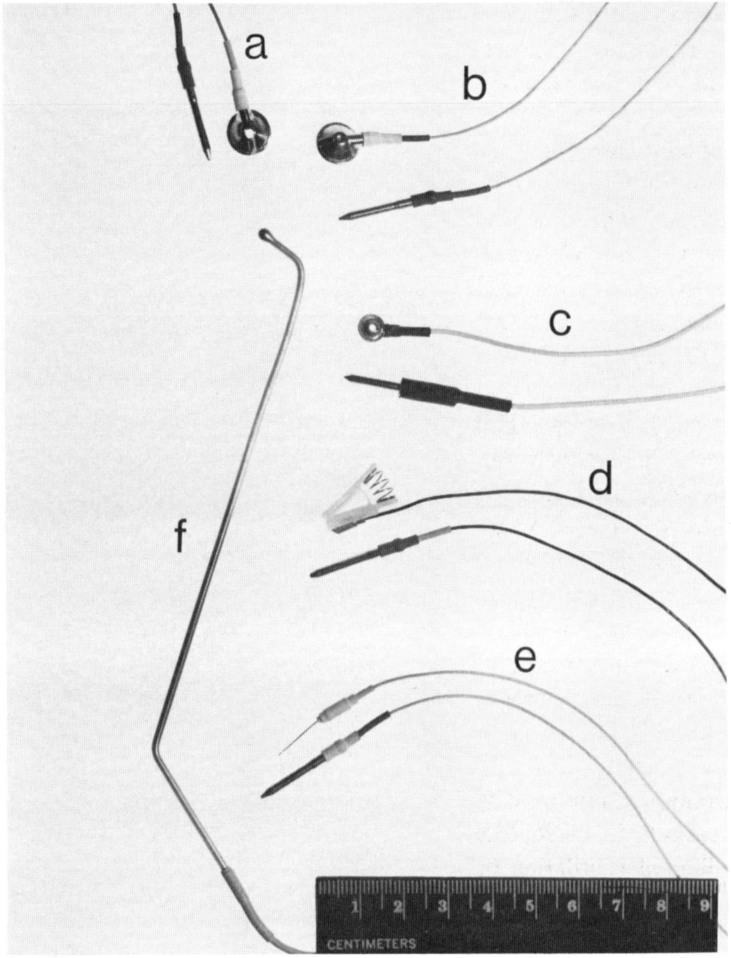


Fig. 2.1. Various types of EEG electrodes, shown with their connector plugs and part of their lead wires. a. Large metal cup electrode with a central hole; b. Large metal cup electrode without hole; c. Small metal cup electrode with central hole; d. Clip electrode; e. Needle electrode; f. Nasopharyngeal electrode.

after each use. Nasopharyngeal electrodes and electrodes penetrating the skin must be autoclaved; penetrating electrodes used on patients with contagious diseases, especially including possible Jakob-Creutzfeldt disease, must be discarded after use.

**2.1.1** *Metal disc and cup electrodes* usually have diameters of 4–10 mm (Fig. 2.1). Smaller or larger electrodes do not make stable mechanical and electrical contact with the scalp. An insulated lead wire is attached to each electrode. The insulation of each wire has a different color for easy identification of each electrode. Mechanical and electrical problems are reduced if the insulations of the lead wires are attached to each other in the form of a stranded cable from which the leads separate only at the two ends. Before electrodes are applied, the application site is determined by measurements (2.3) and prepared by wiping with alcohol or acetone.

Several methods may be used to attach electrodes to the scalp. The collodion technique has the advantage of giving very stable recordings with relatively few artifacts. In this technique, cup electrodes with a central hole are placed onto the prepared scalp site and held in place with a stylus while a few drops of collodion are applied around the edge of the electrode and spread onto the scalp. The spreading and drying of the collodion may be facilitated by a stream of compressed air guided through a tube around the stylus. After the electrode is securely attached, the stylus is removed and the cup is filled with conductive jelly which is injected with a blunt hypodermic needle inserted through the central hole of the cup. If cup electrodes without a central hole are used, they are filled with conductive paste before application to the scalp. Some laboratories place small pieces of gauze soaked with collodion over the electrodes to hold them in place. Electrodes are removed by dissolving the collodion with acetone. Because of the chemicals involved, the collodion method should not be used in areas which have limited ventilation or explosion hazards such as infant isolettes or operating rooms.

Another method of applying electrodes uses a paste which can both hold the electrode in place and provide good electrical contact. After preparation of the scalp site, a piece of this adhesive conductive paste is placed on the scalp and the electrode is pressed into the center of the paste until it makes firm contact. Electrodes with a central hole allow the paste to escape through the hole so that the rim of the cup sits firmly on the scalp. A gauze pad or cotton ball may be placed over the electrode to hold it more securely in place and to delay drying of the paste. This method is fast, but electrodes tend to lose good mechanical and electrical contact more readily than when they are applied with collodion.

Other methods of applying disc or cup electrodes involve the use of: (a) paraffin wax, (b) suction electrodes, or (c) headbands, straps or caps which hold an entire set of electrodes in place. These methods generally give less satisfactory results than the methods described earlier.

Metal disc or cup electrodes may be placed around the eyes, on the chest or other parts of the body to monitor electrical potentials which are generated by eye movements, heart beat, respiration, muscle contraction or body movement and which may contaminate the EEG (4.3). While EEG electrodes may be used to monitor the occurrence of extracerebral activity, they introduce some distortion and special electrodes are required if faithful recordings of such activity are desired.

**2.1.2** *Clip electrodes* are sometimes used for recordings from the earlobes. The clips should contain cups or discs similar to the scalp electrodes to avoid electrical problems caused by recording from dissimilar electrodes.

**2.1.3** *Needle electrodes* are sharp wires, usually made of steel or platinum. They are inserted into the superficial layers of the scalp after thorough disinfection of the insertion site. The advantage of fast application is outweighed by the disadvantages of pain, possible infection and unfavorable electrical characteristics. Some laboratories still use these electrodes for emergency recordings from comatose patients, but most electroencephalographers feel they should not be used.

**2.1.4** *Nasopharyngeal electrodes* are used in addition to scalp electrodes by some laboratories in patients who are suspected of having epileptiform activity in the basal parts of the temporal lobe but who do not show such activity in scalp recordings.

Nasopharyngeal electrodes are made of rigid insulated wire which has z-shape to fit the path of insertion. The tip is an uninsulated metal ball of 2–5 mm diameter. One electrode is inserted through each nostril, slid backwards along the bottom of the nasal cavity near the midline, and then rotated outward. This places the tip against the roof of the nasopharynx and very close to the skull at the base of the middle cerebral fossa, i.e. close to the tip of the temporal lobe.

Because the insertion can cause discomfort, gagging and slight injury to the mucous membranes, it is usually done by a physician. Most patients tolerate the electrodes without discomfort; sleep recordings, which may activate abnormal discharges in the temporal lobes, can usually be obtained with nasopharyngeal electrodes in place.

**2.1.5** *Sphenoidal electrodes* are used in a few laboratories to detect epileptiform activity in the temporal lobes. This electrode consists of a flexible wire with an uninsulated tip which is placed near the sphenoidal wing through a cannula inserted through the temporal and masseter muscles. Electrode placement can be checked by X-ray. The electrodes can be left in place for several days of serial EEG recordings without danger of breaking or injury to the patient.

**2.1.6** *Tympanic electrodes* may be placed near the eardrum to record the EEG from the temporal lobe. Recently, an electrode in the external auditory meatus has been used to record excitation of the acoustic nerve in the study of auditory evoked potentials (7.7.2).

**2.1.7** *Electrocorticographic electrodes* are used during some neurosurgical procedures, usually excision of epileptogenic foci, to record the ECoG from the exposed cortical surface. These electrodes consist of metal balls or saline-soaked cotton wicks which may be mounted on springs and held in place by swivel joints for easy placement.

**2.1.8** *Depth electrodes* are used in a few centers, usually to define the targets for surgical destruction. These electrodes consist usually of a bundle of fine wires which terminate with uninsulated tips at different levels and thus allow for recordings from different depths. The insertion of depth electrodes is guided by determining the position of the target in a three-dimensional reference system and by translating the coordinates of this system to the head of the patient using standard landmarks and X-ray control.

## 2.2 ELECTRICAL PROPERTIES OF RECORDING ELECTRODES

Good recording electrodes should couple the electrical potential changes at the recording site to the input of the recording machine without distortion. To obtain such high fidelity recordings, one must (1) choose recording electrodes of suitable material; (2) measure electrode resistance to ascertain electrical continuity between the two ends of the electrode if in doubt; (3) measure electrode impedance after every electrode application and during the recording to evaluate the electrical contact between electrode and scalp; (4) avoid electrode polarization and bias potentials.

**2.2.1** *Electrode materials* should be those which do not interact chemically with the electrolytes of the scalp. Electrodes coated with gold, silver chloride, tin or platinum are satisfactory.

**2.2.2** *Electrode resistance*, or opposition to direct current flow, is measured occasionally, namely when a break in the electrical continuity between electrode, lead wire and connector plug is suspected. This measurement is made while the electrode is not attached to the scalp. The two uninsulated ends of the electrode are connected to an ohmmeter which passes a weak direct current through the electrode. The resistance of an intact electrode should measure no more than a few ohms.

**2.2.3** *Electrode impedance*, or opposition to alternating current flow, is measured after an electrode has been applied to the recording site to evaluate the contact between electrode and scalp. The impedance of each electrode should be measured routinely before every EEG recording and should be between 100 and 5000 Ω. Electrode impedance is measured with an impedance meter which passes a weak alternating current from the electrode selected for testing through the scalp to all other electrodes connected to the meter (Fig. 2.2). The measured impedance reflects mainly that of the selected electrode, the other electrodes offering multiple return pathways with negligible total impedance.

An alternating current is used for this measurement for two reasons. (a) Alternating current is more representative of the alternating potential changes recorded in the EEG, especially if it alternates at about 10 Hz, a common frequency of EEG potential changes; the opposition to current alternating at this frequency may differ from that to alternating current of other frequencies and, especially from that to direct current. (b) Passage of direct current through an electrode attached to the scalp can electrically polarize the interface between electrode and skin and thereby lead to distortion of subsequent EEG recordings.

Most modern EEG machines have provisions for testing electrode impedance during the recording. This is done by injecting a weak alternating current of constant intensity through a pair of electrodes connected to the input of a recording channel. This causes a pen deflection in that channel with an amplitude

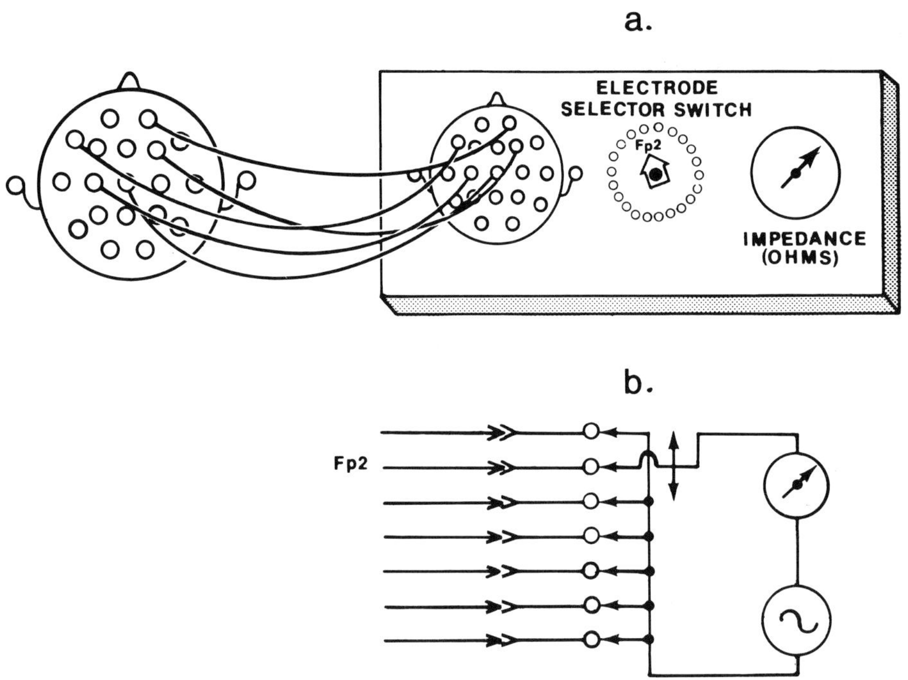


Fig. 2.2. Measurement of electrode impedance. – a. Diagram of the input board with receptacles for the connectors from scalp electrodes (left), selector switch designating electrode Fp2 for impedance measurement (middle), and impedance meter (right). – b. Electrical circuit used for impedance measurement: A weak alternating current is passed through the impedance meter to the electrode selected for measurement (Fp2) and its contact with the scalp (not shown); the current is returned through a combination of all other scalp electrodes. The impedance of the selected electrode is read from the impedance meter; the impedance of the return path is negligible relative to that of the electrode being tested.

proportional to the sum of the impedances of the two electrodes. If the deflection indicated unacceptably high or low impedance, the faulty electrode of the pair must be identified by pairing each electrode with another electrode of acceptable impedance and repeating the current injection.

Both very high and very low impedance are undesirable. Very low impedance acts like a shunt between the recording electrodes and effectively short-circuits the EEG potential differences. It is practically impossible to reduce electrode impedance to less than a few thousand ohms without there being an abnormal pathway of conduction between the electrodes. An electrode showing very low impedance may be making contact with another electrode by an excess of electrolyte jelly or paste, or by saline or sweat forming a conductive bridge between the electrodes on the scalp. Such an electrode should be inspected, cleaned, and reapplied or exchanged if necessary.

Very high impedance is undesirable mainly because connecting an electrode of very high impedance and one of lower impedance to the input of a differential amplifier causes an imbalance which favors the recording of 60 Hz interference* (3.4). Electrodes showing high impedance readings should be checked for good mechanical and electrical contact and the junctions of the lead wire with the metal disc or cup and with the plug terminal should be inspected for possible breaks.

**2.2.4** *Electrode polarization and bias potentials* may occur and distort EEG recordings even when mechanical and electrical recording conditions seem good. Fortunately, the effect of these phenomena on the routine clinical EEG is negligible with modern electrodes, methods of electrode application and recording machines. (1) *Polarization* results from current flow across the interface between electrode and tissue. The current carries positive ions to the more negative part of the junction and

* Interference has a frequency of 50 Hz in countries using alternating current of that frequency.

negative ions to the more positive part. This ion movement polarizes the electrode so that it favors current flow in one direction and resists flow in the opposite direction and thereby distorts the recording of alternating EEG potentials. Polarization is kept to a minimum by (a) a fairly large contact area between electrode and scalp which keeps current density at any one point low; (b) high impedance of the amplifier inputs which keeps the intensity of the current flowing through the electrodes during the recording low; (c) avoidance of steady current flow, especially that used to measure electrode resistance. With these precautions, it is not necessary to use nonpolarizable electrodes such as chlorided silver electrodes for routine clinical EEG recordings, although such electrodes are necessary for other purposes, especially for faithful recording of very slowly changing or steady potential differences. (2) *Bias potentials* result from the exchange of metal ions and electrolytes in the absence of current flow. They interfere with EEG recordings only when they are not steady. Steady bias potentials are the cause of the blocking of amplifiers which occurs immediately after switching to a new selection of electrodes at the input. The effect of bias potentials can be minimized by using (a) electrodes of pure metals with clean surfaces which reduce ion exchange and (b) electrodes of the same kind at the inputs of each amplifier; this neutralizes electrical differences caused by bias potentials.

## 2.3 ELECTRODE PLACEMENT

The International 10–20 System of electrode placement provides for uniform coverage of the entire scalp. It uses the distances between bony landmarks of the head to generate a system of lines which run along and across the head and intersect at intervals of 10 or 20% of their total length. Electrodes are placed at the intersections. The use of the 10–20 System assures symmetrical, reproducible electrode placements and allows comparison of EEGs from the same patient and from different patients, recorded in the same or different laboratories. The system is flexible: additional electrodes, which may be needed to accurately localize an abnormality, can be incorporated by further subdividing the distances between intersections.

The standard set of electrodes for adults (Fig. 2.3) consists of 21 recording electrodes and one ground electrode. The recording electrodes are named with a letter and a subscript. The letter is an abbreviation of the underlying region: prefrontal or frontopolar (Fp), frontal (F), central (C), parietal (P), occipital (O) and auricular (A). The subscript is either the letter z, indicating zero or midline placement, or a number, indicating lateral placement. Odd numbers refer to electrodes on the left, even numbers refer to electrodes on the right side of the head. The numbers increase with increasing distance from the midline except for numbers of temporal and frontopolar electrodes which increase from front to back. The inferior frontal electrodes F7 and F8 are often called 'anterior temporal' electrodes because they fairly faithfully record activity from the anterior temporal area.

Exact measurements are needed to precisely determine the placement of each recording electrode. Measurements are best made with a metric measuring tape of cloth or plastic. A grease pencil is used to mark electrode locations and the intermediate measurements needed to determine them. The measurements refer to three bony landmarks of the skull: (1) the inion, or the bony protruberance in the middle of the back of the head, (2) the nasion, or the bridge of the nose directly under the forehead, and (3) the preauricular point, or the depression of bone in front of the ear canal. Measurements are made in a sequence of five steps (Fig. 3.3).

*Step 1*: The distance between nasion and inion is measured along the midline. Along this line, the frontopolar point, Fp, is marked at 10% above the nasion. Frontal (Fz), central (Cz), parietal (Pz) and occipital (O) points are marked at intervals of 20% of the entire distance leaving 10% for the interval between O and

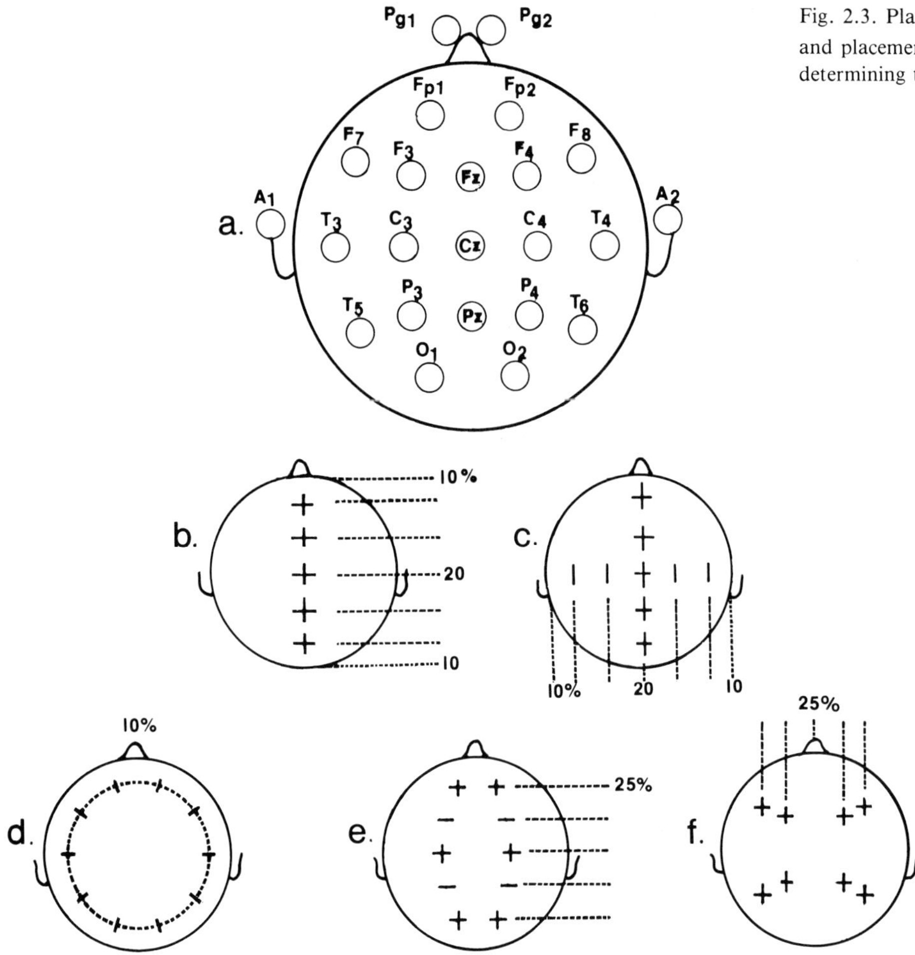


Fig. 2.3. Placement of recording electrodes. – a. Electrode names and placements in the International 10–20 System. – b–f. Steps in determining the electrode placements as described in the text.

inion. The midline points Fp and O are used only for intermediate measurements but receive no electrode and therefore carry no subscript.

*Step 2*: The distance between the two preauricular points across Cz is measured. Along this line, the transverse position for the central points C3 and C4 and the temporal points T3 and T4 are marked 20 and 40% respectively from the midline.

*Step 3*: The circumference of the head is measured from the occipital point (O) through the temporal points T3 and T4 and the frontopolar points Fp. The longitudinal measurement for Fp1 is located on that circumference , 5% of the total length of the circumference to the left of Fp. The longitudinal measurements for F7, T3, T5, O1, O2, T6, T4, F8, Fp2 are at distances of 10% of the circumference.

*Step 4*: The longitudinal distance from Fp1 and Fp2 through C3 and C4 to O1 and O2 is measured on each side. The midpoints of these distances give the longitudinal coordinates of C3 and C4. The midpoints between Fp1 and C3 on the left, and Fp2 and C4 on the right give the longitudinal coordinates for F3 and F4. The midpoints between C3 and O1 on the left, and C4 and O2 on the right give the longitudinal coordinates for P3 and P4.

*Step 5*: Measurements from F7 to F8 through Fz define the transverse coordinates for F3 midway between F3 and Fz, and for F4 midway between Fz and F8; measurements from T5 to T6 through Pz define the transverse coordinates for P3 midway between T5 and Pz and for P4 midway between Pz and T6.

Electrodes are placed at Fz, Cz and Pz, at all lateral points designated above, on or near both ears in positions called $A_1$ and $A_2$ or on the mandibular angles (4.2.4) in positions called $M_1$ and $M_2$, and on the point chosen for the ground electrode, usually in the middle of the head or over one of the mastoids. The use of a smaller number of electrodes in routine EEG is now considered substandard. If needed, additional electrodes may be placed midway between these recording electrodes. In some cases, scalp lesions, skull asymmetries or other abnormalities may make it impossible to place electrodes in the positions of the 10–20 System. In these cases, electrodes should be placed as closely as possible to these positions and as symmetrically as possible on the two sides. The deviations from standard placement should be indicated in a diagram on the EEG record. Other electrode placements may be used for EEG recordings from small infants and for monitoring of extracerebral activity such as eye movements, heart beat, respiratory or other movements (4.3).

## REFERENCES


Arrelano, A.P. (1949) A tympanic lead. Electroenceph. clin. Neurophysiol. 1: 112–113.

Bach-y-Rita, G., Lion, J., Reynolds, J. and Ervin, F.R. (1969) An improved nasopharyngeal lead. Electroenceph. clin. Neurophysiol. 26: 220–221.

Blume, W.T., Buza, R.C. and Okazaki, H. (1974) Anatomic correlates of the ten-twenty electrode placement system in infants. Electroenceph. clin. Neurophysiol. 36: 303–307.

Broughton, R., Hanley, J., Quanbury, A.O. and Roy, O.Z. (1976) Section I. Electrodes. In: Rémond, A. (Ed.), Handbook of Electroenceph. clin. Neurophysiol., Vol. 3A, Elsevier, Amsterdam, pp. 5–27.

Cooper, R. (1963) Electrodes. Am. J. EEG Technol. 3: 91–101.

Craib, A.R. and Perry, M. (1975) EEG Handbook. Beckman Instruments, Fullerton.

De Jesus, P.V. and Masland, W.S. (1970) The role of nasopharyngeal electrodes in clinical electroencephalography. Neurology 20: 869–878.

Ellingson, R.J. (1979) EEGs of premature and full-term newborns. In: Klass, D.W. and Daly, D.D. (Eds.), Current Practice of Clinical Electroencephalography. Raven Press, New York, pp. 149–177.

Geddes, L.A. (1972) Electrodes and the Measurement of Bioelectric Events. Wiley, New York.

Girton, D.G. and Kamiya, J. (1974) A very stable electrode system for recording human scalp electrodes with direct-coupled amplifiers. Electroenceph. clin. Neurophysiol. 37: 85–88.

Grings, W.W. (1974) Recording of electrodermal phenomena. In: Thompson, R.F. and Patterson, M.M. (Eds.), Bioelectric Recording Techniques, Vol. 1C, Academic Press, New York and London, pp. 273–296.

Harner, P.F. and Sannit, R. (1974) A Review of the International Ten-Twenty System of Electrode Placement. Grass Instrument Co., Quincy, Mass.

Ives, J.R. and Gloor, P. (1978) Update: Chronic sphenoidal electrodes. Electroenceph. clin. Neurophysiol. 44: 789–790.

Jasper, H.H. (1958) The ten-twenty electrode system of the International Federation. Electroenceph. clin. Neurophysiol. 10: 371–375.

Kagawa, N. (1962) Electroencephalography in infants with special reference to the newborn: Technique. Am. J. EEG Technol. 2: 99–105.
Mac Gillivray, B.B. (1974) Section I. Electrodes and their use. In: Rémond, A. (Ed.), Handbook of Electroenceph. clin. Neurophysiol., Vol. 3C, Elsevier, Amsterdam, pp. 5–21.
Mavor, H. and Hellen, M.K. (1964) Nasopharyngeal electrode recording. Am. J. EEG Technol. 4: 43–50.
Picton, T.W. and Hillyard, S.A. (1972) Cephalic skin potentials in electroencephalography. Electroenceph. clin. Neurophysiol. 33: 419–424.
Sannit, T. (1963) The ten-twenty system: Footnotes to measuring technique. Am. J. EEG Technol. 3: 23–30.
Silverman, D. (1960) The anterior temporal electrode and the ten-twenty system. Electroenceph. clin. Neurophysiol. 12: 735–737.
Venables, P.H. and Martin, I. (1967) Skin resistance and skin potential. In: Venables, P.H. and Martin, I. (Eds.). A Manual of Psychophysiological Methods. North-Holland, Amsterdam, pp. 53–102.
Werner, S.S., Stockard, J.E. and Bickford, R.G. (1977) Atlas of Neonatal Electroencephalography. Raven Press, New York.
Zablow, L. and Goldensohn, E.S. (1969) A comparison between scalp and needle electrodes for the EEG. Electroenceph. clin. Neurophysiol. 26: 530–533.

# The EEG machine: Parts and functions

# 3

Summary

(3.1) *The input board* is a box which serves to connect the electrodes on the patient's head to the input selector switches of the EEG machine. The terminals of the electrodes are plugged into the receptacles on the input board which are labelled with standard symbols and often arranged in a diagram representing the head. The input board should either contain an impedance meter or provide connections to such a meter. The input board may also contain circuitry which limits the current flow between electrodes.

(3.2) *Input selector switches* on the EEG machine are used to select two electrodes as the input to each amplifier. The selected electrodes, amplifier and writing unit form a system for detection, amplification and display of potential differences between an electrode pair; this system is called 'channel'. In addition to the individual selector switches for each channel, a master selector switch is often provided to choose, with the setting of only one switch, a standard combination of electrodes for all channels.

(3.3) *Calibration pulses* of known voltage are used to measure the amplitude of EEG potentials and to test the functioning of all amplifiers. To further assure that all channels amplify EEG activity in the same manner, one electrode pair recording the patient's EEG may be connected to the inputs of all amplifiers for a brief trial recording and comparison of the write-outs of all channels.

(3.4) *Amplifiers* are the major components of each channel of the EEG machine. Each amplifier has two input terminals, connected to the input selector switches. EEG amplifiers increase only the difference of voltage between the input terminals; identical voltages appearing at the two inputs are not amplified but rejected. This differential amplification serves to distinguish cerebral potentials, which are likely to have different amplitude, shape and timing at recording electrodes in different areas of the head, from electrical artifacts, which are likely to be similar at different recording electrodes. EEG amplifiers are constructed so that a negative potential change causes an upward pen deflection when applied to the first of the two inputs and a downward pen deflection when applied to the second input. Amplification is usually expressed as sensitivity which relates the voltage of a signal to the height of the pen deflection it causes. Less often, amplification is described as gain, i.e. the ratio of output voltage to input voltage.

(3.5) *Filters* selectively reduce the amplitude of voltage changes, or signals, of selected frequencies. A low and a high frequency filter are used to exclude from the EEG very slow and very fast waves and thereby to select the spectrum of frequencies which has the greatest clinical significance. A 60 Hz filter may be used to selectively reduce interference which cannot be controlled by other means. The filters are part of the amplifiers and modify their output before it is connected to the penwriters.

(3.6) *The writing units* are driven by the amplified and filtered potential changes recorded at the scalp. Moving pens or, less often, ink jets or other devices move up and down, writing on chart paper which is moved horizontally at an even speed of usually 3 cm/second.

## 3.1 THE INPUT BOARD

The connectors at the ends of the electrode lead wires are plugged into receptacles in a small input board or box. Each receptacle is labelled with a symbol which indicates the location of the electrode on the head. To aid in selecting the correct receptacle, the receptacles are often arranged in a diagram representing the head. At least 23 receptacles should be available for the standard recording and ground electrodes. Additional receptacles, if available, may be used for additional electrode placements. The wires from each receptacle run in a cable to the EEG machine where they terminate at the input selector switches. In most EEG machines, the input board either contains an impedance meter or has connections for such a meter so that electrode impedance can be measured without changing electrode connections.

Because electrode lead wires should be no longer than 1 meter to minimize artifacts, the input board is kept near the patient. The cable from the input board to the EEG machine may be much longer since it is electrically shielded and less likely to pick up interference. In laboratories using a shielded recording room for the patient, the input board must stay in that room; if the machine is located outside the shielded room, the cable is fed through an opening in the shielding to the EEG machine.

For the safety of the patient, the input board and its connections to the EEG machine should be built so that no more than 20 $\mu$A of current can flow from any one of the electrodes through the patient to ground. Such leakage currents can be kept to a minimum by connecting the patient to the ground of the EEG machine through a ground electrode terminating on the input board. If the EEG machine and the power outlets are properly grounded, this ground electrode is at the same potential as the chassis of the EEG machine and any other grounded piece of metal equipment in the room. To further reduce the chances of accidental current flow through the patient, the patient should be connected to ground through only one electrode. In the ICU or the operating room, patients are often grounded through monitoring equipment, for instance through ECG recording devices. These patients should not also be grounded through an EEG electrode. However, when the ground electrodes of other monitoring equipment are too far from the patient's head to provide a good reference point for the EEG amplifier inputs to discriminate against 60 Hz and other interference (3.4.1), it may be better to disconnect the patient temporarily from the ground of the monitoring equipment and to ground the patient instead through an EEG electrode for the duration of the EEG recording.

## 3.2 INPUT SELECTOR SWITCHES

All EEG machines should have individual selector switches for each channel; as a convenience, many machines also have a master selector switch. These switches are used to connect each channel to the calibration signal, one or more recording electrodes or the ground of the amplifier.

**3.2.1** *Individual channel selector switches* usually consist of rotary, push button, or slide switches with over 21 contact positions. Each channel has two switches, one for each amplifier input.

**3.2.2** *A master electrode selector switch*, if available, may be used to connect a specific combination of electrodes to the input terminals of each amplifier. A master switch has only one position for each combination and can reduce the time spent in setting individual selector switches; this is useful for routine recordings using standard electrode combinations. Individual selector switches must be available for cases where other combinations are needed to demonstrate a particular EEG abnormality.

**3.2.3** *Possible selections* are of four types. (1) The calibration position connects the source of the calibration signal to the amplifier input. (2) Any receptacle of the input board, except that of the ground electrode, can be connected to any amplifier input. The same electrode may be selected at the input of more than one amplifier. However, if the same electrode is selected at both inputs of one amplifier, the inputs are short-circuited, and closed. (3) Combinations of two or more electrodes can be selected at one input to an amplifier on many machines. This selection, often called 'average reference electrode', electrically ties together the selected electrodes so that each one contributes equally to the potential fluctuations recorded from their combination. (4) Ground can be selected as an input to an amplifier, connecting that input to the ground of the amplifier and effectively closing the input regardless of whether or not the ground is connected to the patient.

## 3.3 CALIBRATION

Calibration in clinical EEG has two main purposes: (a) to measure the voltage of the EEG potentials by comparing them with a potential of known voltage; (b) to ascertain whether all channels amplify the same signal in the same way. Both purposes are served by the most commonly used calibration procedure of applying standard voltage pulses simultaneously to the input of all amplifiers. The functioning of the amplifiers can also be compared by using the patient's EEG as a calibration signal.

**3.3.1** *Calibration pulses.* A negative potential of pre-selected voltage is applied to the input of an amplifier by actuating a calibration switch. This results in a sudden pen deflection. Only the initial deflection represents the amplitude of the calibration voltage; even when the calibration voltage is sustained, the pen gradually drifts back to the baseline as the result of the low frequency filter (3.5.1). When the calibration voltage is turned off after the pen has reached baseline, the pen is suddenly deflected in the opposite direction and to the same amplitude as at the beginning of the calibration pulse. For routine calibration, a series of such deflections is recorded in all channels.

The pen deflections of the calibration pulses serve to determine the voltage of EEG potentials recorded at the same amplifier settings. For instance, an EEG potential deflecting a pen to a height of 14 mm at an amplifier setting at which a calibration pulse of 50 $\mu$V produces 7 mm pen deflection has an amplitude of 100 $\mu$V. Although the amplitude of the calibration pulses at different amplifier settings can be derived by multiplying the amplitude of the calibration pulses by the change in amplification, it is good practice to calibrate the amplifiers at the end of a recording for all the settings used during a recording.

**3.3.2** *The patient's EEG* may be used to compare the performance of all amplifiers. To obtain a wide range of EEG frequencies for this comparison, a frontopolar electrode and an occipital electrode on the opposite side are usually selected as input for all amplifiers. The tracings of all pens should be identical.

## 3.4 THE AMPLIFIERS

EEG amplifiers have two main purposes: (1) *Discrimination* is the ability to pick up differences of electrical potential between the electrodes connected to the two inputs

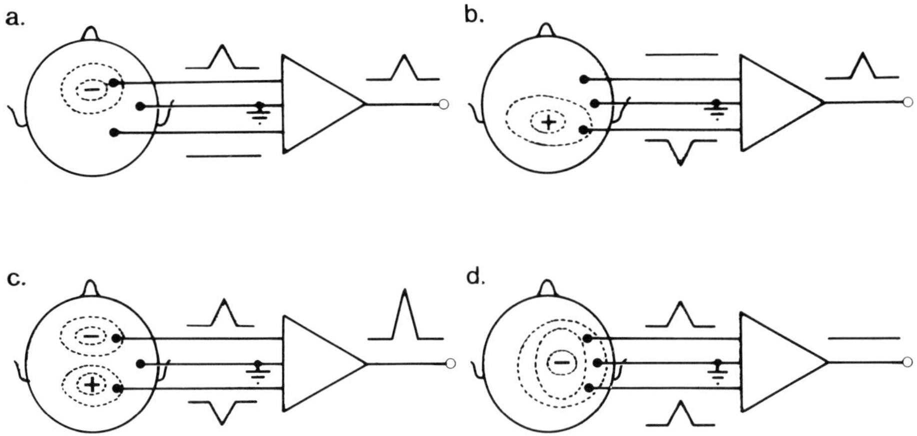


Fig. 3.1. Differential amplification of simple signals, applied to input 1 (top input at the triangular amplifier symbol) and input 2 (bottom input) with respect to an electrical zero level at the ground connection (middle input). Electrical changes at scalp electrodes are indicated by fields on the head diagram; a change towards negative in an electrode is indicated by an upward deflection of the signal above or below the electrode lead; a change towards positive is indicated by a downward deflection. The same polarity convention is used for the signals at the amplifier output which represent pen deflections. – a. A negative signal at input 1 causes an upgoing pen deflection; – b. A positive signal at input 2 is inverted at the ground level and also causes an upgoing pen deflection; – c. Two signals of equal size but opposite polarity appearing simultaneously at both inputs are added to each other and cause a pen deflection twice the size of that caused by each potential alone; – d. Two signals of equal size and the same polarity applied simultaneously to both inputs are subtracted from each other and cause no pen deflection.

while rejecting potentials which are common to the two electrodes; (2) *Amplification* serves to increase the size of potential differences to a level at which they can drive the pens of the EEG machine and be written out on the paper record.

**3.4.1** *Discrimination.* Each amplifier of the EEG machine has two input terminals which are now named ‘input 1’ and ‘input 2’; they were formerly called ‘grid 1’ and ‘grid 2’. Potential changes, or signals, applied to each terminal are amplified to the same degree but in opposite direction with reference to the ground of the amplifier. This is done by inverting the polarity of the signal applied to input 2 so that it is effectively subtracted from the signal applied to input 1. This mode of operation is called ‘differential’ or ‘balanced’ amplification.

The polarity of the output signal of a differential amplifier thus depends not only on the polarity of the input signal but also on the input terminal to which it is applied. EEG machines are wired so that a net negativity at input 1 causes an upward deflection at the output whereas a relative negativity at input 2 causes a downward deflection. Because upward and downward deflections of the pens do not reveal the polarity at either input, up or down deflections should not be called ‘negative’ or ‘positive’.

The results of differential amplification are illustrated by four extreme cases illustrated in Figure 3.1.

(a) A negative signal applied to input 1 causes an upward deflection at the output.

(b) A positive signal applied to input 2 also causes an upward deflection at the output.

(c) Two signals of opposite polarity applied simultaneously to each input produce an output which represents the sum of the outputs caused by either signal alone.

(d) Two signals of the same amplitude, polarity and timing applied to both inputs are subtracted from each other and produce no output. Such signals are said to be in ‘common mode’.

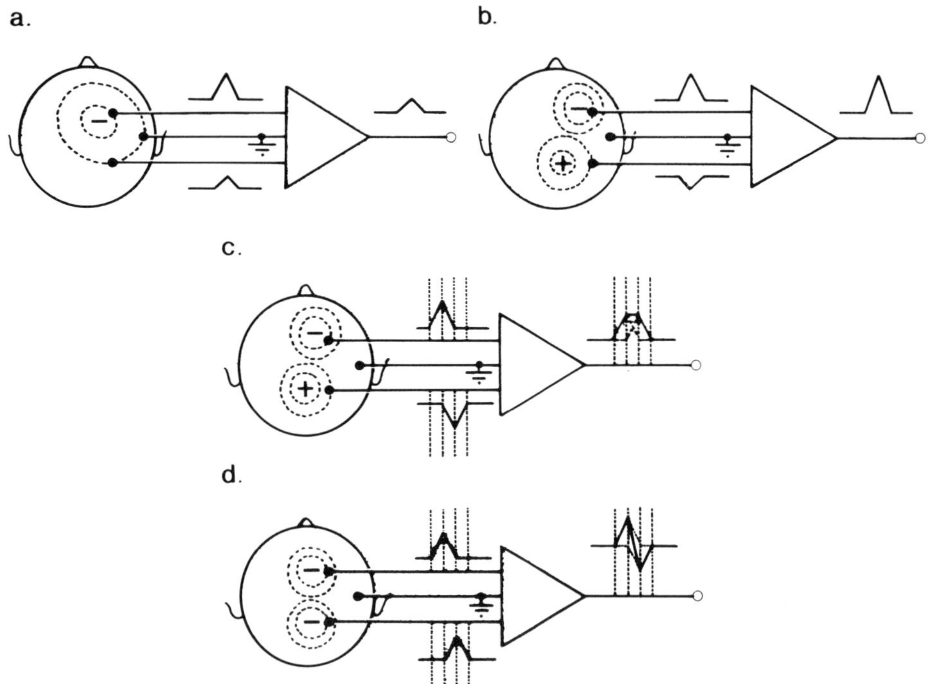



Fig. 3.2. Differential amplification of signals of different amplitude (a and b) and timing (c and d). Symbols are the same as in Fig. 3.1. – a. Simultaneous appearance of a negative potential at input 1 and of a negative potential of half its size at input 2 causes an upgoing pen deflection half the size of that produced by the potential at input 1 alone; – b. Simultaneous appearance of a negative signal at input 1 and of a positive signal of half its size at input 2 causes an upgoing pen deflection of an amplitude one and a half times that produced by the signal at input 1 alone. – c. Appearance of a negative signal at input 1 followed by appearance of a positive signal of the same size at input 2 causes a sustained upgoing pen deflection; – d. Appearance of a negative signal at input 1 followed by a negative signal of the same size at input 2 causes a diphasic pen deflection of a longer total duration and of a faster falling phase than that caused by either signal alone.

The four examples in Figure 3.1 show potentials of identical shape, amplitude and timing. Such potentials are not produced by the brain. However, the simple rules illustrated by these examples can also be applied to more complicated conditions such as shown in Figure 3.2. A change of potential affecting both electrodes to a different degree causes an output of an amplitude corresponding exactly with the difference between the potential at both inputs. For instance, if the potential level at input 1 becomes more negative by 100 μV and that at input 2 more negative by 50 μV or more positive by 50 μV, the amplifier input 'sees' a potential difference between the inputs of 50 μV or 150 μV, respectively (Fig. 3.2a and b). Potential changes involving both inputs in sequence may be offset in time and cause a prolonged output; a potential change which appears at input 2 with some delay in regard to a change at input 1 causes the two changes to be added to each other (Fig. 3.2c) or to be subtracted from each other (Fig. 3.2d). In essence, the output represents an amplification of that part of the input signals which is not common to both input terminals.

Obviously, in differential amplification one type of output can be the result of different kinds of input. The methods used to deduce from the output, namely the EEG, the input, namely the polarity, distribution and relative amplitude of the electrical potentials on the scalp, are discussed in the next chapter.

Discrimination means selection of signals which differ at both inputs and rejection of common mode signals. It is expressed as a ratio comparing differential with common mode amplification of an amplifier. This ratio is measured by applying a signal differentially, i.e. between input 1 and input 2, at a gain setting which produces a measurable output, and by then determining the size of the signal needed to produce the same output when the signal is applied in common mode, i.e. between an interconnection of the two inputs and ground; the ratio of the amplitude of the second input signal over that of the first input signal is the discrimination of the amplifier. Good EEG machines have amplifiers with high discrimination, or rejection ratios, of 10,000 or more.

Differential amplification has the main purpose of eliminating electrical potentials which do not come from the brain. Potentials from the brain are usually not evenly distributed over the scalp and therefore cause different potential levels to appear in at least some of the scalp electrodes connected to the amplifier inputs; these differences are amplified and appear in the EEG. In contrast, potentials from outside the brain usually affect all scalp electrodes in the same manner and are therefore rejected or cancelled by the differential amplifier. This is true especially of 60 Hz interference. However, differential amplification does not always distinguish between cerebral activity and artifacts because some artifacts may produce slightly different potentials at some of the scalp electrodes, and some cerebral potentials may be in common mode at most electrodes. This can lead to (1) failure to reject artifacts and (2) cancellation of cerebral activity.

(1) *Failure to reject artifacts* is usually due to either (a) unequal impedance of the recording electrodes or (b) absence of an effective ground connection to the patient.

(a) *Unequal impedance of the recording electrodes* at the two inputs to an amplifier causes potentials of equal amplitude on the scalp to appear with different amplitude at the inputs. This difference in signal amplitude will then be amplified and appear at the output. The most common result of unequal electrode impedance is the appearance at the output of 60 Hz artifact from alternating current sources. The amplitude of the artifact depends on the severity of the impedance imbalance and the strength of the interference signal. The interference is weak in most EEG laboratories, but may be strong when recordings are made in unshielded locations such as patient rooms, intensive care units and operating rooms; minor imbalances of electrode impedances may then become critical. A common cause of impedance imbalance is partial or complete loss of contact between electrode and scalp. This results in an output reflecting only the difference between a single input and the ground of the amplifier. If the amplifier ground is connected to the patient, the output of such a 'single-ended' amplifier will reflect the potential differences between the input electrode and the ground electrode; the recording usually contains much artifact from 60 Hz interference, heart beat and other sources due to the loss of discrimination against common mode signals. However, if the amplifier ground is not connected to the patient, the output represents the difference between cerebral potential changes and the entirely unrelated potential level of the amplifier ground. This might be called a 'monopolar' recording and is obviously without any use. The term 'monopolar' should not be applied to other recordings, because all other recordings are between two points. This is true regardless of whether the recordings are made with bipolar or with referential montages (4.1).

(b) *Absent or ineffective ground connection to the patient* does not preclude recording of potential differences between input 1 and 2. However, the inputs float without reference to the potential level at which the amplifier inverts input 2 to subtract it from input 1. An amplifier with floating input is therefore more likely to 'see' signals which are equal with reference to the patient's head as being different and to therefore amplify artifacts which would be rejected if the amplifier had an effective ground connection to the patient's head.

(2) *Rejection of cerebral potentials.* Discrimination cancels cerebral potentials that are in common mode. EEG potential changes which appear at exactly the same time and have exactly the same shape and amplitude over all parts of the head would therefore escape detection in recordings from scalp electrodes and would require recordings between one electrode over the head and another electrode elsewhere on the body. Such potential changes probably occur very rarely if at all. More often, even widespread potential changes differ slightly in shape, amplitude and timing at some recording sites over the head.

**3.4.2** *Amplification.* The amplifier increases the voltage difference between the inputs so that the voltage of the output can be used to drive the pens of the EEG machine. This amplifying action can be characterized in terms of sensitivity and gain.

*Sensitivity* is the ratio of input voltage to the pen deflection it produces. Sensitivity is measured in microvolts per millimeter ($\mu$V/mm). A commonly used sensitivity is 7 $\mu$V/mm. At this sensitivity, a calibration signal of 50 $\mu$V causes a pen deflection of about 7 mm. Note that a sensitivity setting of higher numerical value means a lower sensitivity or less amplification: A sensitivity setting of 10 $\mu$V/mm will make a calibration signal smaller than a sensitivity setting of 7 $\mu$V/mm. Conversely, decreasing the setting from 10 $\mu$V/mm to 7 $\mu$V/mm increases the sensitivity of the amplifier.

The sensitivity of each channel can be adjusted between high values of 1 or 2 $\mu$V/mm and low values of at least 1000 $\mu$V/mm. These adjustments are made with switches which increase the sensitivity stepwise by factors of no more than two. A variable control permits equalizing the sensitivity between channels precisely; equalization should be necessary only rarely. In addition to these individual sensitivity controls for each channel, most EEG machines have a master sensitivity switch which controls the sensitivity of all channels.

Because sensitivity can be directly determined by applying a calibration pulse and measuring the pen deflection, sensitivity rather than gain is usually used to describe amplification by EEG machines.

*Gain* is the ratio of signal voltage obtained at the output of the amplifier to the signal voltage applied at the input. For instance, an amplifier set to give an output voltage of 10 V for an input of 10 $\mu$V is said to have a gain of 1 million; this is the usual maximum gain of EEG machines. Gain is sometimes expressed in decibels, the number of decibels amounting to 20 times the $\text{logarithm}_{10}$ of the gain. For instance, a gain of 10 equals 20 dB, a gain of 100 equals 40 dB, a gain of 1 million equals 120 dB. In contrast to sensitivity, gain is defined so that it increases with increasing amplification. However, gain is not a useful measure in clinical EEG because the output voltage of the amplifier is not directly measured.

## 3.5 FILTERS

Filters are used to exclude waves of relatively high or low frequencies from the EEG so that waves in the most important middle range of about 1–30 Hz can be recorded clearly and without distortion. The effect of filters is often illustrated and specified in terms of their actions on electronically generated sine or square waves (Fig. 3.3). It must be stressed that filters affect any component of the EEG to the extent that it raises or falls with a slope corresponding with that of sine waves (Fig. 3.3, right).

Most EEG machines have three kinds of filters. (1) The low frequency filter reduces the amplitude of slow waves. (2) The high frequency filter reduces the amplitude of fast waves. (3) The 60 Hz filter selectively reduces the amplitude of waves of about 60 Hz, the frequency of the most common electrical artifact*. Each of these three filter actions is usually provided by individual channel controls permitting different selections for each channel and by master switches allowing selection of the same settings for all channels.

**3.5.1** *The low frequency filter* can be characterized by its effect either on sine waves, giving the 'low filter frequency', or on square pulses, giving the 'time constant'.

*Low filter frequency* specifies the frequency at which sine waves are reduced in amplitude by a fixed fraction. Figures 3.3 and 3.4 show the effects of different filter settings on sine waves of different frequencies. The first four channels in each figure were recorded with low filter frequencies of 0.1, 0.3, 1 and 5 Hz. The filters reduce the amplitude of sine waves at these frequencies by 20% or 2 dB. Sine waves of lower frequency are reduced more, and even sine waves slightly above the cutoff frequency are reduced some, although by less than 20%. As a result, a sine wave of

* A 50 Hz filter is used in countries using a power line frequency of 50 Hz.

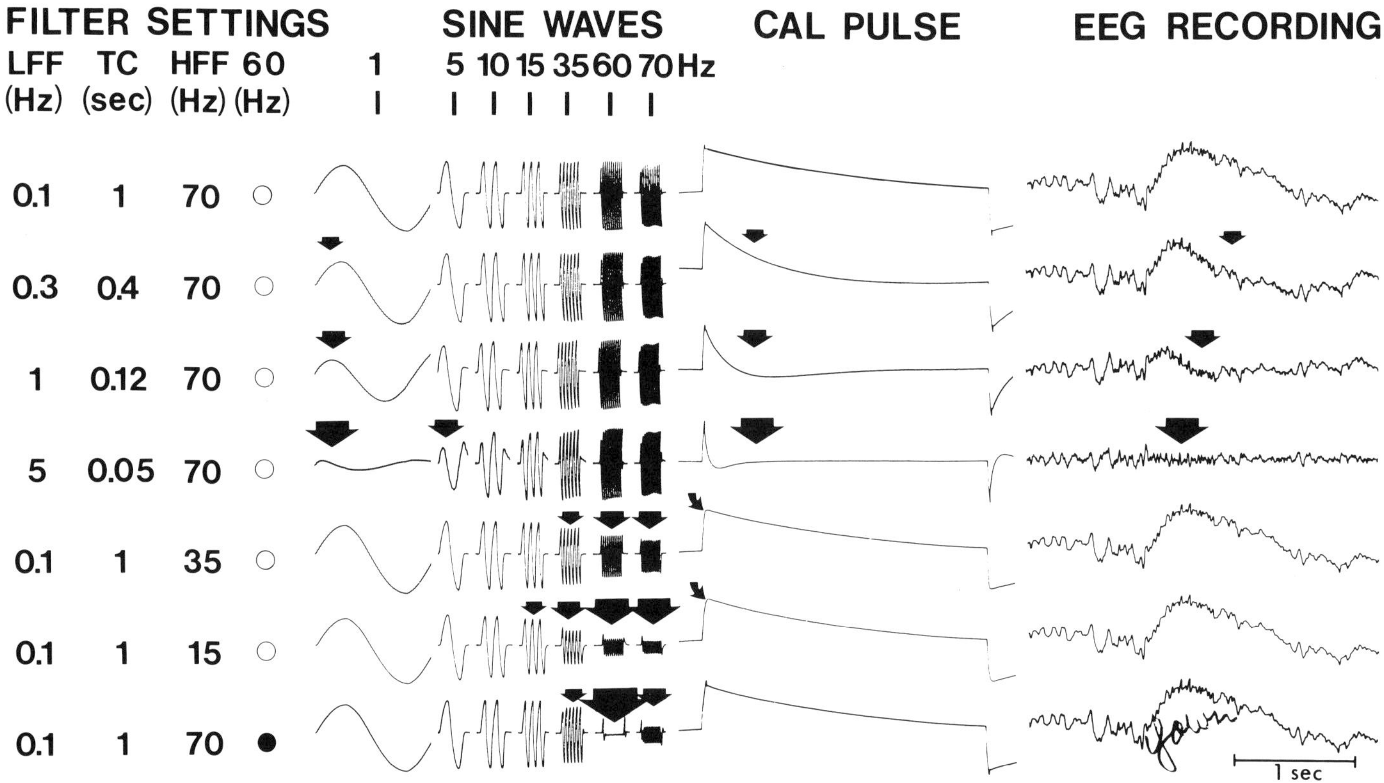
FILTER SETTINGS
LFF (Hz)
TC (sec)
HFF (Hz)
60 (Hz)
SINE WAVES
1 5 10 15 35 60 70 Hz
CAL PULSE
EEG RECORDING
0.1 1 70
0.3 0.4 70
1 0.12 70
5 0.05 70
0.1 1 35
0.1 1 15
0.1 1 70
1 sec

0.3 Hz is nearly abolished by a filter setting of 5 Hz, severly reduced by a setting of 1 Hz, and reduced by 20% by a setting of 0.3 Hz; it can be recorded without amplitude distortion only with a filter setting below 0.3 Hz. It may be noted that filters also distort the time relation between waves of frequencies near the cutoff frequency, each filter delaying these waves by different amounts of time.

The relationship between the amplitude and the frequency of sine waves at different filter settings is summarized in the diagram at the bottom of Figure 3.4. Here, each curve on the left side represents one low frequency filter setting and shows the amount of reduction of amplitude of waves having frequencies below the medium range. This figure makes it clear that filters of EEG machines have no sharp cutoff: Waves of frequencies below the low filter frequency are not entirely eliminated, waves slightly above that frequency are not entirely unaffected.

---

◀ Fig. 3.3. The effect of different filter settings on sine waves of various frequencies, a calibration pulse and a segment of EEG recording. The same signals are applied to the inputs of all channels; therefore, the differences in the outputs, enhanced by arrows, are due to the different filter settings used in each channel. Filter settings are indicated at the left margin. Low frequency filter settings are given both in terms of low filter frequency (LFF) representing the frequency at which sine waves are reduced by 20% in amplitude, and in terms of the corresponding time constant (TC). High frequency filter settings are indicated in terms of high filter frequency (HFF) representing the frequency at which sine waves are reduced in amplitude by 20%. The 60 Hz filter is used only in the last channel. Channels 1–4 show the effect of increasing the low filter frequency, or of decreasing the time constant: The amplitude of sine waves of low frequency is progressively reduced, the calibration pulse returns to baseline faster, and slow waves are reduced in the EEG. Channels 5 and 6 show the effect of decreasing the high frequency filter: Sine waves of high frequency are reduced in amplitude, the calibration pulse is rounded off at its tip, and fast waves in the EEG are reduced in amplitude and increased in duration as compared with channels 4 and 7, although this effect is less noticeable here than in tracings containing fast activity of higher amplitude (Fig. 6.2., Parts 1 and 2). The last channel shows the effect of the 60 Hz filter: Sine waves of 60 Hz are eliminated and those at 35 and 70 Hz are reduced in amplitude, the calibration pulse shows a barely visible deformation in the rising and falling phase, and the EEG tracing loses the slight amount of superimposed 60 Hz activity which is recognizable as the 'hum' or thickness of the tracing in channel 4 and reduced by the high frequency filter settings used in channels 5 and 6; this effect is better appreciated in tracings containing more 60 Hz artifact (Fig. 6.3, Part 1).

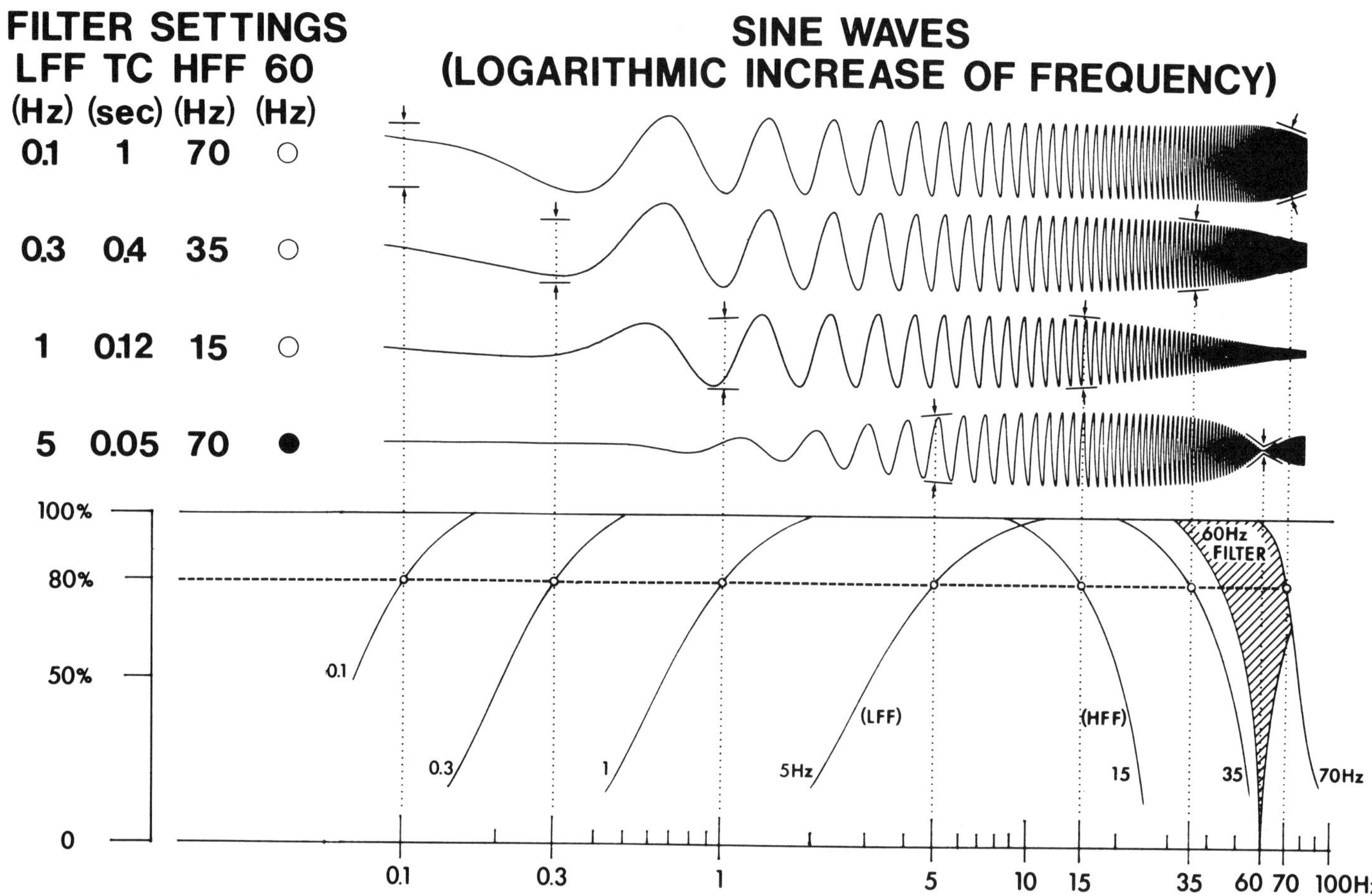

FILTER SETTINGS
LFF TC HFF 60
(Hz) (sec) (Hz) (Hz)
0.1 1 70
0.3 0.4 35
1 0.12 15
5 0.05 70
SINE WAVES
(LOGARITHMIC INCREASE OF FREQUENCY)
100%
80%
50%
0
60Hz FILTER
(LFF)
(HFF)
0.1
0.3
1
5Hz
15
35
70Hz
0.1 0.3 1 5 10 15 35 60 70 100Hz

*The time constant* describes the effect of the low frequency filter on square pulses. The time constant is the time required for the pen to fall to 37% of the peak deflection produced when a steady voltage, such as a calibration pulse, is applied to the input of the amplifier (Fig. 3.5a). The time constant can be easily measured in EEG recordings by drawing a horizontal line at about one-third the height of the calibration signal; the time from the beginning of the calibration pulse to the intersection of the horizontal line with the falling phase of the calibration signal is the time constant (Fig. 3.5a). Figure 3.3 shows the effect of different low frequency filter settings on square pulses. These settings are indicated both in terms of low filter frequencies and of time constants on the left side of the figure. Note that an increase in the time constant means that waves of lower frequency are amplified without distortion, i.e. a *long* time constant, or a time constant of *high* numerical value, corresponds with an effect on waves of *low* frequency. The most commonly used time constant settings fall in the range of about 1 to 0.03 sec.

The values of time constants and low filter frequency can be interconverted. Thus, the time constant TC in a simple network of resistors and capacitors is related to the low filter frequency by the equation $TC = 1/2\ \pi$ f where f is the frequency at

---

◀ Fig. 3.4. The effect of different filter settings on the amplitude of sine waves which have frequencies representative of the spectrum of frequencies recorded in the EEG. *Top*: Sine waves of logarithmically increasing frequency are recorded with filter settings which are indicated at the left margin in the same notation as used for Fig. 3.3. Filter settings for both high and low frequencies are changed between channels 1 to 4 so that the amplitude of slow and fast waves progressively decreases; the 60 Hz filter is used in channel 4. Arrows indicate the frequencies at which the amplitude is reduced by 20%; dotted lines project these values to the graph below. *Bottom*: A graph of filter settings is derived from the recording in the top part and relates the amplitude of sine waves, in percent of total amplification (vertical axis on left), to the wave frequency (horizontal axis with logarithmic scale at bottom). Each curve corresponds with a setting of the low frequency filter (LFF), high frequency filter (HFF) or 60 Hz filter and indicates the reduction in amplitude of sine waves at that setting.

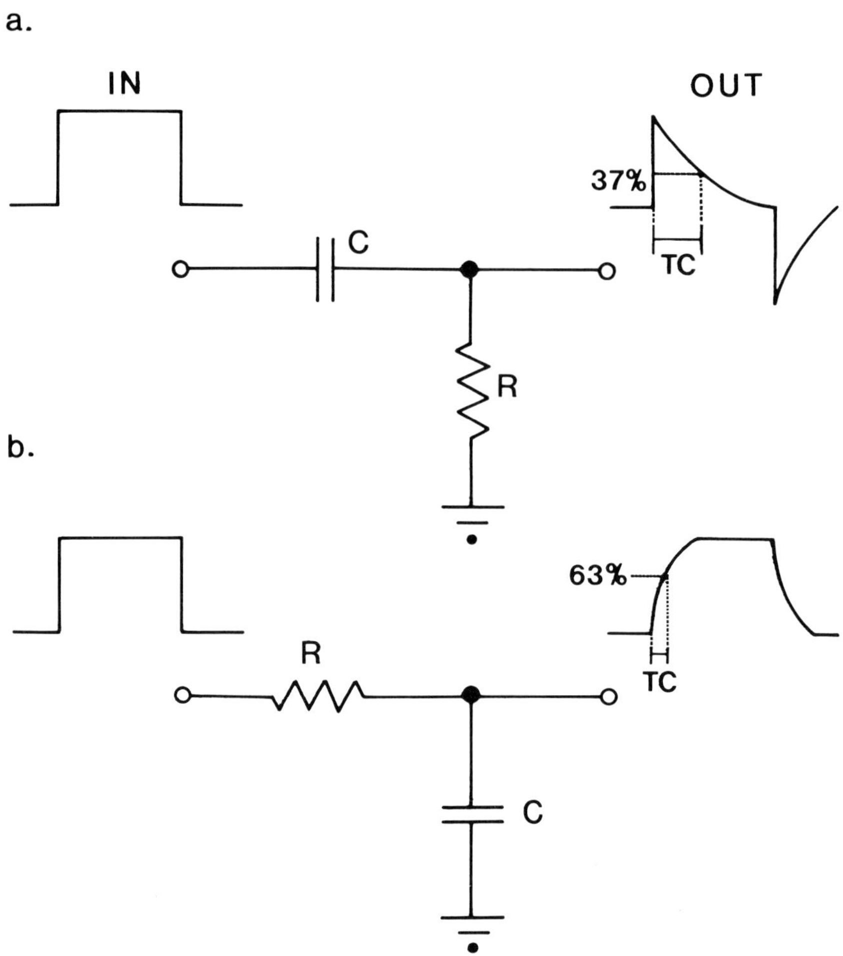
a.
IN
OUT
37%
TC
C
R
b.
63%
TC
R
C

which the amplitude is attenuated by 30% or 3 dB. This means that time constants of 1, 0.3, 0.1 and 0.03 sec, used in some EEG machines, correspond with 30% amplitude attenuation of waves of frequencies of 0.16, 0.53, 1.6 and 5.3 Hz. The low frequency settings producing 20% attenuation at 0.1, 0.3, 1 and 5 Hz, used in some other machines, correspond with time constants of 1, 0.4, 0.12 and 0.035 sec.

*Limits of low frequency* result from the design of EEG machines. Most machines are not designed to record very slow or very long-sustained potential changes. Their inputs do not have direct coupling which is needed to conduct potential changes of zero Hz or direct current (D.C.); instead, they are coupled through capacitors which process alternating signals such as alternating current (A.C.). Direct coupling is not used in clinical EEG because cerebral activity of very low frequency does probably not contain diagnostic information and is very difficult to record without artifacts due to instability of the electrical properties of skin, electrodes, amplifiers and other machine components.

*Electrical construction* of filters often uses a capacitor (C) placed in the path of the signal (Fig. 3.5a) which is separated from ground by a resistor (R). The capacitor opposes slow potential changes more than fast ones. The network in Fig. 3.5a is a low frequency filter, or high frequency pass. It has a time constant of $TC = R \times C$ and a low frequency reduction of 3 dB or 30% at a frequency of $f = 1/2\pi R \times C$.

**3.5.2** *The high frequency filter* reduces the size of fast waves. Its effect is specified

---

◀ Fig 3.5. Circuits of simple low and high frequency filters made of a capacitor (C) and a resistor (R). – a. Low frequency filter consists of a capacitor in the signal path and a resistor connection to ground. The time constant (TC) of this circuit is defined as the time required for a steady input voltage to drop to 37% of its amplitude at the output and equals the product of R × C. – b. High frequency filter consists of a resistor in the signal path and a capacitor connection to ground. The time constant of this circuit is defined as the time required for the output voltage to rise to 63% of a sudden input voltage and is also equal to the product of R × C.

by the frequency of waves which are reduced by a fixed fraction, for instance 30% or 3 dB, or 20% or 2 dB. Figures 3.3 and 3.4 show the effects of high frequency filter settings of 15, 35 and 70 Hz which reduce the amplitude of sine waves at these frequencies by 20% or 2 dB. Sine waves above the cutoff frequencies are reduced more, but sine waves slightly below the cutoff are also reduced, even though by less than 20%. These relations are summarized by the curves on the right side of the diagram at the bottom of Figure 3.4.

The middle part of Figure 3.3 shows the effects of high frequency filters on square waves used for calibration. Square waves contain high frequency components mainly at their peaks. The filtering of high frequencies affects mainly the rise time of the calibration pulses. This effect is barely visible at the normally slow speed of EEG recordings but causes the tips of the calibration pulses to become slightly rounded (curved arrows in Fig. 3.3). This effect becomes more obvious with very low settings of the high frequency filter and very high recording speeds, but measurement of the time constant of the rising phase (TC in Fig. 3.5b) is not practical with the recording methods used in conventional EEG.

High frequency filters must be set to include frequencies faster than those usually considered important in clinical EEG. Although waves of over 35 Hz are of little clinical interest, the use of high frequency filters set at that value can badly distort the EEG. This is especially true of the diagnostically very important fast components contained in spikes and sharp waves; application of high frequency filters can reduce these fast components and thereby transform the spikes and sharp waves into inconspicuous waves. On the other hand, muscle activity, a common contaminant consisting of fast waves, is often not eliminated by filtering as would be desirable, but is instead reduced in amplitude and made to last longer; filtered muscle activity may be more difficult to distinguish from cerebral activity than unfiltered muscle activity (Fig. 6.2).

*Limits of high frequency* are due to the design of the writing units; the commonly used ink pens cannot be driven to write much faster than 70 Hz without significant distortion.

*Electrical construction* of high frequency filters often uses a capacitor (C) to shunt high frequencies from the signal path to ground (Fig. 3.5b). The network in Figure 3.5b reduces the amplitude of waves of a frequency of $f = 1/2\pi R \times C$ by 30% or 3 dB.

**3.5.2** *The 60 Hz filter* is provided in many EEG machines to eliminate the most common type of electrical artifact, namely interference from devices powered by alternating current. This filter sharply reduces the amplitude of sine waves of 60 Hz*, but it cannot accomplish this without also reducing the amplitude of waves of neighboring frequencies to some extent (Figs. 3.3 and 3.4). Although sine waves of 60 Hz are not usually produced by the brain and could be spared from EEG recordings, the 60 Hz filter should not be used routinely for several reasons. (a) Some EEG components, for instance spikes, may contain slopes corresponding with the 60 Hz frequency; filtering at 60 Hz, like filtering with high frequency filters, could reduce these components so that they become unrecognizable. (b) 60 Hz interference may indicate a poor electrode contact or an improper input selection which would go undetected and uncorrected if the 60 Hz filter is used indiscriminately. The 60 Hz filter should therefore be used only in the full knowledge of what it may obscure and after all other efforts to eradicate the cause of the interference have been exhausted.

## 3.6 WRITING UNITS

**3.6.1** *The writing devices* serve to convert the fluctuating potential changes at the

* A 50 Hz filter is used in countries using a power line frequency of 50 Hz.

output of the amplifiers into a vertical movement. In most EEG machines, this is accomplished with oscillographs. An oscillograph consists of a galvanometer coil which is mounted in the field of a permanent magnet so that the coil rotates in response to the electrical potential changes coming from the amplifier output. The shaft of the galvanometer coil protrudes above the writing surface and holds the writing device which moves up and down on the EEG paper with excursions corresponding with the amplitude of the electrical potential changes. The most common writing devices are pens consisting of a metal tube filled with ink from an

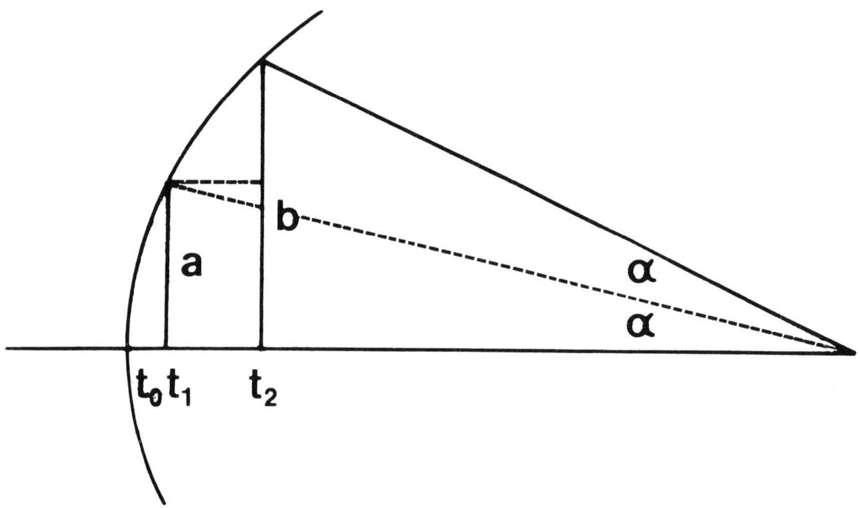


Fig. 3.6. Distortions of the EEG by curvilinear writing movements of pens. The circular movement of the pen around the shaft causes the tracing to deviate from rectangular coordinates both in the horizontal and vertical dimensions. Horizontal error: A pen deflection to the height indicated by line a or b seems to occur at times $t_1$ and $t_2$ even though it is synchronous with $t_0$. Vertical error: The amplitude of b, even though caused by a pen deflection twice that of a, is not twice the amplitude of a.

inkwell. Other writing devices use ink jets, carbon paper, and light or heat sensitive paper.

*Curvilinear distortion* results from the arc-like movement of pens around an axis. The deviation from rectilinear movement causes faulty representation of both vertical and horizontal coordinates (Fig. 3.6). The vertical deflection is neither strictly straight nor strictly proportional to the applied voltage. The horizontal position of a deflected pen depends on the degree of the vertical deflection so that a higher deflection seems to have occurred later in time than a simultaneous deflection of lower amplitude. Both types of distortion increase with the amplitude of the deflection and distort the shape and amplitude of every curvilinear EEG writeout to some degree.

*Vertical and horizontal pen alignment* should be perfect (Fig. 3.7). The pens must have equal distance from each other and point exactly in the direction of the paper movement. The pens must also be aligned so that a signal appearing in all channels at the same time deflects the pens on the same line on the paper, perpendicular to the paper movement; if one pen protrudes to the left or right of the others, a signal written by that pen will seem to have occurred earlier or later than a signal written at the same time by the other pens.

*Faulty pen alignment* may be due to the following:

(1) If the horizontal spacing between the pen tips is uneven regardless of whether or not the pens are connected to the amplifier outputs (Fig. 3.7b), a pen may have been damaged or moved out of its seat; if this is not the case, the pen may have rotated away from its correct position on the galvanometer shaft and should be rotated to the correct position by readjusting its seat on the shaft.

(2) If the horizontal spacing between the pens changes suddenly when they are connected to the amplifier outputs (Fig. 3.7c), the electrical potential level of the output is at fault and should be reset by adjusting the electrical zero potential level of the amplifier outputs. However, minor steps of the baseline may appear during

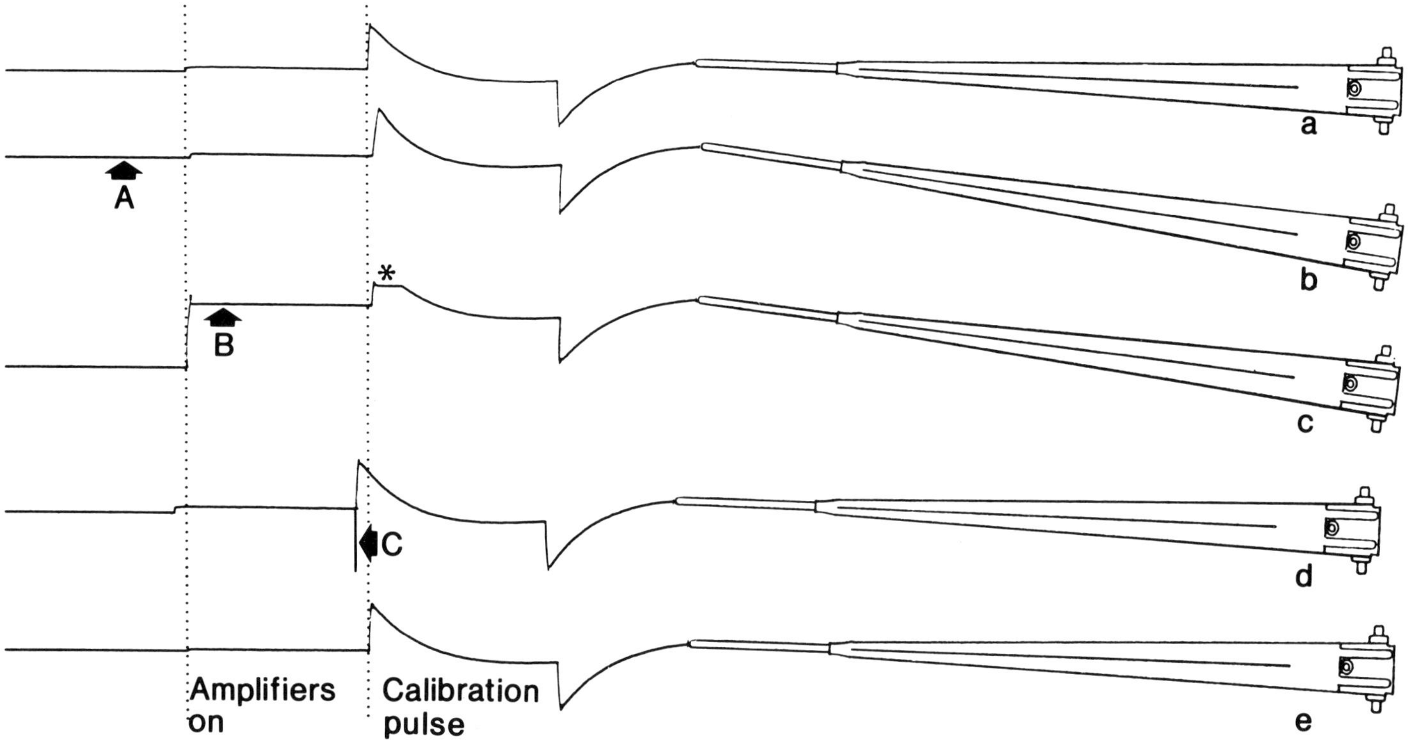


Fig. 3.7. Pen misalignments. Pens a and e are normal: They write tracings that are properly spaced, show only minimal deflections when the amplifiers are turned on ('Amplifiers on'), and do not distort the calibration pulse; the deflections of these pens fall on the same vertical line (dotted lines); Pen b writes a tracing that is displaced upward both before and after the amplifier output is connected to the pens (arrow A); this is due to a mechanical deviation from the zero line, usually caused by an improper adjustment of the pen on its shaft; Pen c writes a tracing that is displaced upward at the moment when the amplifiers are turned on (arrow B) and clips large signals in that direction (*); this is due to an electrical deviation from the zero line caused by faulty adjustment of the voltage level of the amplifier output; Pen d registers deflections that are displaced to the left (arrow C) and seem to occur earlier than those of the other pens; this horizontal deviation is usually due to improper alignment of the oscillograph or of the pen seat.

everyday operation and are tolerable if they are not much larger than the width of the ink tracing (Fig. 3.7a and e). Transient pen deflections may appear suddenly when the amplifier inputs are opened immediately after changing the selection of recording electrodes at the input and are usually due to electrode bias potentials (2.2.4).

(3) If the tips of the pens at rest are not aligned in a straight vertical line on the paper (Fig. 3.7d), the pens deviating from this line can be moved left or right into the correct position by adjusting the position of the pen seat or of the oscillator in the EEG machine. Before making this adjustment, one should be sure that the deviation is not due to improper mounting to the pen in its seat on the galvanometer shaft or to bent or damaged pens.

**3.6.2** *The paper transport* pulls the paper from a folded stack in a storage bin within the machine, moves it at an even speed under the writing pens and across a surface where the ink dries and the record can be inspected and labelled for at least 60 cm, and deposits it into another storage bin where it is folded again. Modern machines use the internationally recommended paper speed of 3 cm/second and usually have additional faster and slower speeds. EEG paper is often imprinted with vertical lines every 3 cm, corresponding with 1 second at regular speed; these intervals may be subdivided. Many EEG machines have time markers producing a pen deflection in an extra channel every 1 second. This should generate intervals of the same length as those printed on the chart paper if the paper is moving at the speed of 3 cm/second.

Physically, the paper transport consists of a motor with gear shift and friction rollers which pull the margin of the paper. The transport mechanism may give rise to various problems.

(a) If the paper slows or stops for a moment during the recording because of a momentary failure of the driving mechanism or because of a momentary resistance of the paper feed, the time base of the recording will be distorted: the pens will deflect up and down with little or no movement to the side and create the impression of very fast and abnormal EEG transients, such as spikes. This artifact can be recognized by the very steep rises and falls of the pen deflections and by the fact that the same phenomenon occurs in all or most channels at the same time (Fig. 6).

(b) When stiff paper with sharp creases is not sufficiently stretched as it is pulled along under the pens, the pens may be bounced up and off the paper at each upward fold. This gives an interrupted, irregular tracing of all pens following each upward fold.

(c) The paper may run not on a straight course or it may track too close to the upper or lower edge. This can be corrected by adjusting the front or rear paper guides and rollers on the machine.

(d) The paper speed may vary due to defects of the friction rollers, gear shift or motor. This distorts the timing of the writeout and makes regular wave shapes appear irregular.

## REFERENCES


Barlow, J.S., Kamp, A., Morton, H.B., Ripoche, A., Shipton, H. and Tchavdarov, D.B. (1978) EEG Instrumentation Standards (revised 1977): Report of the Committee on EEG Instrumentation Standards of the International Federation of Societies for Electroencephalography and Clinical Neurophysiology. Electroenceph. clin. Neurophysiol. 45: 144–150.

Cooper, R., Osselton, J.W. and Shaw, J.C. (1974) EEG Technology. 2nd Ed., Butterworths, London.

Hopps, J.A. (1976) Section V. Shock hazards in electrophysiological recordings. In: Rémond, A. (Ed.), Handbook of Electroenceph. clin. Neurophysiol., Vol. 3A, Elsevier, Amsterdam, pp. 75–79.

Mac Gillivray, B.A. (1974) Section III. Recording the EEG. In: Rémond, A. (Ed.), Handbook of Electroenceph. clin. Neurophysiol., Vol. 3C, Elsevier, Amsterdam, pp. 58–87.

Richey, E.T. and Namon, R. (1976) EEG Instrumentation and Technology. Thomas, Springfield.

Roy, O.Z. and Achorn, E. (1976) Section II. Amplification of bioelectric potentials. In: Rémond, A. (Ed.), Handbook of Electroenceph. clin. Neurophysiol., Vol. 3A, Elsevier, Amsterdam, pp. 28–45.

# 4 Recording strategy

SUMMARY

(4.1) *Multichannel recordings* can be used to determine the distribution of potential changes on the scalp when appropriate electrode combinations, or montages, are used. There are mainly two types of montages, each having different advantages and disadvantages. (1) *Bipolar montages* connect pairs of different electrodes to each amplifier, usually selecting adjacent electrodes for successive channels so that each electrode is common to two channels. Bipolar montages have the advantage of sharply localizing the peaks of potentials, especially of potentials which occupy small areas, but they can create problems by distorting the shape of widely distributed potentials. (2) *Referential montages* connect input 1 of a group of channels to different scalp electrodes and input 2 of all these channels to the same electrode which thus becomes the reference for each channel. Referential montages can provide an undistorted display of amplitude, configuration and distribution of potentials which occupy a wide area, but can cause problems if the reference electrode itself picks up significant cerebral activity.

(4.2) *Specific montages* are usually designed to compare potentials on both sides of the head and in neighboring areas. The best montages use straight chains of equidistant electrodes along and across the head and display the potentials in an orderly sequence of channels. Several simple bipolar and referential montages should be used for routine recordings in all laboratories; to these may be added locally preferred routine montages and montages developed for specific problems. A list of recommended 16- and 8-channel montages for routine recordings, for recordings from newborn infants and for recordings in cases of suspected cerebral death is appended.

(4.3) *Monitoring of extracerebral activity*, for instance of eye movements, heart beat, respiration and muscle activity, is often done to identify artifacts in EEG recordings or to determine sleep stages.

## 4.1 MULTICHANNEL RECORDINGS

As pointed out in the preceding chapter (3.4.1), the output of a single channel does not reveal the polarity, amplitude and timing of potential changes at input 1 and input 2; recordings from a single channel can therefore not indicate the distribution of potentials on the head. This shortcoming can be overcome by simultaneous recording from more than one channel. Multichannel recording can become a powerful instrument in EEG analysis if appropriate montages are used. The most effective electrode combinations, or montages, use straight chains of electrodes in anterior-posterior or transverse rows.

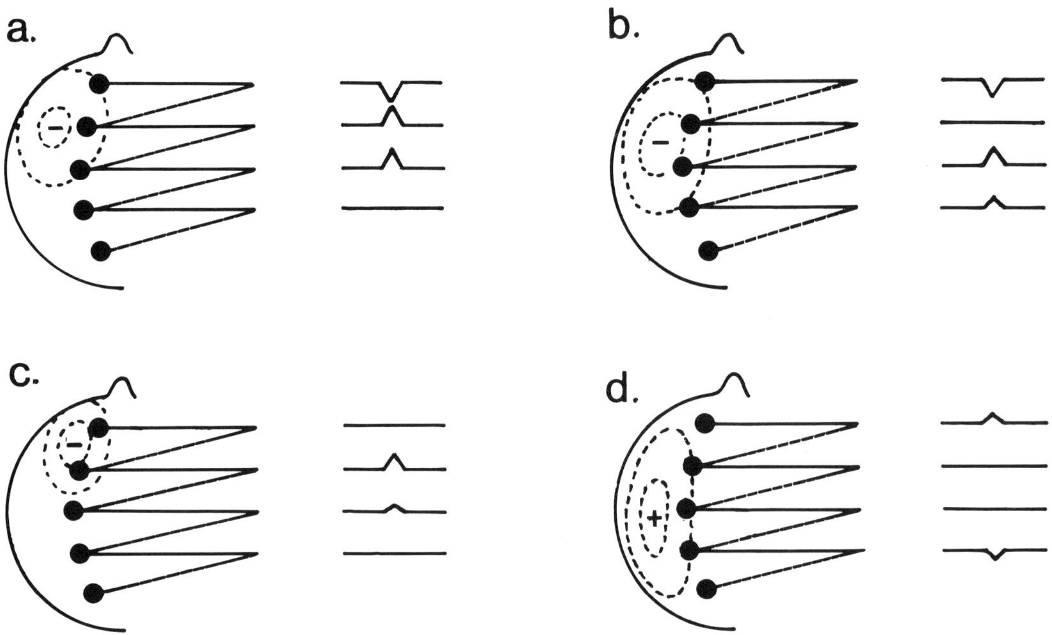


Fig. 4.1. Bipolar montages. a. and b.: Localization of electrical potentials on the scalp by phase reversal; c. and d.: Possible pitfalls of this method.

In general, montages can be divided into two types: bipolar and referential. Although most of the information obtained with one type of montage can be converted into that obtained with the other, each montage has some shortcomings which can be overcome to a degree by the use of the other; both types of montages should therefore be used routinely in every recording.

**4.1.1** *Bipolar montages.* *Strategy*: Bipolar montages connect pairs of different electrodes to the inputs of amplifiers. The best bipolar montages link electrodes in chains so that an electrode at input 2 of one amplifier is also at input 1 of the next amplifier (Fig. 4.1). In this strategy, the origin of a potential is localized not by the amplitude but by the direction of pen deflections. A potential located at an electrode which is common to two amplifiers in a bipolar linkage causes pen deflections of opposite direction, or 'phase reversal' at the output of these amplifiers. Figure 4.1a shows a bipolar montage recording of a negative potential. The top channel shows a downgoing deflection because it is connected to the electrode near the negative potential through input 2, whereas the next channel, being connected to that electrode through input 1, shows an upgoing deflection. It should be obvious that this phase reversal indicates not a reversal of polarity of the potential but only a reversal in the direction of the pen deflection; the potential is negative regardless of the pen deflections. A positive potential would give a phase reversal in the opposite direction, and cause the pens to deflect apart instead of together.

A potential having a maximum between two recording electrodes (Fig. 4.1b) causes no deflection in the channel connected to these electrodes. However, the potential can be detected because these electrodes are also connected to two other channels which will show a phase reversal (channels 1 and 3 in Fig. 4.1b). In the case of a negative potential, the deflections in these channels are towards each other, in the case of a positive potential, they are away from each other.

*Advantages of bipolar recordings*: Bipolar linkages sharply distinguish potential

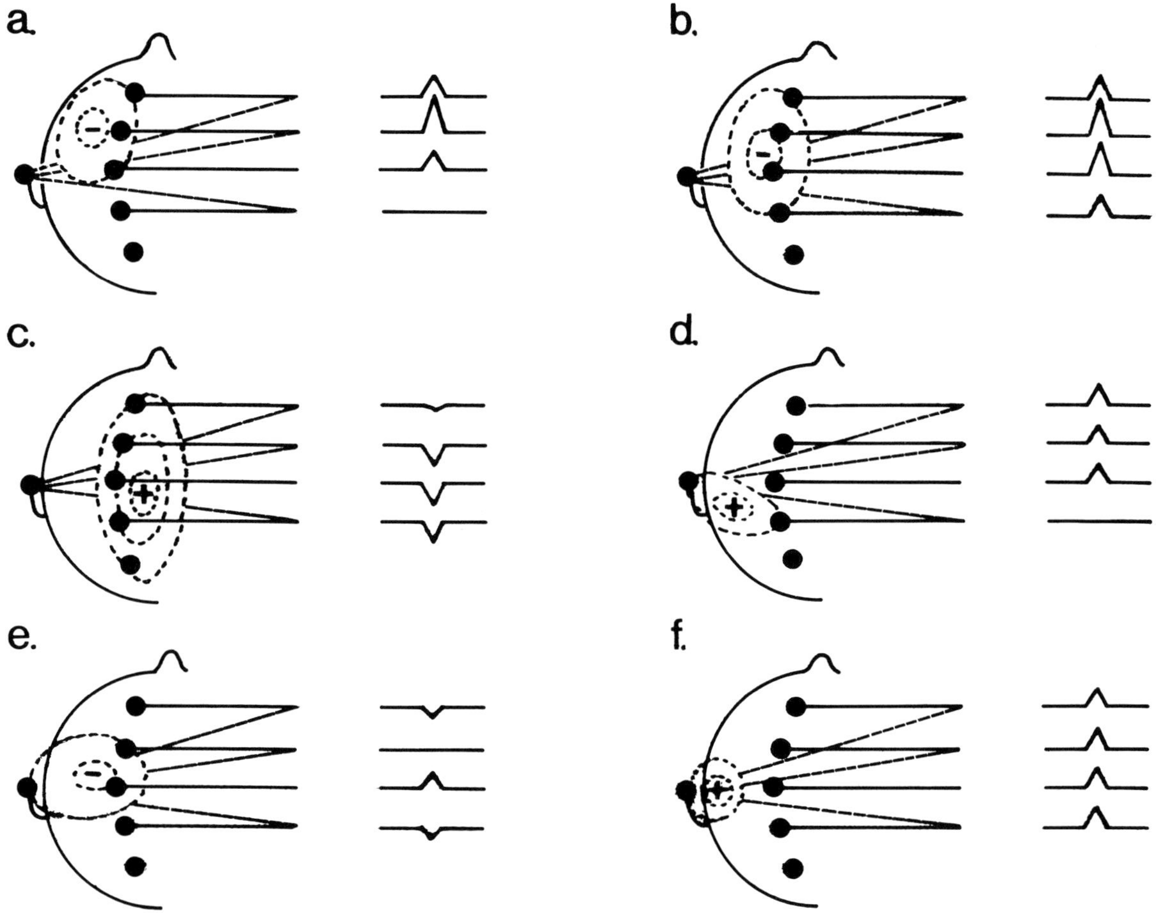


Fig. 4.2. Referential montages. a, b and c: Localization of electrical potentials by amplitude of pen deflections; d, e and f: Possible pitfalls of this method.

changes in neighboring electrodes and thus can localize circumscribed potentials more precisely than can referential montages.

*Disadvantages*: Bipolar montages distort the waveshape and amplitude of potentials which are distributed widely and affect both recording electrodes connected to one channel; in the recording of such a potential, each channel records only that part of the potential which is different at the two electrodes. Potentials between the last two electrodes in a chain may produce confusing pen deflections (Fig. 4.1c), and very widespread potentials may be largely cancelled (Fig. 4.1d).

**4.1.2** *Referential montages. Strategy*: Referential montages connect inputs 1 of a group of amplifiers to electrodes placed on various parts of the head and inputs 2 of these amplifiers to a common electrode placed in an electrically quiet area; this electrode is called the 'reference electrode'. This method records the potential differences between the various points on the head and the reference electrode. Figure 4.2a shows a referential montage recording the same potential as that recorded with a bipolar montage in Figure 4.1a. In the referential montage, the origin of this potential on the head is recognized by the amplitude: The channel which records the potential of highest amplitude is connected to the electrode nearest the origin of the potential. If the output of two channels is of equal amplitude, the origin of the potential is located an equal distance from each of the two electrodes connected to inputs 1 of these channels (Fig. 4.2b). If several channels have similar output, the potential affects input 1 of all these channels (Fig. 4.2c) to an equal degree.

*Advantages*: Referential recording can give an undistorted display of the shape of potential changes and is especially useful for recording of potentials which have a wide distribution.

*Disadvantages*: It is usually impossible to find a reference electrode which is entirely inactive. Potentials at the reference electrode may be large enough to appear in recordings from all channels connected to that electrode. Potentials at such an 'active reference electrode' may produce confusing results and reproduce some of the potential changes usually recorded at the scalp electrodes connected to input 1:

(1) A potential may affect only the reference electrode; for instance a spike in the temporal lobe may appear as a transient positive potential at an ear electrode, a commonly used reference. This will produce an upgoing deflection in all channels connected through input 2 to this electrode (Fig. 4.2f) and appear similar to the potential shown in Figure 4.2b.

(2) A potential located midway between the reference electrode and a scalp electrode may be cancelled in a channel connected to both these electrodes and appear in other channels that are connected to the reference electrode through input 2 (Fig. 4.2d); this is similar to the condition in Figure 4.2a.

(3) A potential may be located between the reference electrode and some scalp electrodes so that it appears as a contribution by input 1 in one channel (channel 3 in Fig. 4.2c), cancels between input 1 and 2 in another channel (channel 2 in Fig. 4.2e) and appears with opposite polarity as a contribution by the reference electrode in input 2 in the other channels (channels 1 and 4, Fig. 4.2c).

It may be difficult to localize the peak of a potential precisely with the referential technique because amplitude, the indicator of a potential peak with this technique, increases with interelectrode distance, i.e. the distance between the scalp and the reference electrode, up to about 10 cm. If the interelectrode distance in different channels of a referential montage varies very much, maximum amplitude may appear not at the electrode nearest the peak but at an electrode located at the greatest distance from the reference electrode.

*An average reference electrode* may be used as a means to reduce the importance of potential changes introduced by the reference electrode (3.2.3). Although this reference reduces the contribution of potential changes by each electrode in proportion to the number of recording electrodes in the average reference, it may show considerable activity if several electrodes in the reference are affected by the same potential changes.

**4.1.3** *Plotting the field* of EEG potentials is not routinely done with pencil and paper, but the steps leading to a picture of the distribution of the contours of potentials in two or three dimensions on the scalp are part of the mental process involved in routine EEG analysis. These plots are based on the idea that the electrode chains laid along and across the head form part of a spatial coordinate system; polarity and amplitude of the potentials at each point are depicted in the vertical direction. The output of all amplifiers at any instant can then be used to plot an electrical field in the form of a picture of mountains and valleys over different parts of the head. The examples of this section use only four channels to define the location of potentials in only one row of electrodes; a three-dimensional picture requires recordings in more than one row of electrodes.

Plots can be made from bipolar and from referential recordings. Figure 4.3a shows the bipolar recording illustrated in Figure 4.1a. The amplitude of each pen deflection is indicated by an arrow to the right of each recording and, because it represents the potential difference between adjacent electrodes, plotted halfway between the recording electrode locations. A line connecting the tips of the arrows outlines the contour of the electrical field in this dimension. Figure 4.3b shows the same potential in a referential recording, also illustrated in Figure 4.2a. The amplitude of each pen deflection, representing the potential difference between each scalp electrode and the reference electrode, is indicated by an arrow to the right of the recordings, and plotted as an elevation above each electrode. The contour of the potential derived from the referential recording is practically identical with the contour obtained from the bipolar recording.

These diagrams show the contour of the field in only one plane. By recording from electrode chains oriented in parallel and at right angles to each other, one can

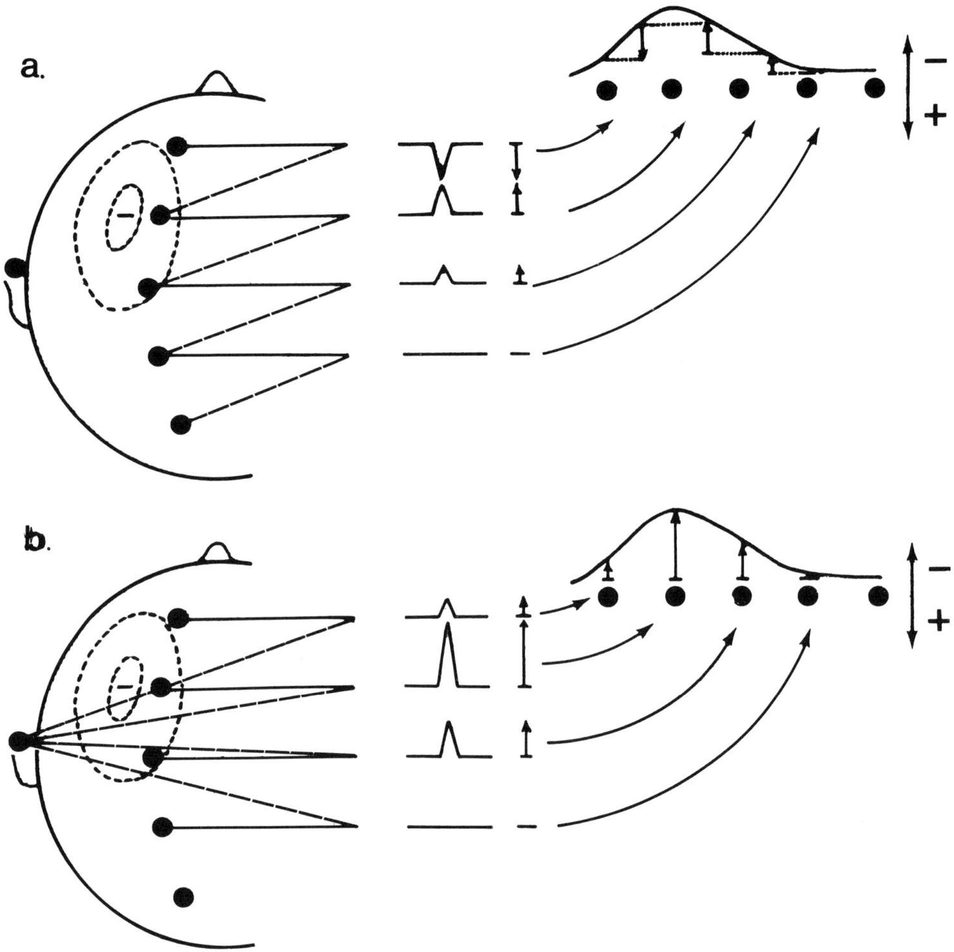
a.
b.

map the distribution of the field in several planes. Points of equal potential levels may be connected with each other and these isopotential lines may be drawn either in a three-dimensional view of peaks and valleys or in a two-dimensional projection of isopotential lines on the surface of the head. Simple two-dimensional views of isopotential lines are used to indicated the distribution of the electrical potentials by the stippled lines in Figures 4.1, 4.2 and 4.3.

*Dipoles* are concepts which are sometimes used to illustrate the distribution of electrical potentials on the scalp. These concepts have a very limited use in clinical electroencephalography. Briefly, the isopotential lines of an electrical field on the scalp may be thought to be generated by an electrical dipole, i.e. a center of two opposing charges. The appearance of a positive or negative field on the scalp may be assumed to be due to a vertically oriented dipole which shows only one pole at the surface, the other pole being buried in the depth of the brain. A horizontal dipole may be invoked in the rare instances where a potential change in one area of the head is consistently associated with an opposite potential change in another area. Although the concept of dipoles may be used to describe the distribution of electrical potentials at the scalp, it should not be mistaken to suggest that EEG potentials are generated by a single source deep in the brain. Dipoles do not correspond with structural components of the brain; the components of the electrical field are generated locally by the sheets of nerve cells in the cerebral cortex (1.1).

---

◀ Fig. 4.3. Plotting the contour line of an electrical field along a chain of electrodes with bipolar (a) and referential (b) montages, both giving the same results. The pen deflections caused by the scalp potential are represented by arrows shown in the middle of the figure; the arrows are used to plot the elevation of the potential above the horizontal electrode chain in the diagram on the right side of the figure. – a. In the bipolar montage, arrows in the diagram are drawn between scalp electrodes and with reference to adjacent arrows; – b. In the referential montage, arrows in the diagram are drawn above scalp electrode locations starting at a common baseline which represents the reference level.

Good montages fulfill a few simple requirements.

**4.2.1** *The number of channels* available is very important. A machine having a large number of channels can be connected to many electrodes simultaneously to record activity from wide areas of the head; such a machine is more useful than a machine with a smaller number of channels. However, even fairly large machines do not have enough channels to record from all useful electrode combinations at the same time; recordings are therefore made using some electrode combinations followed by recordings using other electrode combinations. This poses no problem in the case of potentials which recur frequently and do not change in distribution and shape, but it causes difficulty in the case of potentials which recur infrequently or vary in distribution and shape; the description of such potentials in all dimensions may require very long recording periods or remain incomplete. The chance to get a complete picture in a reasonably short period of time thus increases with the number of recording channels available.

**4.2.2** *Recording strategy* aims at comparing (a) activity in neighboring parts of the head and (b) activity in one area with that in the corresponding area of the other hemisphere. To satisfy both requirements, channels are usually connected to adjacent electrodes, half on one side of the head, and the other half on the other side. The most useful comparisons are made with recordings from chains of equally spaced electrodes connected in bipolar montages of anterior–posterior and transverse electrode linkages and in referential montages.

**4.2.3** *Display of activity* is designed to facilitate comparison of activity in various areas. Two types of display are commonly used. (1) *Block montages* display the activity from neighboring parts of one hemisphere in a block of successive channels, and the activity from the corresponding parts of the opposite hemisphere in another block of channels. This method gives a good overview of the general distribution of patterns. (2) *Alternating montages* show activity from one area of one hemisphere in one channel, and the activity from the corresponding area of the opposite hemisphere in the next channel. This method allows very precise comparison between the two sides. Recordings from the front of the head are commonly displayed above recordings from the back.

**4.2.4** *Specific montages* vary between laboratories, but standard montages used in most large laboratories usually have some features in common. The American EEG Society has developed 'A proposal for standard montages to be used in clinical electroencephalography' which recommends adoption of a minimum set of montages for standard use by all clinical EEG laboratories. This set should include (a) *longitudinal bipolar* (LB) montages, i.e. bipolar montages which connect electrodes in anterior–posterior chains; (b) *transverse bipolar* (TB) montages connecting electrodes in chains across the head; and (c) *referential* (R) montages. Additional montages may be used routinely depending on the needs and preferences of each laboratory; special montages should be designed for individual cases with specific problems not solved by routine montages.

The minimum number of routine montages depends on the number of recording channels available. Recordings with machines having 18 or 16 channels require only three montages, namely one LB, one TB and one R montage. Recordings made with machines having 10 or 8 channels require at least seven montages, namely two LB, three TB and two R montages.

The American EEG Society recommends that recordings from the left side of the head be displayed in channels above those recording from the corresponding areas of the right side. The reference electrode may be placed on the earlobe or the

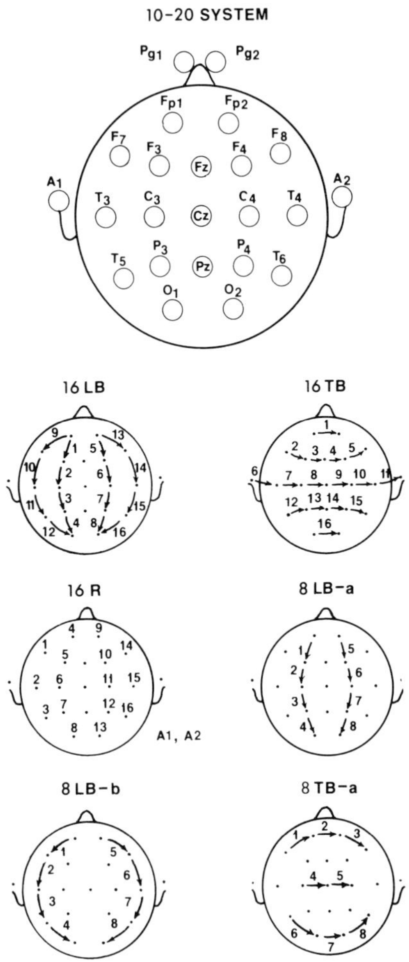


Figs. 4.4 and 4.5. Diagrams of montages for 16-channel and 8-channel EEG machines. All montages use the standard electrode placements of the International 10–20 System. Routine montages use longitudinal bipolar (LB), transverse bipolar (TB) and referential (R) derivations. Recordings of infants (Inf) and recordings made in cases of suspected electrocerebral silence (ECS) combine EEG recordings with monitoring of extracerebral activity (EOG: Electro-oculogram, RESP: respiratory monitor, ECG: heart beat monitor, EMG: surface electromyogram, HAND: hand movement monitor). Each of the small head diagrams represents one montage. The numbers identify the channels. Bipolar montages are indicated by numbers placed near arrows which point from the electrode at input 1 to the electrode at input 2. Referential montages are indicated by numbers placed near the electrode at input 1, input 2 being connected to reference electrodes indicated at the right side of the diagram.

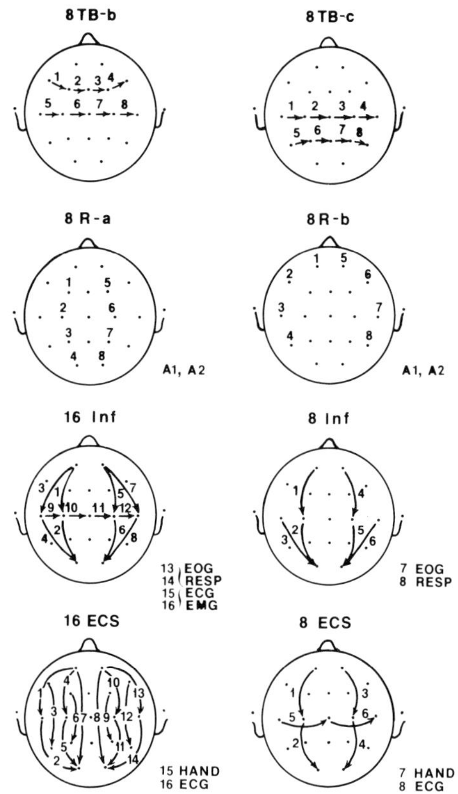

mandibular angle. The mandible may be more suitable especially since an ear electrode (a) tends to pick up spikes and other activity from the temporal lobe and (b) provides insufficient interelectrode distances for recordings from temporal electrodes, causing such recordings to have very low amplitude.

Below is a list of representative montages recommended by the American EEG Society for routine recordings and for recordings from newborn infants with 16-and 8-channel machines; alternatives representing slight variations, for instance referential alternating montages instead of referential block montages, are also included in the recommendations of the American EEG Society. The list also contains montages for 16- and 8-channel recordings in cases of suspected cerebral death or electrocerebral silence. The list is given in two notations. Figures 4.4 and 4.5 show head diagrams using the electrode positions of the 10–20 System. In these figures, bipolar montages are indicated by numbered arrows, each arrow pointing from the electrode at input 1 to the electrode at input 2 of the channel which is indicated by the number of the arrow. Referential montages are indicated by numbers which represent channels and are placed next to the positions of scalp electrodes that are connected to input 1 of these channels while each input 2 is connected to the ipsilateral reference electrode. Tables 4.1, 4.2 and 4.3 give the same montages in the form of lists. Each column represents one montage and lists the pairs of electrodes connected to successive channels.

### 4.3 ELECTRODE COMBINATIONS FOR MONITORING OF EXTRACEREBRAL ACTIVITY

The EEG machine may be used to record physiological activity other than the EEG, for instance eye movements, heart beat, respiration and muscle activity. Although the electrical signals produced by these activities are somewhat distorted in EEG recordings and can be better studied with other methods, they may be included in one or more channels of EEG recording to give an estimate of the occurrence of these activities. One or more of these physiological variables may be recorded intermittently to identify sources of artifacts in the EEG. Two or more of these variables are recorded continuously to identify sleep stages in routine recordings from infants and in special sleep studies in subjects of all ages.

**4.3.1** *Eye movements* are usually recorded in two channels; monitoring in one channel is less reliable. If two channels are available, one electrode is placed slightly above and to the side of one eye, say the left eye (E1), and connected to input 1 of

TABLE 4.1

Tables 4.1–4.3. Lists of the 16- and 8-channel montages shown in diagrammatic form in Figs. 4.4 and 4.5. The same electrode placements and abbreviations of the montage names are used. Under the name of each montage are listed the pairs of electrodes which are connected to input 1 and input 2 of the channels indicated in the column at the left margin

| Channel No. | 16 LB | 16 TB | 16 R |
|---|---|---|---|
| 1 | $Fp_1-F_3$ | $Fp_1-Fp_2$ | $F_7-A_1$ |
| 2 | $F_3-C_3$ | $F_7-F_3$ | $T_3-A_1$ |
| 3 | $C_3-P_3$ | $F_3-F_z$ | $T_5-A_1$ |
| 4 | $P_3-O_1$ | $F_z-F_4$ | $Fp_1-A_1$ |
| 5 | $Fp_2-F_4$ | $F_4-F_8$ | $F_3-A_1$ |
| 6 | $F_4-C_4$ | $A_1-T_3$ | $C_3-A_1$ |
| 7 | $C_4-P_4$ | $T_3-C_3$ | $P_3-A_1$ |
| 8 | $P_4-O_2$ | $C_3-C_z$ | $O_1-A_1$ |
| 9 | $Fp_1-F_7$ | $C_z-C_4$ | $Fp_2-A_2$ |
| 10 | $F_7-T_3$ | $C_4-T_4$ | $F_4-A_2$ |
| 11 | $T_3-T_5$ | $T_4-A_2$ | $C_4-A_2$ |
| 12 | $T_5-O_1$ | $T_5-P_3$ | $P_4-A_2$ |
| 13 | $Fp_2-F_8$ | $P_3-P_z$ | $O_2-A_2$ |
| 14 | $F_8-T_4$ | $P_z-P_4$ | $F_8-A_2$ |
| 15 | $T_4-T_6$ | $P_4-T_6$ | $T_4-A_2$ |
| 16 | $T_6-O_2$ | $O_1-O_2$ | $T_6-A_2$ |

the first channel. A second electrode is placed slightly below and to the side of the other eye (E2) and connected to input 1 of the second channel. Input 2 of both channels is connected to a reference electrode on the ear or mastoid on the same side as the first electrode, namely the left side. Most eye movements produce deflections of opposite direction in the two channels whereas cerebral activity produces deflections of the same direction if it comes from both frontal electrodes or from the reference electrode, or deflections in only one channel if it comes from one frontal electrode.

If only one channel is used for monitoring of eye movements, electrodes E1 and E2 are connected to input 1 and input 2 of that channel. The recording will not

TABLE 4.2

| Channel No. | 8 LB – a | 8 LB – b | 8 TB – a | |
|---|---|---|---|---|
| 1 | $Fp_1 - F_3$ | $Fp_1 - F_7$ | $F_7 - Fp_1$ | |
| 2 | $F_3 - C_3$ | $F_7 - T_3$ | $Fp_1 - Fp_2$ | |
| 3 | $C_3 - P_3$ | $T_3 - T_5$ | $Fp_2 - F_8$ | |
| 4 | $P_3 - O_1$ | $T_5 - O_1$ | $C_3 - C_z$ | |
| 5 | $Fp_2 - F_4$ | $Fp_2 - F_8$ | $C_z - C_4$ | |
| 6 | $F_4 - C_4$ | $F_8 - T_4$ | $T_5 - O_1$ | |
| 7 | $C_4 - P_4$ | $T_4 - T_6$ | $O_1 - O_2$ | |
| 8 | $P_4 - O_2$ | $T_6 - O_2$ | $O_2 - T_6$ | |
| **Channel No.** | **8 TB – b** | **8 TB – c** | **8 R – a** | **8 R – b** |
| 1 | $F_7 - F_3$ | $T_3 - C_3$ | $F_3 - A_1$ | $Fp_1 - A_1$ |
| 2 | $F_3 - F_z$ | $C_3 - C_z$ | $C_3 - A_1$ | $F_7 - A_1$ |
| 3 | $F_z - F_4$ | $C_z - C_4$ | $P_3 - A_1$ | $T_3 - A_1$ |
| 4 | $F_4 - F_8$ | $C_4 - T_4$ | $O_1 - A_1$ | $T_5 - A_1$ |
| 5 | $T_3 - C_3$ | $T_5 - P_3$ | $F_4 - A_2$ | $Fp_2 - A_2$ |
| 6 | $C_3 - C_z$ | $P_3 - P_z$ | $C_4 - A_2$ | $F_8 - A_2$ |
| 7 | $C_z - C_4$ | $P_z - P_4$ | $P_4 - A_2$ | $T_4 - A_2$ |
| 8 | $C_4 - T_4$ | $P_4 - T_6$ | $O_2 - A_2$ | $T_6 - A_2$ |

distinguish between horizontal and vertical eye movements or between eye movements and EEG, but EEG recording is unlikely to interfere at the low sensitivity required to record eye movements from this electrode combination.

**4.3.2** *Heart beat* may be monitored by connecting an amplifier to an EEG electrode placed on the neck or the chest and to another electrode at some distance away. If electrodes with long lead wires are available, standard ECG electrode positions on the extremities may be used.

**4.3.3** *Respiration* is best monitored by recording respiratory body movements or air flow. Respiratory movement may be recorded with a strain gauge or other

TABLE 4.3

| Channel No. | 16 Inf | 8 Inf | 16 ECS | 8 ECS |
|---|---|---|---|---|
| 1 | $Fp_1-C_3$ | $Fp_1-C_3$ | $Fp_1-T_3$ | $Fp_1-C_3$ |
| 2 | $C_3-O_1$ | $C_3-O_1$ | $T_3-O_1$ | $C_3-O_1$ |
| 3 | $Fp_1-T_3$ | $T_3-O_1$ | $F_7-T_5$ | $Fp_2-C_4$ |
| 4 | $T_3-O_1$ | $Fp_2-C_4$ | $Fp_1-C_3$ | $C_4-O_2$ |
| 5 | $Fp_2-C_4$ | $C_4-O_2$ | $C_3-O_1$ | $T_3-C_z$ |
| 6 | $C_4-O_2$ | $T_4-O_2$ | $F_3-P_3$ | $C_z-T_4$ |
| 7 | $Fp_2-T_4$ | EOG | $Fp_1-O_1$ | Hand |
| 8 | $T_4-O_2$ | RESP | $Fp_2-O_2$ | ECG |
| 9 | $T_3-C_3$ | | $F_4-P_4$ | |
| 10 | $C_3-C_z$ | | $Fp_2-C_4$ | |
| 11 | $C_z-C_4$ | | $C_4-O_2$ | |
| 12 | $C_4-T_4$ | | $F_8-T_6$ | |
| 13 | EOG | | $Fp_2-T_4$ | |
| 14 | RESP | | $T_4-O_2$ | |
| 15 | ECG | | Hand | |
| 16 | EMG | | ECG | |

transducer attached to the chest or abdomen; a pressure-sensitive balloon in the esophagus may be used to monitor intrathoracic pressure changes. Respiratory air flow can be monitored with thermistors taped under the nostrils or near the mouth or incorporated in a small face mask collecting air flow from both nose and mouth. While EEG electrodes cannot monitor respiration, they may be of some use in identifying respiratory artifact in EEG recordings. For this purpose, EEG electrodes may be placed on parts of the patient or on any parts of respiratory equipment which move with respiration, for instance ventilator tubing. This should result in recording of movement artifacts corresponding with inspiration and expiration.

**4.3.4** *Muscle activity* can be monitored with EEG electrodes placed over the belly of a muscle. To monitor presence of tonic muscle activity in sleep, electrodes may be placed on the neck below the chin at equal distances of at least 1–2 cm from the midline to record from submental muscles. Needle electrodes inserted into a muscle may be used to record local muscle activity which can be displayed on an EEG tracing within the limitations of the high frequency response and the paper speed of the particular EEG machine.

**4.3.5** *Movement* caused by tremor, myoclonic or convulsive twitching, or movement occurring in coma or sleep, may be monitored by electrodes placed on the moving body parts; such monitoring is likely to indicate the occurrence of movements, but the type of movement must be described on the chart paper during the recording.

**4.3.6** *Blood pressure, galvanic skin response, body temperature, eye position, blood oxygen saturation and other slowly changing or sustained activities* require special electrodes or transducers and can be recorded only with EEG machines and polygraphs equipped with directly coupled amplifiers.

## REFERENCES


Brazier, M.A.B. (1951) A study of the electrical fields at the surface of the head. Electroenceph. clin. Neurophysiol. Suppl. 2: 38–52.

Gloor, P. (1977) Application of volume conductor principles to montage design. Am. J. EEG Technol. 17: 5–20.

Goldman, D. (1950) The clinical use of the 'average' reference electrode in monopolar recording. Electroenceph. clin. Neurophysiol. 2: 211–214.

Harner, R.N. (1977) A recommendation for standard EEG montages. Am. J. EEG Technol. 17: 105–114.

Henderson, C.J., Butler, S.R. and Glass, A. (1975) The localization of equivalent dipoles of EEG sources by the application of electrical field theory. Electroenceph. clin. Neurophysiol. 39: 117–130.

Klass, D.W. (1977) Symposium on EEG montages: Which, when, why and whither. Introduction. Am. J. EEG Technol. 17: 1–3.

Klass, D.W., Bickford, R.G., Ellingson, R.J., Henry, C.E., Knott, J.R., Sharbrough, F., Torres, F., Gloor, P. and Harner, R.N. (1980) A proposal for standard montages to be used in clinical electroencephalography. In: Harner, R.N. (Ed.), Guidelines in EEG – 1980, American Electroencephalographic Society, Willoughby, pp. 36–47.

Knott, J.R. (1977) Commonly used montages in clinical electroencephalography. Am. J. EEG Technol. 17: 85–99.

Mac Gillivray, B.B. (1974) Section II. Derivations and montages. In: Rémond, A. (Ed.), Handbook of Electroenceph. clin. Neurophysiol., Vol. 3C, Elsevier, Amsterdam, pp. 22–57.

Magnus, O. (1961) On the technique of location by electroencephalography. Electroenceph. clin. Neurophysiol. Suppl. 19: 1–35.

Offner, F.F. (1950) The EEG as potential mapping: The value of the average monopolar reference. Electroenceph. clin. Neurophysiol. 2: 215–216.

Osselton, J.W. (1966) Bipolar, unipolar and average reference recording methods. I. Mainly theoretical considerations. Am. J. EEG Technol. 6: 129–141.

Osselton, J.W. (1969) Bipolar, unipolar and average reference recording methods. II. Mainly practical considerations. Am. J. EEG Technol. 9: 117–133.

Schneider, M. and Gerin, P. (1970) Une méthode de localisation des dipôles cérébraux. Electroenceph. clin. Neurophysiol. 28: 69–78.

Schneiderman, N., Dauth, G.W. and VanDercar, D.H. (1974) Electrocardiogram: Techniques and Analysis. In: Thompson, R.F. and Patterson, M.M. (Eds.), Bioelectric Recording Techniques, Vol. 1C, Academic Press, New York and London, pp. 165–200.

Shackel, B. (1967) Eye movement recording by electro-oculography. In: Venables, P.H. and Martin, I. (Eds.), A Manual of Psychophysiological Methods. North-Holland, Amsterdam, pp. 299–334.
Sharbrough, F.W. (1977) The mathematical logic for the design of montages. Am. J. EEG Technol. 17: 73–83.
Tursky, B. (1974) Recording of human eye movements. In: Thompson, R.F. and Patterson, M.M. (Eds.), Bioelectric Recording Techniques, Vol. 1C, Academic Press, New York and London, pp. 99–135.

# The product of the recording: The clinical EEG record

# 5

SUMMARY

The clinical EEG record should represent the electrical activity of the brain as derived from the scalp through recording electrodes, amplified, filtered and written out in a sequence of montages which give a reasonable representation of normal and abnormal patterns such as needed for a clinical interpretation. To serve this purpose, the recording methods must meet certain general technical requirements. Special requirements are made of recordings from infants and small children, of all-night sleep recordings, of recordings evaluating suspected cerebral death, and of recordings transmitted by telephone. Most of these requirements are described in 'Guidelines in EEG' issued by the American EEG Society.

(5.1) *General technical standards* prescribe the use of at least 21 recording electrodes. Electrodes should be placed according to the International 10–20 System and make electrical contact of less than 5000 Ω impedance. The recording should have at least 8 channels; 16-channel recordings are preferable. Both bipolar and referential montages should be used and should be kept as simple as possible. Activity from the front of the head should be displayed at the top of the recording. The sensitivity of the amplifiers should be set at 5–10 $\mu$V/mm at the beginning of the recording. Filters should be set so that they attenuate the amplitude of slow waves of 1 Hz or less and of fast waves of 50 Hz or more by no more than 30% or 3 dB of the amplitude of 8–13 Hz waves. The gain and filter settings should be adjusted during the recording to best display the characteristic features of the patient's EEG. The record should be calibrated at the beginning and the end by calibration pulses and by a test recording using cerebral activity from the same electrode pair in all channels. Calibration at the end of the recording should include calibration pulses recorded at all sensitivity and filter settings used during the EEG recording. Whenever there is any doubt about the proper functioning of an amplifier during the recording, calibration should be repeated. The usual paper speed is 3 cm/sec. Each montage should be run for at least 2 minutes. At least 20 minutes of artifact-free recording should be obtained during wakefulness and should include periods when the eyes are open and when the eyes are closed. In addition, recordings should be made during hyperventilation and photic stimulation. A period of recording during sleep should be obtained when a convulsive disorder is suspected.

The record should be labelled with the patient's name and age, date and time of the recording and other important information. During the recording, notations should be made to indicate the instrument settings, the patient's behavior and any event which could influence the recording or produce artifacts.

(5.2) *Standards for recordings from infants and small children* are the same as the general standards with a few exceptions. A smaller number of electrodes may be used in newborns. Eight-channel machines are barely sufficient for newborns because recordings should include monitoring of eye movements, respiration, heart beat, muscle activity and other physiological variables. Sensitivity and filter settings must be adjusted to display slower and larger potentials than are typical in adult recordings. Recordings in newborns usually require over one hour to include a full cycle of quiet sleep. Waking records from some children may contain so much artifact that only sleep recordings give useful information. Repetitive photic stimulation may be used for activation in some children, but is of no use in newborns. Labelling of the record must precisely reflect the patient's condition, position and all changes during the recording; the gestational and conceptional ages must be indicated for newborns.

(5.3) *Standards for all-night sleep recordings* have not yet been officially formulated. In general, plotting of sleep stages requires recording of EEG, eye movements and tonic muscle activity. Additional recordings of respiration, heart beat and other physiological variables may be required depending on the purpose of the study. The number of channels for EEG recording is often reduced to only one or two when the EEG is used only for monitoring of sleep level and not for detection of cerebral abnormalities.

(5.4) *Standards for recordings in cases of suspected cerebral death* are designed to produce a record which unequivocally answers the question whether or not any electrocerebral activity is present. Determining the patterns and distribution of EEG activity is of secondary concern. Electrocerebral silence or inactivity is defined as the absence of electrocerebral activity over 2 $\mu$V in all areas of the head in recordings made with interelectrode distances of at least 10 cm and with electrode resistances between 100 and 10,000 $\Omega$, or with impedances under 6000 $\Omega$. Recordings demonstrating the absence of electrocerebral activity should not be called 'flat', 'isoelectric' of 'linear' because, if done properly, they are very likely to pick up much activity of extracerebral sources.

At least 8 electrodes should be placed over the cerebral convexity; additional electrodes may be placed on the ears and in other locations. The patient should be grounded through an EEG electrode only if he is not connected to other electrical equipment. High sensitivity and sufficiently wide filter settings must be used. Recordings not showing any electrocerebral activity should be calibrated with pulses of voltages including 2 $\mu$V and contain demonstrations that touching the electrodes causes pen deflections in the corresponding channels. The EEG response to potentially painful stimuli and to loud noise should be checked. Common artifacts such as those caused by heart beat and body or limb movement should be monitored. Recording should be done for at least 30 minutes and should be repeated in case of any doubt about the diagnosis of electrocerebral silence. Recordings for suspected cerebral death should be made only by technicians who are specially trained in these methods and who work under the supervision of a qualified electroencephalographer. Telephone transmission should not be used for these recordings.

(5.5) *Standards for EEG transmission by telephone* require one fully trained technician and one fully equipped EEG machine at both the transmitting and the receiving sites. The recordings at both sites should be identical and include all notes and comments made during the recording by the transmitting technician. These requirements can be fulfilled with current techniques except for some restrictions on high frequencies and limitations on the high sensitivities required for evaluation of cerebral death.

## 5.1 GENERAL TECHNICAL STANDARDS

Good clinical EEG recordings must satisfy many technical requirements. The American EEG Society has issued 'Guidelines in EEG' which contain 'Minimum technical requirements for performing clinical electroencephalography'. These requirements apply to all clinical recordings. Additional requirements are made for some aspects of recordings from infants and small children, from subjects with suspected cerebral death and from patients monitored during all-night sleep. To raise standards above the minimum, the EEG Society has added several recommendations. Standards and recommendations are here presented in a sequence corresponding with the steps of an EEG recording.

(1) *Electrode types.* No particular electrode can be recommended as ideal. Although electrodes are best attached with collodion, electrode pastes are also effective. Needle electrodes should not be used unless absolutely necessary because they may cause infection, pain and poor recordings. They may be used if (a) a recording must be obtained rapidly, (b) the patient is comatose and shows little or no response to pain, (c) the electrodes have been completely sterilized, and (d) the technician is trained in the use of needle electrodes and is aware of the disadvantages and hazards of using these electrodes.

(2) *Electrode placements.* At least 21 recording electrodes should be used and placed according to the International 10–20 System. The head must be measured to determine the location of frontopolar, frontal, central, parietal, occipital, inferior frontal or anterior temporal, middle temporal and posterior temporal positions, all on both sides, and of the frontal, central and parietal midline positions; standard placements include both ears or mandibular angles (2.3). Additional electrodes may be placed between the standard electrodes to localize very circumscribed activity. A ground electrode should be added and connected to the ground input of the EEG

machine unless the patient is connected to ground through other electrical equipment.

If electrode positions were not measured but only estimated, the terms '10–20 System' or 'modified 10–20 System' should not be used, but the term 'estimated 10–20 System' may be applied. Recordings which do not use the 10–20 System should define the relationship between the electrode placements used and those of the 10–20 System.

(3) *Electrode impedance.* The impedance of electrodes should be checked routinely before every recording (2.2). It should not exceed 5000 Ω except for needle electrodes where higher impedances cannot be avoided. Although the EEG Society does not state a particular frequency of alternating current for impedance measurements, a frequency of about 10 Hz is most appropriate. If impedance is not measured routinely, it must be checked at least when an unusual EEG pattern suggests the possibility of an artifact.

(4) *Number of recording channels.* The EEG should be recorded on at least 8 channels at the same time. Sixteen channels are preferable because the chance to correctly localize intermittent abnormalities increases with the number of recording channels.

(5) *Montages.* Recordings should routinely include the bipolar and referential montages recommended by the American EEG Society (4.2.4). Additional montages should also be as simple as possible, easy to describe and easy to interpret. They should use electrodes along straight lines and with equal interelectrode distances. Activity from the front of the head should be displayed at the top of the record, activity from the back at the bottom.

(6) *Sensitivity.* The sensitivity at the beginning of a routine recording should be set at 5–10 μV/mm for all channels. A commonly used sensitivity setting is 7 μV/mm which results in a pen deflection of about 7 mm for a calibration pulse of 50 μV. The sensitivity of all channels should be adjusted during the recording so that

the full range of the pen deflection is used to its best advantage: The EEG should be shown with good resolution and without driving the pens to the extremes or flattening the tracing.

(7) *Filters.* During the recording, the high and low frequency filters should be set so that the amplitude of slow waves of 1 Hz and less, and the amplitude of fast waves of 50 Hz and more, are not attenuated by more than 30% or 3 dB of the amplitude of 8–13 Hz waves. These settings should be changed only to emphasize or clarify unusual patterns in the recording. In general, the filter settings may be changed to increase the range of frequencies recorded, but they should not be used to narrow this range beyond the limits specified above except for good reason because such a limitation may eliminate or deform important cerebral activity. Filters should not be used to 'clean up' artifacts and produce a 'pretty record'.

(8) *Calibration.* Each record should be calibrated by applying known voltages to all channels at the beginning and the end of the recording. The calibration at the end should include calibration pulses recorded at each of the various combinations of sensitivity and filter settings used in the recording. The calibration pulses should have voltages strong enough to produce pen deflections of 7 mm or more, so that differences of 5% or more between channels can be detected; the pulses should not be so strong that they overdrive the pen deflection. Calibration pulses of different voltage need to be used for different sensitivity settings. If the amplitude, shape, horizontal and vertical alignment of the calibration pulses differs between channels, the cause for these differences must be determined and eliminated.

Although not required by the guidelines of the American EEG Society, it is good practice to further ascertain that all channels have the same recording characteristics over the range of EEG frequencies by connecting the inputs of all recording channels to the same pair of scalp electrodes and recording a few pages at the beginning and end of each record (3.3.2). The guidelines recommend that this procedure and recalibration with square pulses be used at any time during the recording when there is reason to suspect a malfunction of the recording equipment. Another useful test when electrode malfunction is suspected is the injection of a weak alternating current signal through the electrodes and recording the pen deflection; high electrode impedance is indicated by a high deflection, low impedance by a low deflection (2.2).

(9) *Paper speed*. This is not specified by the guidelines of the EEG Society. A speed of 30 mm/sec is recommended internationally and used routinely in most laboratories (3.6.2). Slower speeds may be used intermittently, for instance while the EEG shows slow waves or while waiting for a patient to fall asleep. Faster speeds may be used to resolve fast events, for instance to determine time relationships between similar waves in different channels to evaluate the shape of spikes, or to distinguish between 60 Hz and muscle artifact.

(10) *Length of the recording.* Each montage should be recorded for at least 2 minutes. The waking record should contain at least 20 minutes of artifact-free recording at rest including brief periods when the eyes are open (11.1.6). This period does not include the time required for hyperventilation, photic stimulation and sleep recordings.

(11) *Hyperventilation.* Overbreathing should be used routinely except when contraindicated by diseases of heart and lungs, acute cerebral disorders, coma or conditions causing pain during hyperventilation. The technician should explain and demonstrate hyperventilation and encourage the patient to hyperventilate for at least three minutes. The EEG should be recorded during and for one minute after hyperventilation, and longer if hyperventilation induces abnormalities.

(12) *Photic stimulation.* This activation procedure is not among the recommendations of the American EEG Society. However, it is used in many laboratories because it can induce diagnostically important abnormalities. It is not used routinely in all laboratories because it may, on rare occasions, induce generalized seizures; this may happen both in patients with a history of seizures and, extremely rarely, in

patients without such a history. However, the development of seizures can usually be avoided if photic stimulation is stopped as soon as seizure activity appears.

Photic stimulation is performed with a stroboscopic lamp producing bright flashes of diffuse light. The lamp is placed about 30 cm from the patient's eyes. Flashes are given at rates including 1, 3, 8, 10, 15, and 20 Hz in trains of about 10 seconds. Thorough testing includes periods when the eyes are closed, open, and while they are being opened and closed. The occurrence of each flash is monitored using either a synchronizing pulse of the flash generator or a photocell attached to the patient's body near the eyes. The latter method has two advantages. (a) It records the actual appearance of the flash and thus avoids false indications which may be given by a synchronizing pulse if the flash bulb does not work or if the flash is not directed at the patient. (b) Movements by the patient, sometimes elicited by the flash, are picked up by the leads of the photocell. The monitor pulse is displayed on an auxiliary channel, if available, or on a recording channel.

(13) *Sleep.* A period of EEG recording during sleep should be obtained as part of the routine record in patients with suspected or known convulsive disorders whose waking record shows no focal epileptiform activity (14.2.1). The sleep recording should not shorten the minimum period of the waking record. To increase the chance of obtaining a sleep recording, many laboratories ask patients to sleep little the night before the recording.

If sleep does not occur spontaneously, some laboratories induce sleep with a sedative, such as chloral hydrate. This has obvious legal implications, including the need to warn the patient not to drive while sedated.

(14) *Special procedures* which are of risk to the patient should be carried out only for specific indications and then only in the presence of a qualified physician, in an environment with adequate resuscitation equipment, and with the informed consent of the patient, responsible relative or guardian.

(15) *Labelling and editing of the record.* Proper labelling of the record is of the

greatest importance; even a technically perfect EEG is useless without written comments by the technician. The technician must describe (a) the patient's medical characteristics, (b) the patient's behavior during the recording, (c) the montages, and (d) the instrument settings.

(a) *The description of the patient* should be written on the record and include at least the patient's name and age, the date and time of the recording, a list of all current medications, the time of the last meal, the name, amount and time of administration of any sedative taken during or shortly before the recording. Failure to document this information on the record can lead to serious medical and legal problems.

In addition to these minimum requirements, the technician should write down other important information. Cranial defects or abnormalities, scalp lacerations and contusions should be identified in a head diagram explaining the spatial relation between the abnormalities and the recording electrodes, especially where the abnormalities necessitated deviations from the electrode placements of the 10–20 System. The technician may obtain important information from the patient or the patient's chart, and thus complement the information given by the referring physician. Items of special importance are a history and description of seizures, head injuries and significant diseases, the provisional diagnosis, reason for the EEG recording, abnormal laboratory test results, etc. Previous EEG recordings of the same patient should be available at least at the time of the interpretation.

(b) *The description of the patient during the recording.* The technician should indicate the patient's level of alertness, namely awake, drowsy, asleep or comatose, and any change of that level occurring during the recording. Unusual behavior such as restlessness, agitation, confusion, failure to cooperate, abnormal speech, hearing and vision should be noted. The technician should try to recognize every movement of the patient, especially eye movements including eye blinks, eye opening and closing, movements of the face and head, swallowing, chewing, talking, coughing, sneezing, etc.; each movement should be indicated on the record at the time it occurs, especially if it causes an artifact in the recording. If there is any doubt whether an artifact is due to any such movement, the technician should ask the patient to repeat the movement and mark the request and the patient's response on the record. If seizure activity is suggested by a movement of the patient or by the appearance of epileptiform activity in the EEG, the technician should test the responsiveness of the patient by asking him how he feels and, if there is no answer, giving him a test word to remember. Later, when the patient is responsive, the technician should ask the patient if he remembers something being said and if he remembers the test word; these questions and the answers should be written on the record. If epileptiform activity appears frequently or if it can be triggered by stimulation, the technician may ask the patient to count or to recite a nursery rhyme and note any interruptions by spontaneous or triggered epileptiform activity.

The technician should rate the patient's performance of hyperventilation as good, fair or poor. After hyperventilation, the patient should be asked how he felt during hyperventilation and, especially, whether hyperventilation reproduced or intensified any of his usual symptoms. The patient's response should be written on the chart.

In essence, the technician should continuously monitor the patient's behavior and document every movement and every word spoken during the recording. This is necessary because most artifacts can be positively identified only during the recording by correlating pen deflections with movements or other events. The technician is in the unique position of being able to make the diagnosis of a seizure by demonstrating a loss of responsiveness or documenting other, sometimes subtle, behavioral seizure manifestations during the occurrence of epileptiform activity in the EEG. The reader, if unaware of the patient's behavior, may be unable to identify many artifacts or to diagnose a seizure. The technician's attempt to identify every possible source of artifacts will also help to faster recognize and eliminate artifacts during the recording.

(c) *Description of montages.* The electrode combinations selected for each channel must be clearly indicated at the beginning of each run. This may be done in one of several ways. (1) Abbreviations of the electrode placements used as input 1 and input 2 may be written in front of the tracing of each channel as in Tables 4.1–4.3. (2) Using a head diagram, the tracing of each channel may be connected to two electrode placements in the diagram; a solid line is commonly used to indicate the electrode connected to input 1, and a broken line is used to indicate the electrode connected to input 2; this method is used for EEG illustrations in this text. (3) Electrode placements in the head diagram may be connected with arrows, each arrow being labelled with the number of the channel it represents and pointing from the electrode at input 1 to the electrode at input 2; this method is used in the illustration of montages in this text (Figs. 4.4 and 4.5). (4) Rubber stamps giving a list of the electrodes or a diagrammatic representation of a montage are used in some laboratories, but they can lead to errors more easily than other, less automatic methods. Montages should not be labelled with code names such as 'montage A' or 'run 1' because the meaning of the code may be unknown to the EEG reader.

(d) *Description of instrument settings.* The settings of master and individual channel switches controlling sensitivity and filters should be indicated at the beginning of each run and during calibration; the voltage of the calibration pulse must be identified. Every change of these settings and of chart speed must be indicated on the record when it is made and the affected channels must be clearly specified.

## 5.2 STANDARDS FOR RECORDINGS FROM INFANTS AND SMALL CHILDREN

Most of the general technical standards also apply to this age group. However, there are a few exceptions which are summarized in the guidelines of the American EEG

Society on 'Minimal technical standards for pediatric electroencephalography' and are detailed below.

(1) *Electrode types.* Silver-silver chloride electrodes in the shape of a cup with a central hole for injection of conductive jelly (2.2.1) are best. Application with collodion is recommended because children are more likely than adults to move and produce artifacts. Collodion and acetone should not be used in isolettes and other areas with limited air circulation or explosion hazards; electrodes may be applied with electrode paste under these circumstances.

(2) *Electrode placements.* Newborn infants, especially those with small heads, do not need the full number of electrodes prescribed by the 10–20 System. A minimum reduced array includes the following electrodes: Fp1, Fp2, C3, Cz, C4, T3, T4, O1, O2, A1 and A2. If the baby's earlobes are too small, mastoid electrodes M1 and M2 may be substituted for A1 and A2. Suitable alternatives for Fp1 and Fp2 in the reduced array are Fp3 and Fp4, placed midway between the Fp1 and F3 and the Fp2 and F4 positions; however, these placements yield unequal interelectrode distances when used in bipolar montages.

(3) *Number of recording channels.* Instruments with more than 8 channels, preferably 16 channels, should be used especially in newborns because two or more channels must be used to monitor extracerebral activity.

(4) *Montages.* Recordings from newborns need continuous monitoring of extracerebral electrical activity to indentify alertness and sleep states and to recognize artifacts and abnormalities of breathing and heart rate. Most important is monitoring of respiration, eye movement, and heart beat; neck muscle activity is monitored in some instances (4.3).

Montages for 16-channel instruments usually devote at least 4 channels to extracerebral activity; montages for 8-channel instruments reserve 2 channels for monitoring of eye movements and respiration and use 6 channels for EEG. Examples of montages are listed in Chapter 4 (4.2.4).

(5) *Sensitivity.* The sensitivity needs to be adjusted more often in infants and young children; their EEG may have fairly high amplitude so that sensitivity needs to be reduced to 10 or 15 $\mu$V/mm. The sensitivity of channels monitoring extracerebral activity of newborns must be adjusted according to the output; eye movements and submental EMG should be recorded at 7 and 3 $\mu$V/mm respectively.

(6) *Filters.* EEG recordings from infants should use time constants between 0.25 and 0.6 sec, i.e. low filter frequency settings which reduce the amplitude of sine waves of 0.3 to 0.6 Hz by 30% or 3 dB. Eye movements should be monitored with the same filter settings. EMG recordings should be made with higher settings of the low frequency filter and with the highest setting of the high frequency filter. Respiration should be monitored with very low settings of the low frequency filter but not with direct coupling.

(7) *Length of the recording.* Newborns require usually over one hour of recording to show both active sleep and a full cycle of quiet sleep. The chances of obtaining such a recording are best when the EEG is scheduled at feeding time and the baby is fed after application of the electrodes. Sedation should not be used to obtain a sleep record in newborns. Shorter recording periods than one hour are acceptable only when the EEG is grossly abnormal; even then, a period of one hour may be required to demonstrate the absence of variability.

Children may produce so many artifacts by moving and other mechanisms that satisfactory waking records of the length recommended for adults cannot be obtained; recordings during sleep may then provide the only useful information. In patients over three months of age, the technician should attempt to obtain recordings during wakefulness when the patient's eyes are open and when they are closed; passive eye closure, accomplished by placing the technician's hand over the patient's eyes, may be used to demonstrate the reactivity of EEG rhythms (11.1.6).

(8) *Photic stimulation.* Flashes of 1–30 Hz should be used during wakefulness if indicated for activation in children. Repetitive photic stimulation is not useful for newborns.

(9) *Labelling and editing the record.* In addition to the requirements described for EEG recordings in general, recordings from infants must state the baby's gestational age at birth and conceptional age, i.e. gestational age plus time since birth, in weeks, together with the chronological age since birth. Other relevant information, such as levels of blood gases and serum electrolytes, should be noted for the use of the electroencephalographer. Before recording EEGs of infants and young hospital patients, especially those requiring bedside recording, the technician should consult with the nursing staff concerning the patient's condition and any limitations on recording procedures. The patient's condition should be clearly indicated at the beginning of every montage; the position of head and eyelids of infants should be noted. Changes of position and other movements must be monitored as carefully as in adults. Stuporous or comatose patients and patients showing an invariant EEG pattern should be given visual, auditory and somatosensory stimulation. The stimuli and the patient's responses should be indicated on the recording paper at the time of their occurrence; absence of responses must also be noted. Infants should be stimulated only at the end of the recording period to avoid interruption of sleep cycles.

## 5.3 STANDARDS FOR ALL-NIGHT SLEEP RECORDINGS

All-night sleep recordings are made to study a variety of sleep disorders and of other conditions associated with abnormal bodily functions during sleep. These studies require monitoring of extracerebral activity in addition to recording of the EEG. Although minimum technical standards have not yet been officially established, it is generally agreed that identifying and plotting of sleep stages requires recording of EEG, eye movement and submental muscle activity. Other variables may also need to be recorded depending on the purpose of the study. For instance, investigations of sleep apnea require additional monitoring of respiratory air flow, respiratory movements of chest or abdomen and, if possible, of blood oxygenation. If the EEG is recorded only to monitor the depth of sleep and not to look for cerebral abnormalities, the number of channels used for EEG recording may be reduced to one or two.

### 5.4 STANDARDS FOR RECORDINGS IN CASES OF SUSPECTED CEREBRAL DEATH

The EEG is an important tool in the evaluation of cerebral death, a diagnosis often considered in victims of severe cerebral damage characterized by coma, absent or insufficient spontaneous respiration and absent brain stem reflexes. This diagnosis requires, amongst other criteria, repeated demonstrations of the absence of electrocerebral activity of over 2 $\mu$V in amplitude. For adults and older children, electrocerebral silence found in two recordings at an interval of 24 hours is usually considered conclusive, unless one or both recordings were made in the presence of drugs depressing the central nervous system, of significant hypothermia or circulatory shock. In infants and younger children, especially those under three years of age, this rule cannot be applied (a) because they can survive longer periods of electrocerebral silence without cerebral death and (b) because they may show persistent EEG activity in the absence of cerebral blood flow, i.e. in the absence of cerebral functioning.

Recording techniques in cases of suspected cerebral death must be designed to search for any trace of cerebral activity and take special precautions to avoid the possibility that failure to record EEG activity is due to faulty methods or equipment rather than to absent cerebral activity. The American EEG Society has issued guidelines of 'Minimum technical standards for EEG recording in suspected cerebral death'; the guidelines are presented and discussed here.

(1) *Electrode placements.* At least 8 scalp electrodes should be used and placed in the frontopolar (Fp1, Fp2), central (C3, C4), temporal (T3, T4) and occipital (O1, O2) positions on both sides. Additional electrodes may be placed in the frontal areas (F3, F4), at the vertex (Cz) and on the earlobes (A1, A2), mastoids, mandibular angles or noncephalic reference points. A ground electrode should be added but not connected if other electrical equipment is attached to the patient (3.1). Applying only the minimum number of electrodes may be not the best strategy, because if the recording shows electrocerebral activity, a complete recording using all routine placements should be obtained. To be prepared for this possibility, the full set of recording electrodes may be applied at the start of the recording.

(2) *Electrode impedance.* The impedance of electrodes should be between 100 and 6000 Ω for reasons discussed elsewhere (2.2.3). Although the definition of electrocerebral silence also contains a statement about electrode resistance, this measurement requires application of direct current and should not be made unless non-polarizable electrodes are used. The impedance of all electrodes should be similar to reduce the chance of artifacts due to imbalance of amplifier inputs.

Higher impedances may have to be accepted for needle electrodes which may be used in cases of suspected cerebral death if a record must be obtained fast.

(3) *Number of recording channels.* The guidelines of the American EEG Society do not specify a minimum number of channels except to say that more than one channel is necessary and that the major brain areas should be covered. It would seem that an 8-channel machine would be the minimum and would allow 6 channels of EEG recording in addition to 2 channels for recording of heart beat and body movements.

(4) *Montages.* Interelectrode distances of at least 10 cm should be used because recording at shorter distances may attenuate amplitude. Bipolar montages should therefore use twice the distance between neighboring electrode placements in the

10–20 System. Referential montages may use the ear opposite to the scalp electrodes for long interelectrode distances. The heart beat artifact is often seen in such linkages and may be reduced by changing the position of the head or by using both ears as an average reference. More than one montage should be used; examples of useful 16-channel and 8-channel montages are illustrated in Chapter 4 (4.2.4). If occipital leads are difficult to attach or pick up too much movement artifact induced by artificial respiration, the combinations F7-T5, F3-P3, Fz-Pz, F4-P4 and F8-T6 may give better results.

(5) *Sensitivity.* A sensitivity of at least 2 μV/mm, or a higher sensitivity such as 1 μV/mm, should be used during all or most of the minimum recording period (see below). This is very important because activity of 2 μV, i.e. the critical amplitude for electrocerebral silence, cannot be clearly distinguished at lower sensitivities.

(6) *Filters.* Filter settings should not attenuate any electrocerebral activity, especially very slow waves which are likely to occur in deep coma. Attempts should be made to record with low frequency filters at 0.3–0.5 Hz, i.e. time constants of 0.3–0.4 seconds; however, this strategy may be without value if it obscures the recording with low frequency artifacts such as those produced by respiratory movement, perspiration, etc. The 60 Hz filter should be used as needed.

(7) *Calibration.* Calibration should follow the recommendations for general standards of recording. In addition, recordings in cases of suspected cerebral death should include calibration pulses having the size of electrocerebral activity recorded; if no electrocerebral activity can be recorded, calibration should include 2 μV at the highest sensitivity used. This recommendation intends to assure that even low amplitude electrocerebral activity, if present, would cause a pen deflection the size of the calibration pulse. Recordings with all channels connected to the same electrode pair, recommended by the general guidelines, are useful only if these recordings show activity sufficiently large for a valid comparison between channels.

(8) *Verifying the integrity of the recording system.* If a recording at high

sensitivity and wide interelectrode distances shows no electrocerebral activity, it is necessary to demonstrate that this is not due to a fault of the recording system. The recording of calibration pulses does not entirely exclude this possibility because it tests the recording system only between the inputs of the amplifiers and the penwriters whereas the fault may lie between the electrodes and the amplifier input. To test this part of the recording system, each electrode should be touched gently with a pencil or cotton swab during the recording; the electrode touched and the moment of touching should be indicated on the chart. Touching an electrode should create an artifact in the recording channels connected to that electrode. This artifact verifies that (a) the electrode is capable of recording, and (b) the correct electrode is selected for that channel.

(9) *Stimulation of the patient.* The reactivity of the EEG of comatose patients should be tested by stimulation with sudden loud sounds and by stimuli which produce pain in wakeful persons, for instance pinching of the skin. Flashes of bright light may also be used. The type and moment of stimulation and the behavioral reaction of the patient, including the absence of a reaction, should be noted on the chart. The tracing may show different types of reactions: Transient EEG activity may be induced in some patients who have no spontaneous EEG activity; extracerebral responses may be elicited, for instance frontal potentials representing the retinal response to light flashes; artifacts may appear as the result of active or passive movements of the patient or of other mechanisms.

(10) *Monitoring sources of artifacts.* Because of the high sensitivity and wide interelectrode distances, recordings in suspected cerebral death are very likely to pick up artifacts. Possible sources of artifacts should be monitored (4.3). As a minimum, heart beat and movement should be included in the recordings (4.2.4).

(a) *Artifacts arising from heart beat* are very common and consist of ECG components, pulse waves and ballistic movements transmitted to the head and electrode wires.

(b) *Movement* of the patient may cause artifact which can be monitored with two electrodes on the back of the right hand, separated by 6–7 cm.

(c) *Respiratory artifact*, if impossible to eliminate by positioning of the patient and equipment, should be monitored during at least part of the recording. Stopping the respirator momentarily may help to identify respiratory artifact that cannot be eliminated.

(d) Electrical interference may be evaluated by connecting a resistor of 10,000 Ω between the inputs of one amplifier and placing it near the patient. This 'dummy patient' is representative of the electrical impedances of the EEG electrodes on the patient and can indicate the amount and type of interference from sources other than the patient.

(e) *Muscle artifact* may obscure the tracing. If it cannot be eliminated by repositioning of the patient or massaging the muscles near the contaminated recording electrode, a neuromuscular blocking agent may be used under the supervision of a physician.

(11) *Length of the recording.* At least 30 minutes of recording at a high sensitivity are needed to demonstrate electrocerebral silence; this period includes the time for the procedures of stimulating the patient and checking the integrity of the recording system.

(12) *Repeat recordings.* If technical or other problems leave any uncertainty about the diagnosis of electrocerebral silence, the entire recording should be repeated after a few hours.

(13) *Qualification of technician.* Recordings in cases of possible cerebral death should be made only by technicians who have had supervised instruction and recording experience in intensive care units and who work under the direct supervision of a qualified electroencephalographer.

(14) *Telephone transmission.* Recordings made for the determination of cerebral death should not be transmitted by telephone because telephone networks at present can introduce artifacts preventing reliable interpretation (5.5).

## 5.5 TELEPHONE TRANSMISSION

Since transmission of EEGs by telephone from smaller hospitals to larger centers is now being used more and more often, recommendations for telephone transmission of EEGs have been included in the guidelines of the American EEG Society and in the report of the Committee on EEG Instrumentation Standards of the International Federation of Societies for EEG and Clinical Neurophysiology. The recommendations generally stipulate that technical standards of EEG recording should not be lowered by telephone transmission. This requires two fully trained technicians and two complete EEG recording machines. The machines should be connected so that the EEG at the transmitting site is completely and faithfully duplicated at the receiving site; at present, this requirement cannot be entirely fulfilled because currently used conventional telephone systems limit transmission of high frequencies for an 8-channel EEG to about 50 Hz and may introduce artifacts into recordings of low amplitude. However, these limitations may be acceptable in most cases. Specific recommendations for telephone transmission are listed below.

(1) *Technicians* at both the transmitting and receiving laboratories should be fully trained and qualified EEG technicians. In addition, they should be familiar with telephone transmission techniques and, if possible, with each other's laboratories.

(2) *Duplicate EEG records* should be produced. Recording a copy at the transmitting site is required so that the transmitting technician can correlate ongoing EEG activity with the patient's behavior and identify and eliminate artifacts. The requirement for a copy at the transmitting site may be eliminated in the future if acceptable alternative methods of monitoring the EEG at the transmitting site become available.

The comments of the transmitting technician, especially those which are vital for the identification of artifacts, should be transmitted simultaneously with the EEG to the receiving site. This can be done by signals in a standard code which temporarily replace the EEG recorded in one channel. Such a signalling system may be supplemented by intermittent voice communications between transmitting and receiving sites. A fail-safe code should be included to indicate technical problems, especially the loss of signal at the receiving site during transmission.

(3) *Fidelity of the recording*: The tracing at the transmitting and receiving sites should be identical. As mentioned above, this is currently possible for recordings not including frequencies over 50 Hz and not consisting of very low amplitude activity.

(4) *Cerebral death* cannot be evaluated appropriately by recordings transmitted over the telephone because artifacts from telephone networks may appear and obscure or mimick electrocerebral activity of low amplitude.

## REFERENCES


Anders, T., Emde, R. and Parmalee, A. (1971) A Manual of Standardized Terminology, Techniques and Criteria for Scoring of States of Sleep and Wakefulness in Newborn Infants. ULCA Brain Information Service, NINDS Neurological Information Network.

Ashwal, S. and Schneider, S. (1979) Failure of electroencephalography to diagnose brain death in comatose children. Ann. Neurol. 6: 512–517.

Bennett, D.R., Hughes, J.R., Korein, J., Merlis, J.K. and Suter, C. (1976) An Atlas of Electroencephalography in Coma and Cerebral Death. Raven Press, New York.

Green, J.B. and Lauber, A. (1972) Return of EEG activity after electrocerebral silence: Two case reports. J. Neurol. Neurosurg. Psychiat. 35: 103–107.

Guilleminault, C. and Dement, W. (1978) Sleep Apnea Syndromes. Liss, New York.

Harner, R.N., ed. (1980) Guidelines in EEG – 1980. American Electroencephalographic Society, Willoughby.

Jacobson, A., Kales, A., Zweizig, J.R. et Kales, J. (1965) Special EEG and EMG techniques for sleep research. Am. J. EEG Technol. 5: 5–10.

Klem, G.H. (1979) Some problems of bedside EEG recording. Am. J. EEG Technol. 19: 19–29.

Montoya, M.L. and Hill, G. (1968) EEG recording in intensive care units. Am. J. EEG Technol. 8: 85–95.

Pajot, N. (1974) EEG recording techniques in full-term and premature infants. Am. J. EEG Technol. 14: 108–120.
Rechtschaffen, A. and Kales, A. (1968) A Manual of Standardized Terminology, Techniques and Scoring System for Sleep Stages of Human Subjects, U.S. Government Printing Office, Washington.
Werner, S.S., Stockard, J.E. and Bickford, R.G. (1977) Atlas of Neonatal Electroencephalography, Raven Press, New York.
Williams, R.L., Karacan, I. and Hursch, C.J. (1974) Electroencephalography (EEG) of Human Sleep: Clinical Applications. Wiley, New York.

# 6 Artifacts

SUMMARY

Artifacts are pen deflections caused not by cerebral activity. They may be due to (6.1) *other physiological activity* originating from the patient, for instance eye or body movement, muscle contraction and heart beat, (6.2) *interference* from power lines and other electrical sources affecting the recording electrodes, or (6.3) *malfunctioning of the recording system* which includes the recording electrodes, amplifiers, pen motors and paper drive. Artifacts must be avoided as much as possible because they may mimick or obscure cerebral activity. Because even perfect application of electrodes and correct settings of machine controls do not guarantee an artifact-free recording, the technician must constantly observe the patient and the paper record during the recording, looking for any unusual feature in the record that could be an artifact. If artifacts do occur, their source should be identified and eliminated promptly. This may require stopping the recording, checking electrode contact and impedance, interelectrode distances, machine settings and other possible causes of artifact. Although many artifacts can be recognized by their characteristic shape, a positive identification can be made only during the recording by correlating pen deflections suspected of being artifacts with concomitant events which may be causing artifacts.

## 6.1 ARTIFACTS FROM THE PATIENT

**6.1.1** *Blinking and other eye movements.* These movements cause potential changes which are picked up mainly by frontal electrodes, although they may extend into central and temporal electrodes. Vertical eye movements cause pen deflections mainly in channels recording from electrode pairs in longitudinal chains near the midline, for instance Fp1-F3, Fp2-F4; lateral eye movements cause deflections mainly in channels recording in lateral or transverse chains, for instance Fp1-F7, Fp2-F8, F7-F3, F8-F4. Blinking or eye closure causes large downgoing pen deflections; eye opening produces an upward deflection (Fig. 6.1). Rapid eye move-

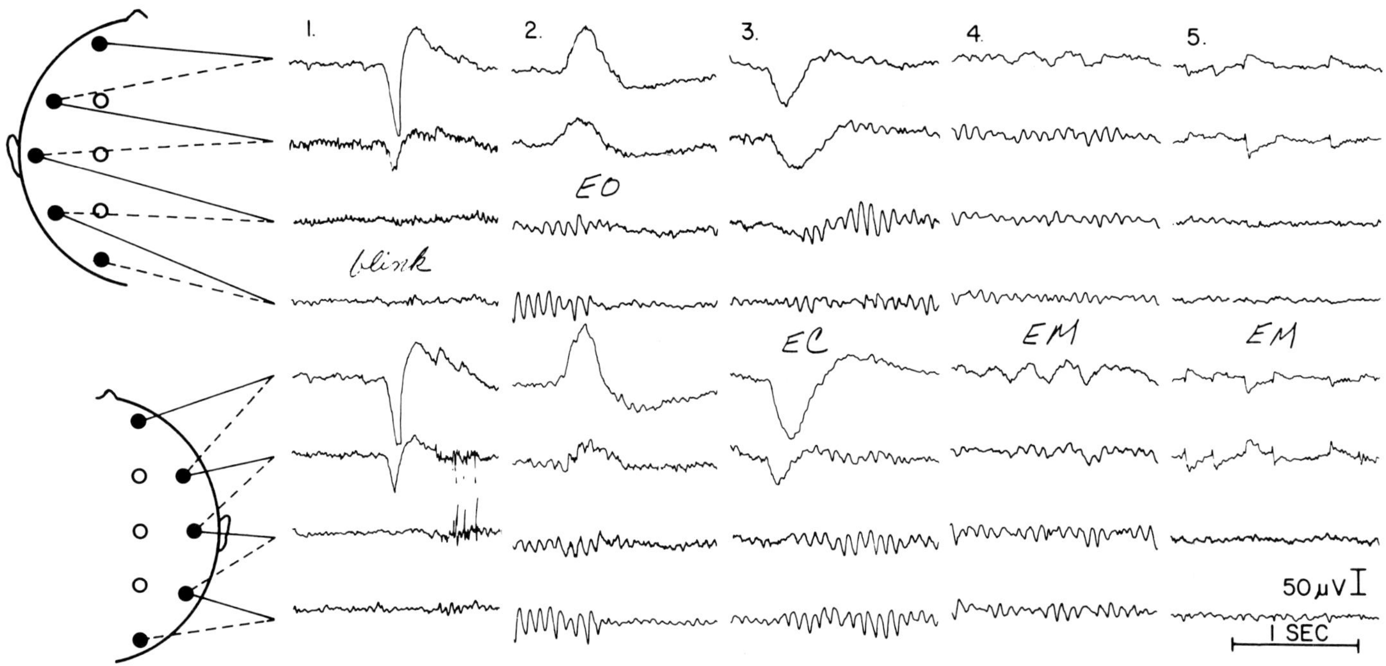


Fig. 6.1. Eye movement artifacts. 1. Blink, 2. eye opening (EO), 3. eye closing (EC), 4. rhythmical slow eye movements (EM), 5. saccadic eye movements (EM) preceded by spicules due to contraction of lateral eye muscles. Tracings show the technician's notations made during the recording to identify the cause of the artifacts.

ments cause jagged artifacts (Fig. 12.2). Muscle artifact may appear along with eye movements. Lateral eye movements may be preceded by a single sharp muscle potential which may resemble a cerebral spike and, in combination with the eye movement artifact, form a spike-and-wave artifact.

Eye movement artifacts have long been believed to be due to movement of the eyeball which carries a steady electrical charge, the cornea being about 100 mV positive with respect to the retina. However, it seems that movement of this corneo-retinal dipole is not necessary to produce blink artifacts: movements of the lids across the eyeball appear sufficient. Moreover, eye movement artifacts can be recorded even after removal of the eye including cornea and retina, suggesting that movement of residual membranes deep in the orbit can cause artifacts.

Eye movement artifacts in the EEG can usually be identified by their frontal distribution, their symmetry on the two sides and their characteristic shape. However, several exceptions to these rules may make identification of eye movements difficult. The frontal origin of eye movement artifacts may remain unclear in referential montages, particularly those using ear electrodes which may be contaminated by eye movements. Eye movement artifacts may be asymmetrical in patients with disconjugate eye movements, for instance in patients who have only one eye. Repetitive eye movements may mimick cerebral rhythms; slowly repetitive eye movements may closely resemble bilaterally synchronous frontal slow waves, and repetitive eye movements associated with lid flutter during eye closure may cause frontal rhythms of about 10 Hz.

Eye movement artifacts can be identified during the recording by observing the patient and correlating eye blinks and movements with pen deflections. Even eye movements during eye closure can usually be seen through the eyelids. These movements can be further identified by their disappearance when the patient complies with the instruction to keep his eyes closed and still. If unable to do this, the patient may be told to place his fingertips on his eyes, or the technician may hold the eyelids

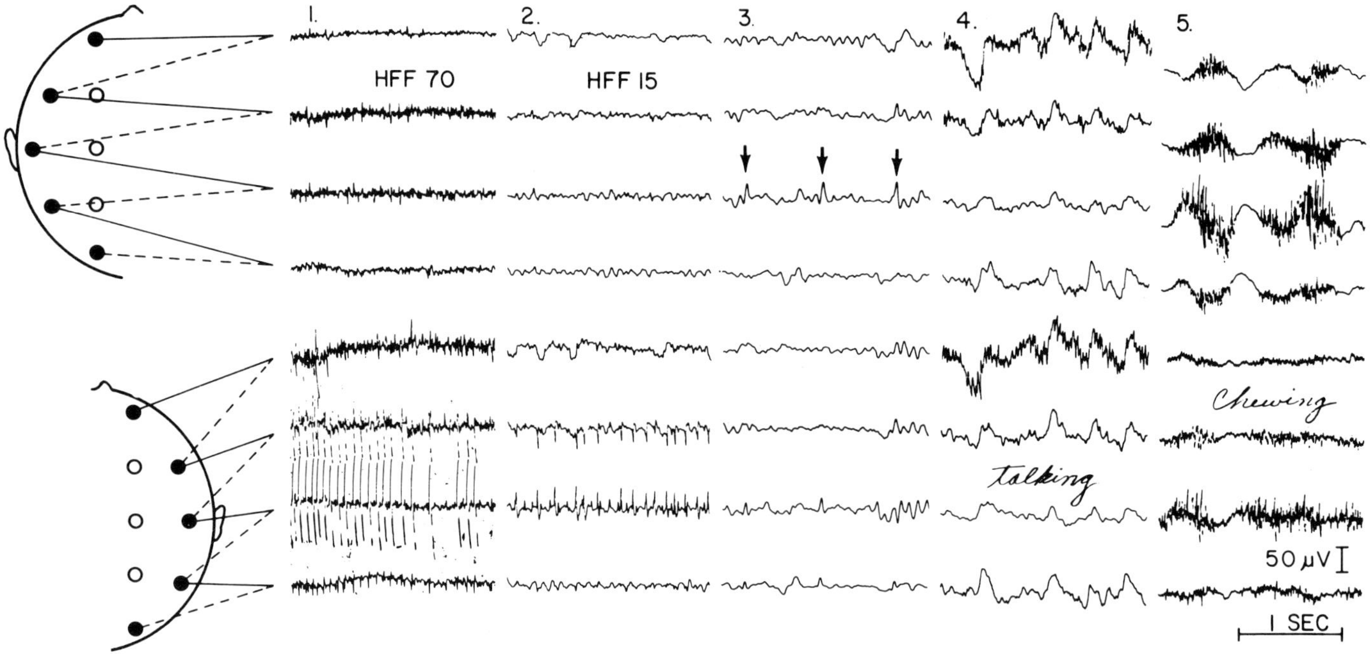


Fig. 6.2. Common artifacts generated by extracerebral physiological activity. 1. Continuous muscle artifact in all channels with superimposed intermittent muscle artifact of high amplitude in channels 6 and 7; the recording is made with a high frequency filter setting of 70 Hz; 2. Continuation of the recording shown in part 1., but with a high frequency filter setting of 15 Hz; 3. Heart beat artifacts (arrows); 4. Artifacts due to talking and frontal muscle contraction; 5. Compound artifact caused by chewing movements and associated muscle artifact.

and at the same time monitor eye movements felt through the eyelids. Taping cotton balls over the eyes may stop eye movements but obscures observation of eye movements and precludes recording the effect of eye opening and closing on the EEG. If eye movements cannot be stopped and cannot be distinguished from frontal slow waves in the EEG, eye movements may be monitored by electrodes placed near the eyes and linked so that eye movements can be distinguished from cerebral activity (4.3.1). Recordings from these linkages should be displayed simultaneously with, and next to, the recordings of frontal slow waves. Comparison of these recordings usually allows clear distinction between eye movement artifact and cerebral slow waves.

**6.1.2** *Muscle artifact.* Muscle activity causes very short potentials which usually recur. If they recur as discrete potentials with the same shape and in the same distribution (Fig. 6.2), they may resemble cerebral spike discharges except that most cerebral spikes are of much longer duration than muscle action potentials. If they recur in rapid bursts of discharges (Fig. 6.2), they usually consist of several different types of potentials which merge and obscure the recording of cerebral activity. Muscle artifacts from scalp and face muscles occur mainly in the frontal and temporal regions but may be recorded by electrodes nearly anywhere on the head. Reducing the settings of the high frequency filter will reduce the amplitude of these fast potentials, but will also change their form (3.5.2) so that single muscle potentials may look more like spikes, and repetitive potentials may look like cerebral fast waves (Fig. 6.2).

Muscle artifact, even if not related to recognizable movement by the patient, is usually easily identified by its shape and repetition. It can be reduced and often eliminated by asking the patient to relax, drop the jaw or open the mouth slightly, or change position. Artifact from a single electrode can sometimes be stopped by gently pushing on that electrode, by stroking or massaging the skin near the electrode, or by reapplying the electrode. Reducing high frequency filter settings is only of limited value because of the aforementioned distortion.

A few specific conditions cause special electrographic patterns. Repetitive movements such as chewing, blinking or tremor may give rise to a combination of fast muscle and slow movement artifacts which may resemble cerebral discharges, especially if the combinations repeat with similar shape. Such rhythmical combinations may occur in tremor of Parkinson's disease, photomyoclonic responses, and other nonepileptic myoclonic contractions. On the other hand, seizures may lead to muscle activity so that a recording electrode picks up mixtures of cerebral seizure activity and muscle activity caused by the seizure. Bursts of muscle potentials of one kind may be followed by bursts of muscle potentials of a different amplitude and shape in the rare facial myokymia which is often associated with brain stem lesions causing no other EEG signs.

**6.1.3** *Movement artifact.* Movements of the head and body or of the electrode wires can cause artifacts even if all electrodes make good mechanical and electrical contact. Movement artifacts are often erratic and not repetitive unless the movement is rhythmical as, for instance in tremor, chewing and sucking (Fig. 6.2).

Movement artifacts are usually easily recognized during the recording by their association with visible movements and should be identified meticulously by indicating the moment and kind of movement on the chart. Many movement artifacts can be abolished by asking the subject to stop moving. In persons who do not comply, for instance in restless or confused patients, infants and children, patients having seizures, tremors or other movement disorders, the movements must be reduced as far as possible. Rarely is there need to use a recording channel for monitoring of movements (4.3.5).

**6.1.4** *The heart beat artifact.* Potential changes generated by the heart are picked up in the EEG mainly in recordings with wide interelectrode distances, especially in linkages across the head and to the left ear, and in subjects with short necks. The artifact may appear in all channels using a common reference, or only in one or a few channels. Small artifacts reflect mainly the R-wave of the electrocardiogram (Fig. 6.2). Larger artifacts may reflect additional components of the electrocardiogram. Very large artifacts are often produced by interference from a cardiac pacemaker (Fig. 6.3).

In contrast to most other artifacts, the heart beat artifact cannot usually be eliminated by corrective actions during the recording. It is rarely the only manifestation of a bad electrode contact and can therefore not usually be abolished by improving the contact or replacing the electrode. Referential recordings combining both ears as a reference tend to show less heart beat artifact than referential recordings to one ear. If necessary, heart beat can be eliminated from a referential recording by using a balanced noncephalic reference. This consists of one electrode on the neck and one on the sternum, connected through a variable resistor which may be adjusted to null the ECG components affecting both these electrodes. If there is any doubt whether sharp waves are due to the heart beat artifact or to cerebral activity, the technician should record the heart beat in one channel and compare it with the timing of the suspected sharp waves (4.3.2).

If the heart beat has not been monitored during the recording and the EEG reader has difficulty in distinguishing heart beat artifact from cerebral activity, it is sometimes useful to measure the interval between suspected heartbeat artifacts and apply this measure to subsequent suspicious events to determine whether they have equal intervals and therefore are likely due to heartbeat, or fall into the interval between events and are less likely of cardiac origin. However, this method may fail in extrasystoles and other cardiac arrhythmias, especially those altering the shape of the heartbeat artifact.

**6.1.5** *Pulse wave artifact.* Periodic waves of smooth or triangular shape may be picked up by an electrode on or near a scalp artery as the result of pulse waves producing slight changes of the electrical contact between electrode and scalp. This is more likely to happen with electrodes in the frontal and temporal areas than with electrodes in the posterior head regions.

This artifact is recognized by its usually regular recurrence. If the heartbeat artifact is picked up in the same recording, it precedes the pulse wave artifact by a constant interval (Fig. 24.2). If necessary, the pulse wave artifact may be identified by simultaneous recording of the heartbeat. If it is eliminated by reapplication of the electrode at some distance from the pulsating artery, the new electrode position should be indicated on the chart.

**6.1.6** *Perspiration.* Very slow drifting of the pens, lasting up to several seconds in duration, may occur as the result of sweating which changes the electrode impedance and skin potential. This artifact is most common in frontal electrodes and usually occurs in several channels at the same time. It can be reduced by cooling the subject's head with a fan or by airconditioning. If this does not succeed, the affected electrodes may need to be replaced and the scalp should be cleaned and dried by wiping with acetone or alcohol. An increase of the low frequency filter setting should be used only as the last resort.

**6.1.7** *Movements of the tongue and other oropharyngeal structures.* These movements may produce intermittent or repetitive slow waves in a wide distribution, often with a maximum in the middle of the head. Tongue movement causes a 'glossokinetic' artifact because the tip of the tongue has a negative electrical charge with respect to the root. Tongue movement explains part of the artifacts generated by speaking, swallowing, chewing, sucking, coughing and hiccoughing; movements of other structures probably contribute to these artifacts (Fig. 6.2) and account for those seen with sobbing. Artifacts from temporal, facial and scalp muscles may be mixed with the movement artifact. Palatal myoclonus causes rhythmical muscle artifacts at rates of about 100–200 per minute which are best seen in referential montages to an ear electrode and persist in sleep.

Many of these artifacts may be identified during the recording if they are associated with visible movements and if they disappear when these movements stop. The artifacts may be further identified by having the subject repeat the movement suspected of having caused the artifact, for instance by having the subject swallow, cough or say the words 'lilt' or 'Tom Thumb'.

**6.1.8** *Dental restorations with dissimilar metals.* Spike-like artifacts may be produced by dental fillings with dissimilar metals whenever the metal pieces are moved against each other, for instance in chewing, swallowing or speaking.

## 6.2 INTERFERENCE

The most common artifact due to electrical interference comes from power lines and equipment. It has a frequency of 60 Hz in North America and of 50 Hz in many other countries. A slight amount of this interference is unavoidable wherever alternating current is used. While this background interference may be picked up by faulty electrodes and may appear in one or a few channels, inordinately strong interference can cause artifacts even with good recording electrodes and equipment; these artifacts are then likely to appear in all channels of all recordings made in the same recording room (Fig. 6.3). The artifacts may be introduced either electrostatically by unshielded power cables and regardless of current flow, or electromagnetically by strong currents flowing through cables and equipment such as transformers and electromotors. Electrostatic interference can be reduced by

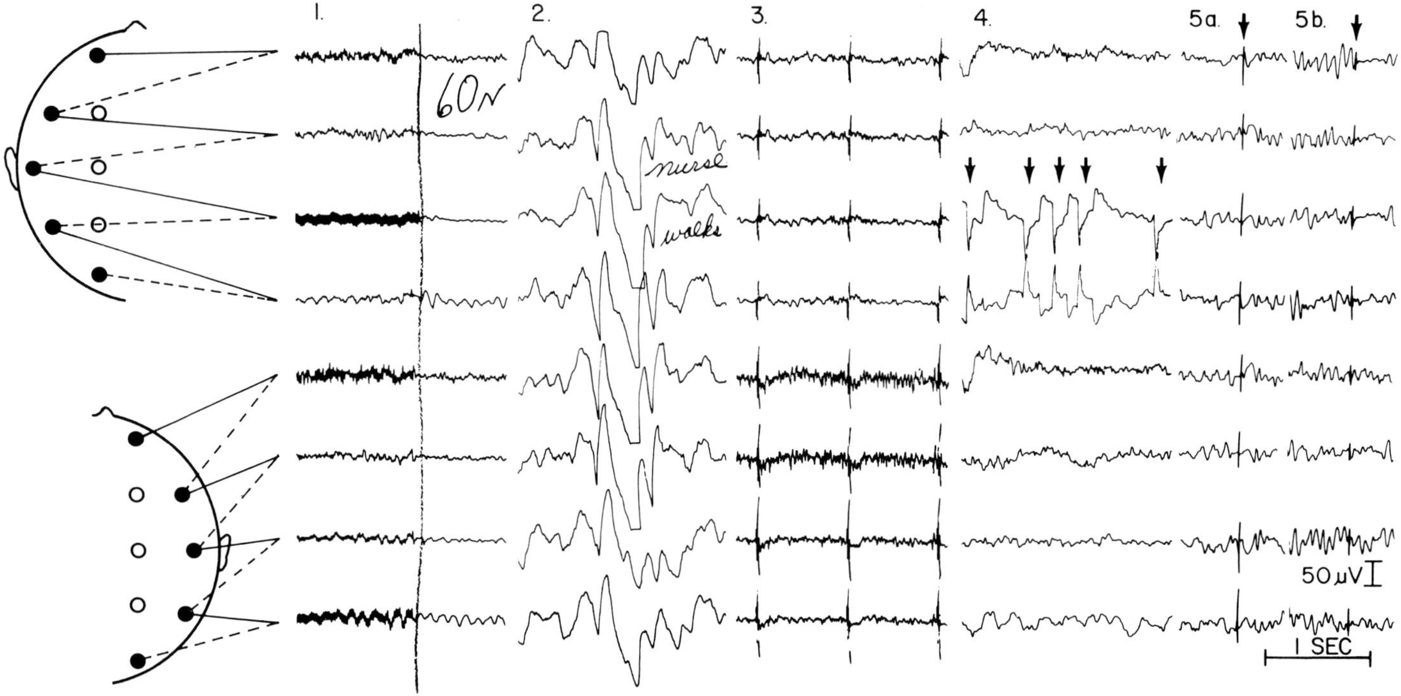


Fig. 6.3. Nonbiological artifacts. 1. 60 Hz interference before and after turning on the 60 Hz filter (60∼); 2. Artifacts induced by a nurse walking near the patient; 3. Cardiac pacemaker artifacts; 4. 'Electrode popping' artifacts (arrows) from the left posterior temporal electrode making poor contact; 5a. and 5b. 'Paper stop' artifacts (arrows) due to intermittent failure of paper drive.

shielding the offending power cables and by using a shielded room for the recording; electromagnetic interference can be reduced by proper wiring of the power cables. Other types of interference include signals from nearby television stations, radio paging, telephone ringing, cardiac pacemakers (Fig. 6.3), or any movement of a charged body near the recording electrodes; electrostatic artifacts may be produced by a person walking through the recording room (Fig. 6.3) or by drops falling in an intravenous drip. However, modern EEG machines have such high discrimination and input impedance that they reject all but the most powerful sources of interference from the environment. In setting up a laboratory, it is therefore not necessary to shield the recording room unless a trial recording from a patient or a 10,000 Ω resistor, placed at the prospective recording site, shows strong interference.

When recordings are made in an environment with much interference such as an intensive care unit or an operating room, the patient's head and the connections to the EEG machine should be kept as far from power cables as possible. Any swaying of electrode wires and movement of tubing or of other charged objects should be minimized. Equipment other than the EEG machine should be unplugged if feasible; even the respirator may be stopped for short periods to obtain artifact-free recordings or to determine the cause of interference.

## 6.3 ARTIFACTS ARISING FROM RECORDING ELECTRODES AND EQUIPMENT

**6.3.1** *Artifacts arising from electrodes, electrode terminal board, input cable and selector switches.* Most artifacts in this category are distinguished from cerebral activity in that they differ radically from previously recorded activity, do not blend with other simultaneously recorded activity but seem to be superimposed on it, and appear only in channels connected to one electrode. However, not all of these artifacts are easily recognized. Although some of them have characteristic shapes, others lack such features and may resemble cerebral activity. A common artifact is 'electrode popping' which is due to a sudden change of electrode contact causing pen deflections which rise or fall abruptly and may mimick spike discharges (Fig. 6.3). Other electrode artifacts rise and fall more slowly and may resemble cerebral slow waves.

Identification and correction of artifacts in the distribution of one electrode requires checking electrical and mechanical continuity. Because the artifact is often due to faulty contact between the electrode and the scalp, the first step is to look at that junction: The electrode may be partly or completely detached, the lead wire may be broken, or the conductive paste or jelly may have dried up. As a next step, electrical impedance should be measured (2.2.3); if it is high, the electrode should be refilled with conductive jelly or paste, reapplied, or replaced if it is defective. If the artifact persists, the receptacle jack or the wiring of the input terminal board may be at fault; this can be investigated by changing the connections between electrodes and receptacles of the faulty channel so that the electrodes and the receptacles of that channel are presented in different channels: The electrodes of the faulty channel are connected to receptacles giving good recordings when connected to other electrodes, and electrodes not giving artifacts when connected to other receptacles are connected to receptacles of the faulty channel. If the artifact changes channels corresponding with the electrodes from the faulty channel, one of these electrodes is at fault and can be identified by connecting the two electrodes to different channels and observing in which channel the artifact then appears. However, if the artifact remains at one receptacle, the input board or subsequent components of the recording channel may be at fault. In practice, the technician at this point or earlier will examine a piece of recording made while the inputs are closed. If the artifact persists under this condition, it arises from the recording machine and should be investigated accordingly (6.3.2). However, if the artifact is present only when the input is open, and if an electrode fault has been excluded, the source of the artifact may be further determined by replacing the input board and input cable if replacements are available, and by checking the input terminals and selector switches if they are accessible.

**6.3.2** *Artifacts arising from the recording machine.* Like artifacts from the electrodes, artifacts from the machine may often be recognized by the sudden appearance of waveforms very different from cerebral activity. The source of the artifacts can often be traced to one functional component of the machine. Trouble-shooting is facilitated by two features of modern EEG machines. (a) Many components have indicator lights and electrical contact points with prescribed voltage readings which can be checked easily. (b) Components of individual channels are made of modules which can be exchanged. Artifacts due to faults of components that are common to all channels often cause lack of power or 60 Hz interference. Power failure may be caused by a faulty outlet or a blown fuse in the EEG machine. If a replacement fuse also blows, the power supply may be at fault. Sixty hertz interference in all channels may be due to (a) a powerful source of interference in the recording room (6.2), (b) a faulty or absent connection of the subject with the ground of the EEG machine (3.4.1), (c) defects in the power supply or other parts of the machine.

Artifacts caused by components of individual channels appear only at the output of the defective channels and persist independently of the input selection. The causes of these problems can be traced by exchanging modular components of one channel with the corresponding components of another channel. For instance if 60 Hz artifact in one channel suggests a problem in its amplifier, this can be investigated by exchanging the amplifier for an amplifier of another channel not showing that artifact.

# REFERENCES


Barry, W. and Jones, G.M. (1965) Influence of eyelid movement upon electro-oculographic recording of vertical eye movements. Aerospace Med. 36: 855–858.

Beaussart, M. and Guiev, J.D. (1977) Section III. Artefacts. In: Rémond, A. (Ed.), Handbook of Electroenceph. clin. Neurophysiol., Vol. 11A, Elsevier, Amsterdam, pp. 80–96.

Bickford, R.G. and Klass, D.W. (1964) Eye movement and the electroencephalogram. In: Bender, M. (Ed.), The Oculomotor System. Harper and Row, New York, pp. 293–302.

Brittenham, D. (1974) Recognition and reduction of physiological artifacts. Am. J. EEG Technol. 14: 158–165.

Espinosa, R.E., Klass, D.W. and Maloney, J.D. (1978) Contribution of the electroencephalogram in monitoring cardiac dysrhythmias. Mayo Clin. Proc. 53: 119–122.

Harlan, W.L., White, P.T. and Bickford, R.G. (1958) Electric activity produced by eye flutter simulating frontal electroencephalographic rhythms. Electroenceph. clin. Neurophysiol. 10: 164–169.

Joynt, R.J. (1959) An EEG artefact in palatal myoclonus. Electroenceph. clin. Neurophysiol. 11: 158–160.

Lehtonen, J.B. and Koivikko, M.J. (1971) The use of non-cephalic reference electrode in recording cerebral evoked potentials in man. Electroenceph. clin. Neurophysiol. 31: 154–156.

Mac Gillivray, B.B. (1974) Section IV. Artefacts, faults, and fault-finding. In: Rémond, A. (Ed.), Handbook of Electroenceph. clin. Neurophysiol., Vol. 3C, Elsevier, Amsterdam, pp. 88–102.

Matsuo, F., Peters, J.F. and Reilly, E.L. (1975) Electrical phenomena associated with movements of the eyelid. Electroenceph. clin. Neurophysiol. 38: 507–511.

Milnarich, R.F., Tourney, G. and Beckett, P.G.S. (1957) Electroencephalographic artifact arising from dental restorations. Electroenceph. clin. Neurophysiol. 9: 337–339.

Pasik, P., Pasik, T. and Bender, M.B. (1965) Recovery of the electro-oculogram after total ablation of the retina in monkeys. Electroenceph. clin. Neurophysiol. 19: 291–297.

Redding, F.K., Wandel, V. and Nasser, C. (1969) Intravenous infusion drop artifacts. Electroenceph. clin. Neurophysiol. 26: 318–320.

Stephenson, W.A. and Gibbs, F.A. (1951) A balanced non-cephalic reference electrode. Electroenceph. clin. Neurophysiol. 3: 237–240.

Westmoreland, B.F., Espinosa, R.E. and Klass, D.W. (1973) Significant prosopo-glossopharyngeal movements affecting the electroencephalogram. Am. J. EEG Technol. 13: 59–70.

# Other methods of recording and analysis

# 7


SUMMARY

(7.1) *Oscilloscope displays* may be used to monitor the EEG; they are especially useful in ascertaining proper functioning of other recording and analyzing equipment.

(7.2) *Telemetry and portable tape recordings* are used to record the EEG as the patient moves about. Telemetric recording of the EEG is often combined with television monitoring of behavior.

(7.3) *Magnetic tape recording* is used for electronic analysis of the EEG after the actual recording is completed.

(7.4) *Computer analysis* uses either small 'special purpose' or 'hard wired' computers which are capable of only one or a few types of analysis, or 'general purpose' computers which may be programmed for a greater variety of analyses.

(7.5) *The spontaneous EEG* may be analyzed in several ways. *Power spectral analysis* shows the power of EEG wave components which occur at different frequencies. *Compressed spectral arrays* illustrate how the distribution of power at different frequencies changes with time. *Cross-correlation* can indicate similarities in the EEG recorded simultaneously from different areas of the head. *Autocorrelation* compares components recorded from the same area at different times. *Spatial relations* may be analyzed by maps showing the momentary distribution of potentials on a diagram of the head or by maps depicting isopotential lines between a chain of electrodes as a function of time.

(7.6) *Evoked potentials* are elicited by stimulation of the visual, auditory or somatosensory system and can be extracted from the background EEG by computer summation of a large number of individual responses. These potentials are used clinically to search for abnormalities of conduction through the sensory pathways.


## 7.1 OSCILLOSCOPE DISPLAYS

An oscilloscope may be used to display one or more channels of EEG when there is no need to write a permanent record. This method is often used to inspect electrical recordings as they are stored on, or played back from, magnetic tape or computer memory. For example, oscilloscope tracings are commonly used to monitor the recording of evoked potentials (7.6) to ascertain that they are free of artifact. Oscilloscopic monitoring is especially useful for this purpose because it displays a much wider range of frequencies than a paper record and thus facilitates recognition of artifacts and of response components.

The oscilloscope cannot replace the conventional paper record in the interpretation of clinical EEGs because the tracing vanishes and produces no permanent record to allow for comparison of successive recordings. Therefore, oscilloscopic tracings may be used only to monitor disposable parts of the recording such as periods spent while waiting for a person to go to sleep.

## 7.2 TELEMETRY AND PORTABLE MAGNETIC TAPE RECORDINGS

These methods are used to record the EEG while subjects are free to move about, especially in studies which require long recording periods to investigate intermittent disturbances such as seizures. Electrodes with very short lead wires are attached to the scalp and connected to miniature battery-powered amplifiers on or near the head. Calibration, change of montages and correction of artifacts are more cumbersome than in routine recordings.

**7.2.1** *Telemetry* transmits the EEG either through a long cable or through a portable radiofrequency transmitter to the recording machine. To reduce the number of transmitting elements, the outputs of all channels are electronically mixed into a single channel before transmission and then separated again at the receiving site. Telemetric EEG recordings may be combined with closed circuit television recordings of the subject's behavior; both recordings may be stored on magnetic tape for later analysis and correlation of EEG with behavior.

**7.2.2** *In portable tape recordings*, amplifiers are connected to a cassette recorder or other light tape recorder which stores the EEG for later playback and oscilloscope display or EEG writeout. This method has the disadvantage that it offers no provisions for recognition and correction of artifacts and for behavioral correlations during the recording.

## 7.3 MAGNETIC TAPE RECORDING

This technique is indispensable when EEGs are to be analyzed electronically at some time after the recording, i.e. 'off-line'. For visual analysis of clinical EEGs, a paper record is also made at the time of the original recording. Important considerations regarding magnetic tape recordings are (1) modulation techniques, (2) bandwidth and recording speed, (3) number of channels and tape width.

**7.3.1** *Modulation techniques* must be used because potential changes as slow as those of the EEG cannot be recorded directly by open reel or cassette tape recorders conventionally used for audiorecordings. The EEG is therefore encoded by making it modulate a fast event. A common technique is frequency modulation (FM) which uses a fast sine wave as a carrier and increases or decreases its frequency in proportion to the amplitude of the EEG potentials. These sine waves are recorded on tape and are demodulated on playback, to reconstruct the slower voltage changes of the original EEG.

**7.3.2** *The bandwidth of the recording and the tape speed* are directly related to each other, faster tape speeds being required for recordings of a wider frequency range. The frequencies of the conventional EEG, falling well within the range of 0–100 Hz, can be recorded at tape speeds as low as those used for audiorecordings, namely $1\frac{7}{8}$ inches per second. Higher frequencies, such as those studied in some types of computer analysis of the spontaneous EEG and evoked potentials, require faster tape speeds. Calibration pulses, which must be stored on tape with each EEG recording, are used to determine the amplitude and to evaluate the fidelity of the recording.

**7.3.3** *The number of channels and the tape width* are directly related to each other. Eight channels of EEG can be stored on 1/4 inch tape of open reels and audiocassettes, sixteen channel recordings require wider tape. One channel of recording should have provisions to record vocal comments or a code which identify the subject, the recording conditions, montages, machine settings, behavioral correlates and sources of artifact during the recording.

## 7.4 COMPUTER ANALYSIS

Computers are used to extract information from the EEG which is not obtainable with visual analysis. Because no computer programs are available which can replace the conventional visual analysis of paper records, good practice requires that all clinical EEG recordings to be analyzed by computer should be written out as a paper record. Other EEG recordings should at least be monitored on an oscilloscope to recognize and eliminate artifacts and malfunctions.

Most computer methods now use digital techniques which transform the continuous voltage changes of the EEG into segments of equal length and measure the voltage of each segment. These voltages, which are an analogue of the amplitude of the EEG potentials on the scalp, are converted into sequences of digital numbers in a process called 'analog-to-digital conversion'. The numbers are manipulated by computer programs and the results are either presented in numerical form or, after reconversion to analog form, displayed in the form of a continuous curve.

Two types of digital computers can be distinguished by the method of programming. 'Hard-wired' or 'special purpose' computers have one or a few programs permanently stored in their memory. Parameters of the analysis can be selected by front-panel controls. These small computers perform a limited number of operations very efficiently. They are often used for averaging of evoked potentials. In contrast, 'general purpose' computers are programmed for each task by sequences of instructions given in a specific code or 'language'. Once a program has been developed, it is stored on paper tape, magnetic tape or magnetic disc and loaded into the computer when needed. Parameters of analysis are selected by giving keyboard commands. Although general purpose computers are more versatile, they require more time for setting up and running a program than a special purpose computer. However, most analyses of the spontaneous EEG are rather complex and require general purpose computers.

## 7.5 COMPUTER ANALYSIS OF SPONTANEOUS EEG

**7.5.1** *Power spectrum.* Any waveform in the EEG, regardless of whether it is sinusoidal or not, can be considered to be composed of a set of sine waves of specific frequency and amplitude. A sample of EEG recording can therefore be represented by its component sine waves; the amount of sine waves at each frequency in the EEG sample may be represented by plotting the amount versus the frequency of the sine wave components. The amount of waves in a spectrum of frequencies is usually expressed not as amplitude but as the square of amplitude, or power; the plot of power versus frequency is a power spectrum (Fig. 7.1). Although power spectra can be calibrated in terms of absolute power, the relative representation of different frequencies is generally of greater practical importance. For instance, power spectra

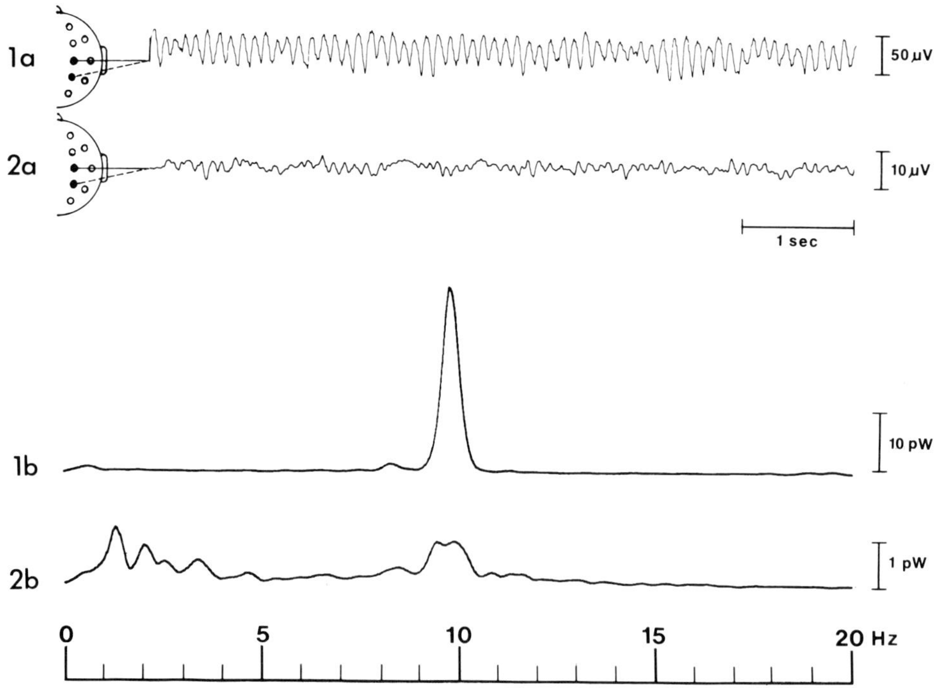


Fig. 7.1. Power spectra of normal (1) and abnormal (2) EEGs. The top two tracings (a) show strips of the paper tracing recorded between the right central and parietal electrode in a normal subject (1a) and a patient (2a). The bottom section shows power spectra (b) computed from about 13 seconds of the same recordings. The power spectrum of the normal subject (1b) shows activity mainly at 10 Hz, representing the 10 Hz waves seen in 1a; the power spectrum from the patient in 2b shows activity at about 1–4 Hz and at 10 Hz, reflecting the combination of slow waves and 10 Hz waves in 2a. Vertical calibration is in picowatts (pW).

made from one area of the head at different times, or from different parts of the head at the same time, may show clinically significant differences.

Power spectra may be plotted of successive segments of the continuously recorded EEG and stacked one above the other in the form of a compressed spectral array. Figures 7.2 and 7.3 show compressed spectral arrays of the EEG recorded in eight channels simultaneously.

Power spectrum analysis is a useful way to demonstrate slight differences in the preponderance of waves of different frequencies and slight shifts of frequency. This can be helpful especially in the detection of abnormal amplitude and frequency of slow waves. However, it should be remembered that other important information may be lost in this method of analysis. Most important are (a) the phase relationships between waves in different areas; and (b) spikes which occur infrequently and have relatively little power; additional spike-detecting programs are therefore sometimes used in conjunction with power spectral analysis.

**7.5.2** *Correlation analysis.* *Cross-correlation* evaluates the similarity between signals from two different sources recorded simultaneously. Similarities of both amplitude and shape are measured as the covariance of the signals; similarities of shape regardless of amplitude are expressed by the correlation coefficient which varies between +1, indicating that the signals have identical shape and polarity, and −1, indicating that they have identical shape but opposite polarity. If the two sources generate signals which have similar shape but different timing, the correlation coefficient will vary if the signals are displaced against each other in time; the dependence of the correlation coefficient on the time interval is represented by the correlation function. The correlation coefficient also varies with the frequency of the EEG components; the dependence of the correlation coefficient on the EEG frequency is the coherence function.

*Autocorrelation* compares amplitude and shape of the EEG from one area of the

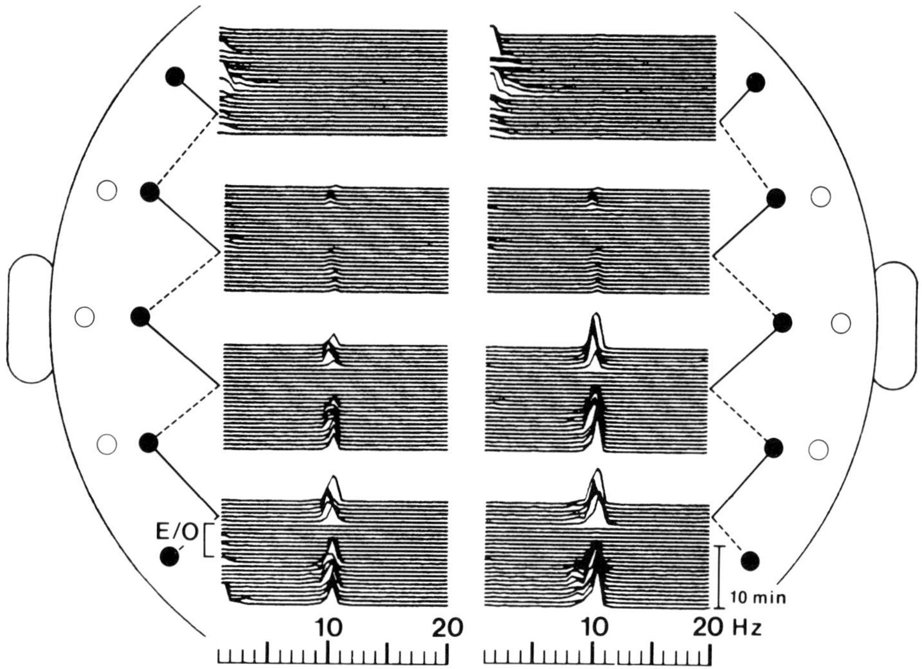


Fig. 7.2. Compressed spectral array of a normal EEG. Each of the eight blocks of tracings represents power spectra computed from simultaneous EEG recordings derived between the electrodes indicated on the head diagrams at the sides of the illustration. Each line in the blocks represents one power spectrum plotted for a recording period of about 35 seconds; successive spectra are stacked vertically. The posterior head regions show power mainly at about 10 Hz which disappears with eye opening (E/O) midway in the recording and reappears after the eyes are closed. The power in the low frequency range in the frontal regions is due to eye movement artifacts.

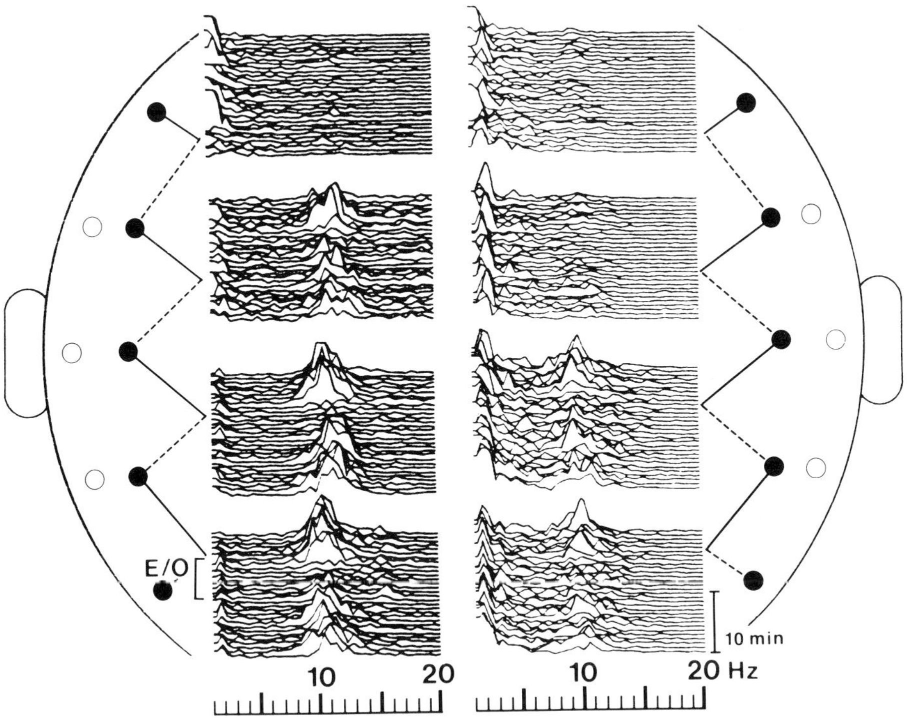


Fig. 7.3. Compressed spectral array of an abnormal EEG. Power spectra are plotted with the same methods as used in Fig. 7.2. The spectra from the right posterior head regions differ from those from the left side in that they show a considerable amount of power below 8 Hz with a maximum at 1–3 Hz. Power at 10 Hz is reduced on the right side as compared to the left, especially in the fronto-central region. Eye opening (E/O) reduces power at 10 Hz noticeably on the left side but hardly at all on the right.

head at different times. Essentially, the analysis displaces the EEG against itself in time and measures correlation at different time intervals. This method is especially suited to reveal periodic components.

**7.5.3** *Spatial analysis.* Several methods serve to depict the changing distribution of potential fields. Most use isopotential lines which were discussed earlier (4.1.3). One method plots the distribution of potential lines superimposed on a diagram of the head; because each such plot represents only one moment, successive plots must be made at different times and viewed one after another. Another method plots isopotential lines between a chain of electrodes versus time, generating a spatio-temporal map, sometimes referred to as 'chronotopogram'.

## 7.6 COMPUTER AVERAGING OF EVOKED POTENTIALS: GENERAL TECHNIQUES

Sensory stimulation produces electrical responses in the relay stations of the sensory pathways including the cortical receiving areas. These responses may be distinguishable in the EEG recorded from the overlying scalp, but they are often small and buried, indistinguishable from the EEG. These responses can be extracted from the EEG, and their details can be enhanced, by administering repetitive stimuli and averaging the EEG recording following each stimulus (Fig. 7.4). By this method, EEG components related to the stimulus are enhanced while components unrelated to the stimulus, also considered 'noise' in this context, are decreased and tend to average to zero.

To average evoked potentials with a computer, a stimulus is delivered to the subject at the onset of each averaging period. Stimuli are usually spaced far enough apart that responses do not overlap and interact with each other; however, the interaction of responses is made the subject of some studies which use fast stimulus rates. The analysis period, or epoch, is chosen to last for only a fraction of the interval between stimuli. The length of the epoch is determined by the type of the response; it varies between 10 msec for auditory far-field potentials and 250 msec or more for visual evoked potentials.

Recordings are usually made with ordinary EEG electrodes, but electrode placements depend on the sensory system under study and do not usually coincide with those of the 10–20 System. Generally, recordings are made using one electrode closer to the site of the response and one farther away; these electrodes are connected to the inputs of an amplifier as in usual EEG recording. The bandwidth of the amplifier may need to be wider than that of routine EEG recordings so that very fast or very slow components of the response are not attenuated. The output of the amplifier is connected to the input of the computer, and usually also to a monitoring oscilloscope (7.1). A synchronizing pulse between the stimulator and computer serves to start the computer operation shortly before or at the beginning of the stimulus. On receiving the synchronizing signal, the computer samples the voltage of the recording at successive intervals of the epoch. Most computers offer 1024 averaging intervals or addresses the contents of which are displayed as an oscilloscope sweep after each stimulus. The digital values of the amplitudes of the recording at each interval during the epoch are stored at the corresponding address of the computer memory. During successive epochs, the amplitude is again sampled and digitized. Each number representing an amplitude at a different interval after the onset of the stimulus is added to the collected numbers stored at the corresponding interval during the preceding epochs. In this manner, successive responses are added to each other (Fig. 7.4). To obtain the average from this sum, the amplitude may be divided by reducing the gain. True averaging computers perform a division at the time of each addition of a response so that the addresses contain the average values at all times. This keeps the oscilloscope display from increasing in amplitude during the averaging procedure. Many computers have provisions for simultaneous averaging in more than one channel.

*Clinical use of evoked potentials.* Potentials evoked by stimulation of a sensory path are used to test conduction through that path. Abnormalities of conduction are recognized by comparing the responses of the patient under study with values obtained in the same laboratory from a group of normal subjects. Normal values vary both between individuals and in the same individual with time. To reduce variability and thereby to increase the ability to detect abnormalities, stimulus and recording conditions must be rigidly standardized. Also, normative data should be obtained for different age groups and for other variables of significance. Clinically, the most important abnormal finding is an increase of the latency of response components; this indicates a delay in conduction and implies damage to nerve fibers of the sensory system under study. Reduction of amplitude, changes in shape and even complete absence of components are less reliable signs because they can be caused by factors outside the pathway of the nervous system.

Evoked potentials can be divided by sensory modality into (1) visual, (2) auditory, and (3) somatosensory. Visual evoked potentials can be subdivided by stimulus type into potentials elicited by flashes of diffuse light ('flash response'), potentials evoked by reversal of a checkerboard pattern ('pattern reversal' or 'pattern shift response'), and potentials provoked by other visual stimuli. Auditory and somatosensory responses can be subdivided into 'cortical evoked potentials' which, like visual evoked potentials, are presumably generated at the sensory receiving areas of the cerebral cortex, and into 'brain stem' or 'far field' responses, presumably generated by relays of the sensory pathways in the brain stem. Auditory and somatosensory responses can be further subdivided by the stimulus type.

**7.6.1** *Visual evoked potentials: general strategy.* Visual stimulation excites retinal pathways and initiates impulses which are conducted through the central visual path to the primary visual cortex, largely buried in the mesial surface of the occipital hemispheres. Fibers from this area project to the secondary visual cortical areas on the occipital convexity. Through this path, a visual stimulus to the eyes causes an electrical response in the occipital regions which can be recorded with electrodes placed over occipital points. Clinical recordings are often made between electrodes placed in the midoccipital and mid-central areas; these recordings do not attempt to separate contributions from each hemisphere. However, electrode placements vary between different laboratories and may include lateral placements.

Because of the particular anatomy of the central visual pathway, two types of abnormalities can be distinguished by visual stimulation. (a) A prechiasmal defect, namely a defect of the eye or optic nerve, may alter the response to stimulation of the eye on that side, regardless of whether responses are recorded from the left or right side of the head. (b) Post-chiasmal defects, namely defects of the optic tract, lateral geniculate body, optic radiations or visual cortex may produce abnormalities of responses recorded from the affected side of the head regardless of which eye is stimulated. Experience has shown that visual evoked potentials are much more effective in discovering prechiasmal conduction defects than postchiasmal defects. For this reason, visual evoked potentials are particularly sensitive indicators of abnormalities in patients with multipe sclerosis which commonly affects the optic nerves. Abnormal visual evoked potentials may be found in patients without history of retrobulbar neuritis and without findings of optic atrophy or visual field defects. In contrast, many patients with proven damage to the postchiasmal part of the visual path, even with visual field defects, may have evoked potentials which are normal by conventional standards; future investigations may develop criteria which permit better identification of postchiasmal lesions.

*Pattern reversal or pattern shift* responses are elicited by having the subject look at a pattern of checkerboard squares in which all black squares suddenly turn white and all white squares turn black. Each of these reversals or shifts causes a response with a major peak at a latency of about 100 msec. The response varies with the retinal area stimulated, the location of the recording electrodes, the luminance of

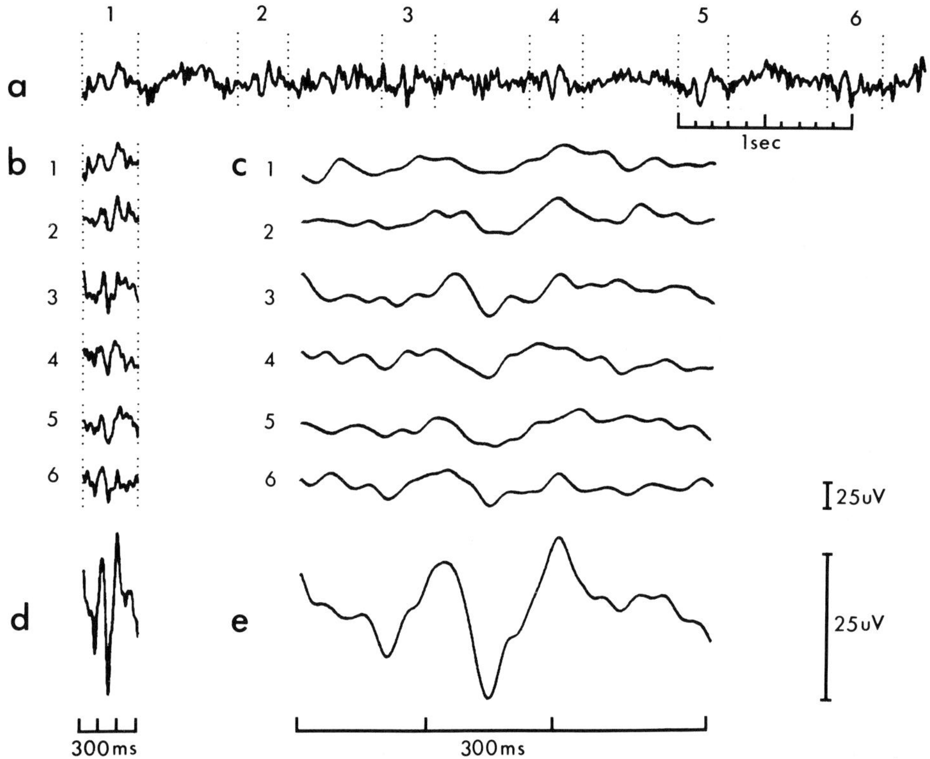


Fig. 7.4. Computer averaging of evoked potentials. The top line a shows continuous EEG recorded between the right occipital and ear electrode in a normal subject while light flashes were presented at intervals slightly shorter than 1 second (dotted lines at the beginning of periods 1 to 6). The computer sampled the voltage changes during periods of 300 msec after each flash (segments between dotted lines). These segments are arranged vertically in b with the same time scale as in a; they are show in c with an expanded time scale. The samples are added in d and e. The summation enhances features which are common to the individual responses. The sum can be converted into an average by dividing the gain by the number of samples.

the pattern and other factors including the patient's visual acuity and ability to focus on the stimulus pattern. However, if these variables are kept constant, response latencies vary only within very narrow limits between normal subjects. Generally, good results can be obtained by presenting checkerboard patterns on a television screen at 1 m distance in a dark room; squares should have sidelengths of about 4–8 mm, i.e. subtend 15–30′ of visual angle; squares of much larger size produce local flash effects on the retina when they shift.

*The flash response* is elicited by delivering a bright flash of diffuse light at a distance of 30–50 cm from the subject's eyes. This produces a series of potential changes, or components, recordable in the occipital regions. The major component, often having positive polarity at the occiput and a peak latency of 50–100 msec, may be seen in the continuously recorded EEG (Fig. 7.4a) and in single oscilloscope sweeps (Fig. 7.4b and c); however, the entire response, which has many components and lasts over 100–200 msec, cannot be seen without computer averaging (Fig. 7.4d and e). Because flash responses vary widely between subjects, this response type is not very effective in detecting abnormalities. This is the major reason why pattern reversal responses are now used with increasing frequency.

*Other visual stimuli* can be used to elicit visual evoked potentials. One stimulus consists of gratings of black and white bars with sharp borders or with sinusoidal transitions of light intensity; both the intervals between the gratings and the intensity of the contrast can be varied to investigate defects of visual channels carrying information on specific spatial frequencies. Stimulus rates of flashes or reversing patterns may be increased to include frequencies at which individual responses fuse to patterns akin to the photic driving response seen in the routine EEG recordings from many normal subjects (Fig. 14.2). This 'steady state' response does not identify latency of components but may show differences of amplitude at different frequencies. Some investigators have reported examining procedures using patterns of continuously varying size; these methods are said to be able to measure visual acuity and degree of amplyopia and may be helpful to examine persons with short attention span, especially children.

**7.6.2** *Auditory evoked potentials.* Special recording and stimulating methods have been developed which permit recording of signals generated by subcortical structures in the auditory path; these signals are often called 'far field auditory evoked potentials' or 'brain stem auditory evoked responses'. Stimulation of either ear evokes potentials which can reveal lesions in the brain stem that involve the auditory pathway without affecting hearing. Evoked potentials of this type are also used to evaluate hearing in infants ('electrical response audiometry'). In contrast to the short-latency brain stem evoked potentials, the potentials elicited after longer latency in the auditory cortex are difficult to obtain and have not become useful diagnostic tools.

Brain stem auditory evoked responses are recorded between widely spaced electrodes, usually placed on the vertex and the mastoid. Stimuli are delivered to one ear through earphones. Because the sound waves delivered to one ear can travel through the skull to the opposite ear, a continuous masking sound is often simultaneously delivered to the opposite ear. Stimulus rates of 10 Hz are commonly used because the responses of brain stem structures have very short latency and duration. Several thousand stimuli are usually given because of the small amplitude of the individual responses. Stimuli usually consist either of clicks or of tone bursts.

*Click stimuli* of about 60 dB above the subject's hearing threshold elicit a sequence of up to seven components (I–VII) which occur within the first 10 milliseconds after the click and are probably generated mainly by: I. the acoustic nerve, II. cochlear nucleus, III. superior olivary nucleus, IV. lateral lemniscus, V. inferior colliculus, VI. medial geniculate nucleus and VII. auditory radiations. A lesion in one of these structures produces an abnormality of the response beginning at the component which represents excitation of that structure. Thus, a lesion involving the inferior colliculus would increase the latency and reduce the amplitude of components V, VI and VII, while a lesion of the acoustic nerve would affect all components of the response. Some difficulty of interpreting brain stem evoked potentials may arise in the case of patients with peripheral hearing deficits that alter the evoked potentials.

*Tone bursts* are brief trains of sine waves of rapidly increasing amplitude which are used by some laboratories instead of click stimuli. The frequency of the stimulus is made a variable in some studies attempting to assess hearing ability at different frequencies.

Frequency following responses are elicited by repetitive square or sine wave stimuli. If spaced closely enough, these stimuli make individual responses fuse into a rhythm similar to the steady state response to rapidly repetitive visual stimuli. The diagnostic value of these responses is under study.

**7.6.3** *Somatosensory evoked potentials.* 'Far field somatosensory evoked potentials' are now recorded in many laboratories to study the conduction of impulses through the lower parts of the somatosensory pathway. The recording techniques vary between laboratories. Generally, electrical stimuli are applied to the median nerve at the wrist at an intensity near that which produces thumb twitches. Stimulus rates of up to 10 Hz and stimulus numbers of several thousand are used. Recordings are usually made between several electrode pairs simultaneously. One electrode of each pair may be placed in a midline position on the scalp, other electrodes record the ascending volley over the brachial plexus, and over the neck or inion; the cortical evoked potential may be recorded between an electrode over the parietal cortex opposite to the stimulated side and a distant electrode. Little agreement exists between different laboratories as to the latency, shape and origin of the individual components. These differences will probably be resolved as stimulating and recording techniques are standardized.

**7.6.4** *Spinal evoked potentials.* These potentials can be recorded with EEG or other surface electrodes placed on skin at different levels of the spine. Stimulation of the peroneal nerve elicits potentials with peak latencies which increase with the distance from the stimulus site. Conduction velocity in the spinal cord can be calculated by dividing the distance between recording points by the difference in peak latencies recorded at these points. This method may become useful for the evaluation of spinal defects.

**7.6.5** *The contingent negative variation (CNV)* is elicited by presentation of paired stimuli. It consists of a long-sustained negative potential with a maximum at the vertex which follows the evoked potential elicited by the first stimulus. It builds up with the subject's expectation of the second stimulus and has therefore also been called 'expectancy wave'. The CNV differs from other evoked potentials in that (a) it represents an electrical correlate not of sensory conduction but of the psychological process of expectation, and (b) it is such a slow potential change that it needs to be recorded with special electrodes and amplifiers capable of recording very low frequencies. The CNV has been used mainly in psychological and psychiatric research, but it has not yet become an important diagnostic tool.

## REFERENCES


Bickford, R.G. (1979) Newer methods of recording and analyzing EEGs. In: Klass, D.W. and Daly, D.D. (Eds.) Current Practice of Clinical Electroencephalography. Raven Press, New York.

Binnie, C.D., Batchelor, B.G., Bowring, P.A., Darby, C.E., Herbert, L., Lloyd, D.S.L., Smith, D.M., Smith, G.F. and Smith, M. (1978) Computer-assisted interpretation of clinical EEGs. Electroenceph. clin. Neurophysiol. 44: 575–585.

Bodis-Wollner, I., Hendley, C.D., Mylin, L.H. and Thornton, J. (1979) Visual evoked potentials and the visuogram in multiple sclerosis. Ann. Neurol. 5: 40–47.

Bourne, J.R., Miezin, F.M., Ward, J.W. and Teschan, P.E. (1975) Computer quantification of electroencephalographic data recorded from renal patients. Computers and Biomedical Research 8: 461–473.

Bricolo, A., Turazzi, S., Faccioli, F., Odorizzi, F., Sciarretta, G. and Erculiani, P. (1978) Clinical application of compressed spectral array in long-term EEG monitoring of comatose patients. Electroenceph. clin. Neurophysiol. 45: 211–225.

Burger, D. and Lairy, G.C. (1978) Multivariate analysis of drug-effects on electrophysiological signals in man. Neuropharmacol. 17: 891–904.

Celesia, G.G., Soni, V.K. and Rhode, W.S. (1978) Visual evoked spectrum array and interhemispheric variations. Arch. Neurol. 35: 678–682.

Chiappa, K.H., Burke, S.R. and Young, R.R. (1979) Results of electroencephalographic monitoring during 367 carotid endarterectomies. Use of a dedicated minicomputer. Stroke 10: 381–388.

Chiappa, K.H., Harrison, J.L., Brooks, E.B. and Young, R.R. (1980) Brainstem auditory evoked responses in 200 patients with multiple sclerosis. Ann. Neurol. 7: 135–143.

Cracco, R.Q. and Cracco, J.B. (1976) Somatosensory evoked potential in man: Far field potentials. Electroenceph. clin. Neurophysiol. 41: 460–466.

Cracco, J.B., Cracco, R.Q. and Stolove, R. (1979) Spinal evoked potential in man: A maturational study. Electroenceph. clin. Neurophysiol. 46: 58–64.

Desmedt, J.E. (1977) Visual evoked potentials in man: New developments. Clarendon Press, Oxford.

Dimitrijevic, M.R., Larsson, L.E., Lehmkuhl, D. and Sherwood, A. (1978) Evoked spinal cord and nerve root potentials in humans using a non-invasive recording technique. Electroenceph. clin. Neurophysiol. 45: 331–340.

Duffy, F.H., Burchfiel, J.L. and Lombroso, C.T. (1979) Brain electrical activity mapping (BEAM): A method for extending the clinical utility of EEG and evoked potential data. Ann. Neurol. 5: 309–321.

Ertekin, C. (1978) Comparison of the human evoked electrospinogram recorded from the intrathecal, epidural and cutaneous levels. Electroenceph. clin. Neurophysiol. 44: 683–690.

Goff, W.R. (1974) Human average evoked potentials: Procedures for stimulating and recording. In: Thompson, R.F. and Patterson, M.M. (Eds.) Bioelectric Recording Techniques, Vol. 1B, Academic Press, New York and London, pp. 101–156.

Gotman, J., Gloor, P. and Ray, W.F. (1975) A quantitative comparison of traditional reading of the EEG and interpretation of computer-extracted features in patients with supratentorial brain lesions. Electroenceph. clin. Neurophysiol. 38: 623–639.

Gotman, J. and Gloor, P. (1976) Automatic recognition and quantification of interictal epileptic activity in the human scalp EEG. Electroenceph. clin. Neurophysiol. 41: 513–529.

Halliday, A.M., McDonald, W.I. and Mushin, J. (1973) Visual evoked response in diagnosis of multiple sclerosis. Br. Med. J. 4: 661–664.

Hjorth, B. (1973) The physical significance of time domain descriptors in EEG analysis. Electroenceph. clin. Neurophysiol. 34: 321–325.

Isaksson, A. and Wennberg, A. (1975) Visual evaluation and computer analysis of the EEG. A comparison. Electroenceph. clin. Neurophysiol. 38: 79–86.

Ives, J.R., Thompson, C.J. and Gloor, P. (1976) Seizure monitoring: A new tool in electroencephalography. Electroenceph. clin. Neurophysiol. 41: 422–427.

Jewett, D.L. and Williston, J.S. (1971) Auditory-evoked far fields averaged from the scalp of humans. Brain 94: 681–696.

Kellaway, P. and Petersén, I. (1973) Automation of Clinical Electroencephalography. Raven Press, New York.

Lehmann, D. and Skrandies, W. (1979) Multichannel evoked potential fields show different properties of human upper and lower hemiretina systems. Exp. Brain Res. 35: 151–159.

Lieb, J.P., Woods, S.C., Siccardi, A., Crandall, P.H., Walter, D.O. and Leake, B. (1978) Quantitative analysis of depth spiking in relation to seizure foci in patients with temporal lobe epilepsy. Electroenceph. clin. Neurophysiol. 44: 641–663.

Matousek, M., Arvidson, A. and Friberg, S. (1979) Serial quantitative electroencephalography. Electroenceph. clin. Neurophysiol. 47: 614–622.

Otto, E., Brauer, D. and Wilhelm, M. (1977) Characterization of EEG activity patterns in human sleep by means of variance and discriminant analyses. Acta Biol. med. germ. 36: 1113–1131.

Parker, D.M. and Salzen, E.A. (1977) Latency changes in the human visual evoked response to sinusoidal gratings. Vision Res. 17: 1201–1204.

Praetorius, H.M., Bodenstein, G. and Creutzfeldt, O.D. (1977) Adaptive segmentation of EEG records: A new approach to automatic EEG analysis. Electroenceph. clin. Neurophysiol. 42: 84–94.

Ragot, R.A. and Rémond, A. (1978) EEG field mapping. Electroenceph. clin. Neurophysiol. 45: 417–421.

Regan, D., Milner, B.A. and Heron, J.R. (1976) Delayed visual perception and delayed visual evoked potentials in the spinal form of multiple sclerosis and in retrobulbar neuritis. Brain 99: 43–66.

Roy, O.Z. (1976) Section III. Biotelemetry and telephone transmission. In: Rémond, A. (Ed.), Handbook of Electroenceph. clin. Neurophysiol., Vol. 3A, Elsevier, Amsterdam, pp. 46–66.

Schlag, J. (1973) Generation of brain evoked potentials. In: Thompson, R.F. and Patterson, M.M. (Eds.), Bioelectric Recording Techniques, Vol. 1A, Academic Press, New York and London, pp. 273–316.

Shahrokhi, R., Chiappa, K.H. and Young, R.R. (1978) Pattern shift visual evoked responses. Arch. Neurol. 35: 65–71.

Sokol, S. (1976) Visually evoked potentials: Theory, techniques and clinical applications. Survey of Ophthalmology 21: 18–44.

Starr, A. (1978) Sensory evoked potentials in clinical disorders of the nervous system. Ann. Rev. Neurosci. 1: 103–127.

Stockard, J.E., Stockard, J.J., Westmoreland, B.F. and Corfits, J.L. (1979) Brainstem auditory-evoked responses. Normal variation as a function of stimulus and subject characteristics. Arch. Neurol. 36: 823–831.

Storm van Leeuwen, W., Lopes da Silva, F.H. and Kamp, A., eds. (1975) Part A. Evoked responses. In: Rémond, A. (Ed.), Handbook of Electroenceph. clin. Neurophysiol., Vol. 8A, Elsevier, Amsterdam.

Tharp, B.R. and Gersch, W. (1975) Spectral analysis of seizures in humans. Computers and Biomedical Research 8: 503–521.

Tyler, C.W., Apkarian, P., Levi, D.M. and Nakayama, K. (1979) Rapid assessment of visual function: An electronic sweep technique for the pattern visual evoked potential. Invest. Ophthalmol. Visual Sci. 18: 703–713.

Vaughan, H.G. (1974) The analysis of scalp-recorded brain potentials. In: Thompson, R.F. and Patterson, M.M. (Eds.), Bioelectric Recording Techniques, Vol. 1B, Academic Press, New York and London, pp. 157–207.

Walter, D.O., ed. (1972) Part B. Digital processing of bioelectric phenomena. In: Rémond, A. (Ed.), Handbook of Electroenceph. clin. Neurophysiol., Vol. 4B, Elsevier, Amsterdam.

# Part B
# The normal EEG

# Definition of the normal EEG, relation to brain function

# 8

SUMMARY

(8.1) An EEG is usually called normal not because it contains normal patterns but because it lacks abnormal patterns.

(8.2) A normal EEG does not guarantee the absence of cerebral pathology because not all abnormalities of brain structure and function produce abnormalities of the EEG.

(8.3) An abnormal EEG does not always indicate cerebral abnormality. A few specific mild EEG abnormalities can be seen in some instances in otherwise normal persons.

## 8.1 DEFINITION OF THE NORMAL EEG

A wide variety of normal EEG patterns can be seen in different persons of the same age, and an even greater variety of normal patterns can occur in different age groups; the waking record generally shows more variability between subjects than the sleep EEG. It is therefore not practical to define the normal EEG by listing all normal patterns and their variations; such a list would be too long. Nor can the normal EEG be defined by requiring that specific normal components be present; in this regard, the EEG differs from other tests such as the electrocardiogram. The problem of defining the normal EEG is therefore better approached in a different way. In contrast to the great variety of normal patterns, there are only a few EEG components, such as spikes and sharp waves, certain slow waves and amplitude changes, which are known to be definitely abnormal in each age group. The normal EEG can therefore be defined more effectively by the absence of abnormal components than by the presence of normal patterns. Conversely, an EEG is considered abnormal if it contains abnormal components regardless of whether or not it also contains normal components. The EEG reader therefore has to know the major features of the normal EEG at different ages and to distinguish from them abnormal components by using a set of precise descriptors (9).

**8.1.1** *The normal EEG up to the age of 19 years.* The normal EEG undergoes enormous changes from the early premature period to about the age of 19 years. Characteristic patterns appear at fairly predictable ages and later disappear or change into more mature patterns. The variety of patterns which are accepted as normal is greater during this period than during adulthood. Even abnormalities such as spikes and slow waves have clinical implications which differ from those of similar components in adults. Little is known about the clinical significance of the failure of normal patterns to appear and disappear at expected ages; failure of electrographic maturation is suggestive but not indicative of behavioral retardation.

**8.1.2** *The normal EEG of adults.* Between the ages of 20 and 60 years, the normal EEG shows only few changes; these changes have little clinical importance. The limits between normal and abnormal patterns are better defined in this age group than in younger persons and abnormal patterns correspond fairly well with basic types of brain lesions, although not necessarily with specific diseases.

**8.1.3** *The normal EEG above the age of 60 years.* The normal EEG at this age is similar to that of younger adults except that a few specific patterns which would be considered abnormal at a younger age become acceptable as normal.

## 8.2 A NORMAL EEG DOES NOT ALWAYS MEAN NORMAL BRAIN FUNCTION

Although acute, severe and large abnormalities of the brain are likely to cause EEG abnormalities, normal EEGs may be seen in some cases of long-standing, mild and small cerebral abnormalities. For instance, a small infarct in the internal capsule far from the recording electrodes may cause a catastrophic hemiplegia but no EEG abnormality. A large infarct near the recording electrodes may cause EEG changes which last for a few weeks or months but then disappear even though the neurological deficit persists. The EEG may remain normal for a long period in slowly progressive, widespread brain diseases, such as senile dementia, which lead to cerebral atrophy and mental changes. An epileptogenic focus may escape detection if it does not fire during the recording or if it is too far from the recording electrodes.

## 8.3 AN ABNORMAL EEG DOES NOT NECESSARILY MEAN ABNORMAL BRAIN FUNCTION

Most abnormal EEG patterns indicate abnormal brain function. However, abnormal patterns occur occasionally in persons not showing evidence of brain disease. The type and incidence of these patterns is fairly well known in adults. A slight excess of a certain kind of slow waves (21.1.2), and an EEG of unusually low amplitude (24.2.2), occur in about 5–15% of normal persons after the age of 20 years. One might be inclined to call these patterns normal, especially since they occur most commonly in apparently normal persons; however, the same patterns can be seen in patients with mild forms of diseases which, in their more severe stages, are associated with more pronounced expressions of the same EEG patterns. This suggests that in at least some persons, mild manifestations of these patterns indicate mild cerebral abnormalities. In order not to overlook the possibility of such cerebral abnormalities, one should therefore categorize even the mild forms of these patterns as EEG abnormalities. This attitude finds some support in the observation that the incidence of these mild EEG abnormalities decreases in groups of persons who have passed strict examinations, for instance tests used for the selection of flying personnel.

## REFERENCES


Goldensohn, E.S. and Koehle, R. (1975) EEG Interpretation: Problem of Overreading. Futura, Mount Kisco, New York.

Hawkes, C.H. and Prescott, R.J. (1973) EEG variation in healthy subjects. Electroenceph. clin. Neurophysiol. 34: 197–199.

Hill, D. (1952) EEG in episodic psychotic and psychopathic behaviour. Electroenceph. clin. Neurophysiol. 4: 419–442.

Torres, F. and Blaw, M.E. (1968) Longitudinal EEG-clinical correlations in children from birth to 4 years of age. Pediatrics 41: 945–954.

Van Dis, H., Corner, M., Dapper, R., Hanewald, G. and Hok, H. (1979) Individual differences in the human electroencephalogram during quiet wakefulness. Electroenceph. clin. Neurophysiol. 47: 87–94.

Williams, D. (1941) The significance of an abnormal electroencephalogram. J. Neurol. Psychiat. 4: 257–268.

# 9 Descriptors of EEG activity

SUMMARY
To analyze the EEG, the reader needs to distinguish: 1. *Wave form*; 2. *repetition*; 3. *frequency*; 4. *amplitude*; 5. *distribution*; 6. *phase relation*; 7. *timing*; 8. *persistence*; and 9. *reactivity*. These features allow the EEG reader to recognize different patterns.

## 9.1 WAVE FORM

*Wave form* or *shape* are simple terms used to describe the *configuration* or *morphology* of a wave. Any change in the difference of the electrical potential between two recording electrodes is called a *wave*, regardless of its form. Any wave or sequence of waves is called *activity*. Many waves are *regular*, i.e. they have a fairly uniform appearance due to symmetrical rising and falling phases (Fig. 9.1, Part 1). Some regular waves are similar to sine waves and are called *sinusoidal* (Fig. 9.1, Part 2) while other regular waves may be arch-shaped or saw-toothed. *Irregular waves* have uneven shapes and durations (Fig. 9.1, Part 4).

A *monophasic* wave is a single deflection either up or down from the baseline. A *diphasic* wave has two components on opposite sides of the baseline while a *triphasic* wave has three components alternating about the baseline. A *polyphasic* wave has two or more components of different direction. These terms do not indicate whether a wave has positive or negative electrical polarity (3.4.1) nor whether it was recorded with bipolar or referential electrode montages (4.1).

A *transient* is an event which clearly stands out against the background. It consists of either a single wave or a *complex*, i.e. a sequence of two or more waves which have a characteristic form or recur with a fairly consistent shape (Fig. 9.1, Part 5).

A *sharp transient* is a wave of any duration which has a pointed peak at conventional EEG recording speed. A sharp transient with a duration of 70 to 200 msec is called a *sharp wave* (Fig. 9.1, Part 6). A *spike* is a sharp transient with a duration of 20 to 70 msec (Fig. 9.1, Part 7). The terms 'spike' and 'sharp wave' are usually further restricted in three respects. (1) These terms are not used for waves having the duration and sharpness of spikes or sharp waves if these waves form part of a background rhythm, for instance mu rhythm (Fig. 11.3), even if they are occasionally isolated from the rhythm and then stand out against the background. (2) These terms are not applied to some well-defined elements of normal patterns, for instance lambda waves (Fig. 11.3) and vertex sharp transients or V waves (Fig. 12.1). (3) These terms are usually reserved for sharp transients which recur with similar shape at different times in the same recording. A single sharp transient of less than 70 msec can be safely called 'spike' only if it has a very characteristic shape. Spikes and sharp waves which occur only once in a recording or recur only with varying shapes are often referred to as 'sharp transients' because they have less significance in the diagnosis of seizure disorders than do stereotyped spikes or sharp waves (17.3).

A spike may be followed by a slow wave and form a *spike-and-wave complex* (Fig. 9.1, Part 8) which may repeat at regular intervals. Spike-and-wave complexes recurring at rates below 3 Hz are called *slow-spike-and-wave complexes*. A sharp wave may be followed by a slow wave and form a *sharp-and-slow-wave complex;* complexes of this kind usually last longer than a third of a second and therefore do not repeat at rates over 3 Hz. In some cases, two or more spikes occur in sequence, forming *multiple spike complexes*, also called *polyspike complexes* (Fig. 9.1, Part 9). These complexes may be followed by a slow wave and thus form part of a *multiple spike-and-slow-wave complex* or *polyspike-and-slow-wave complex* (Fig. 9.1, Part 10). Spikes recorded in the EEG should not be confused with action potentials of single nerve cells which are recorded through microelectrodes inserted into the brain and which last only about 1 msec (1.1.3); they too are often called spikes but are never observed in the surface EEG.

Spikes and sharp waves are abnormal except for certain types which appear under well defined conditions described later (11.9.1; 19.4). Single spikes and sharp waves, and complexes which contain spikes and sharp waves and last for less than a few seconds are called *interictal epileptiform activity*; longer lasting activity of this type and of some other types is called *seizure pattern* or *ictal pattern* (17.1). Although seizure patterns are often associated with clinical seizure manifestations, they may

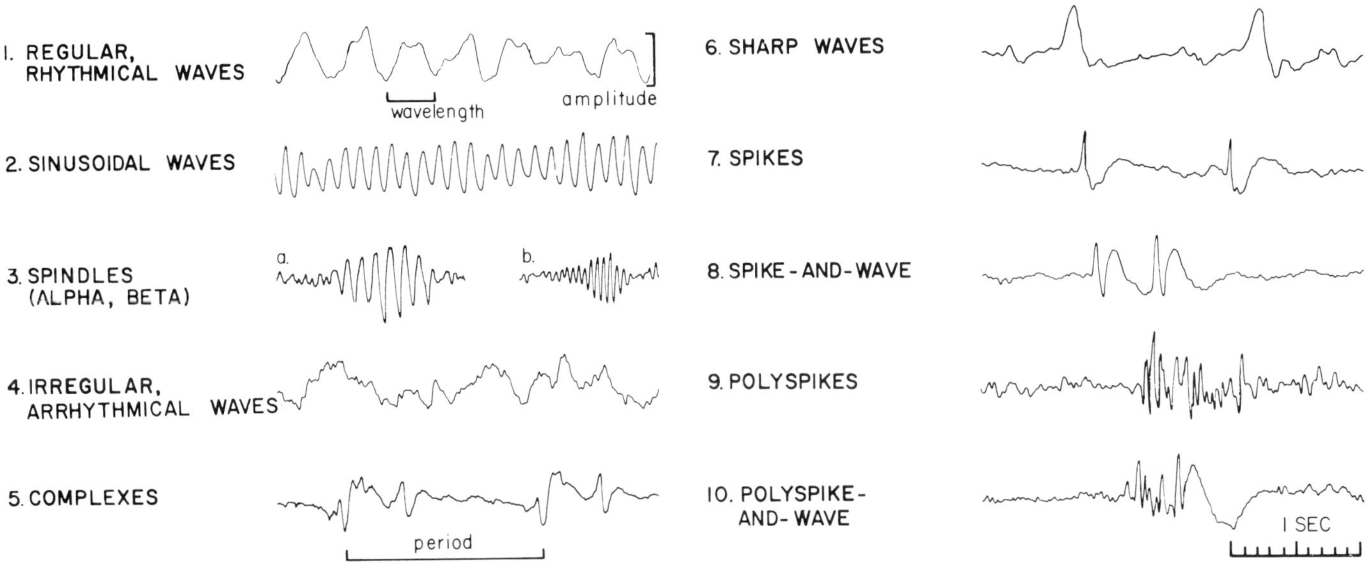


Fig. 9.1. Characteristic wave forms.

occur without such correlates and are then called *subclinical seizure pattern*. Both interictal and ictal patterns are here called *epileptiform* in contrast to the definition in the glossary of the International Federation of Societies for Electroencephalography and Clinical Neurophysiology which uses the term 'epileptiform' only for interictal patterns.

*A paroxysm* consists of one or more waves which begin abruptly, reach maximum amplitude rapidly, and disappear suddenly. These waves clearly stand out against the background, are usually abnormal, and are often seen in epileptiform patterns. Paroxysms often consist of complexes (Fig. 9.1, Part 5), but not all complexes begin and end abruptly, and not all paroxysms recur with a similar shape.

## 9.2 REPETITION

*Repetition* of waves may be rhythmical or arrhythmical. *Rhythmical* repetitive waves have similar intervals between individual waves; they are usually regular and often sinusoidal in shape (Fig. 9.1, Parts 1–3). *Spindles* are groups of rhythmical repetitive waves which gradually increase and then decrease in amplitude (Fig. 9.1, Part 3). Rhythmical repetitive waves were formerly called 'monorhythmic' or 'monomorphic'. *Arrhythmical* repetitive waves are characterized by variable, irregular intervals between individual waves (Fig. 9.1, Part 4). They can be considered to be a sequence of waves of different frequency. They often have irregular shape. Arrhythmical irregular waves were formerly called 'polyrhythmic' or 'polymorphic'.

## 9.3 FREQUENCY

*Frequency* refers to the number of times a repetitive wave recurs in one second. A wave completing three cycles in one second is called a wave of 3 Hertz (Hz) or of 3 per sec. The frequency of single or repetitive waves can be determined by measuring the duration of an individual wave, the *wavelength* (Fig. 9.1, Part 1), and calculating the reciprocal. For instance, a wave lasting 250 msec or 1/4 second is said to have a frequency of 4 Hz, regardless of whether or not it repeats. Single waves and complexes may repeat at intervals longer than the wavelength and are then called 'periodic', the *period* being the time interval between them (Fig. 9.1, Part 5).

The frequency of EEG waves is often divided into four groups or *frequency bands*, namely:

- delta frequency band: under 4 Hz
- theta frequency band: from 4 to under 8 Hz
- alpha frequency band: from 8 to 13 Hz
- beta frequency band: over 13 Hz (Fig. 9.2).

These divisions are somewhat arbitrary; many EEGs contain waves of frequencies

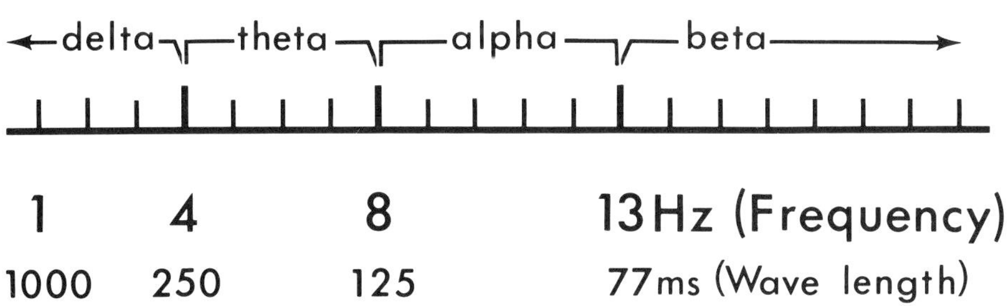


Fig. 9.2. Frequency bands. Delta, theta, alpha and beta frequency bands, defined by wave frequency and length.

extending across the boundaries of the bands, for instance waves of 3–5 Hz. Nonetheless, the frequency bands help to set apart the most important normal and abnormal waves in the EEG, and frequency is one of the most important criteria for assessing abnormality in clinical EEG. Waves under 8 Hz are commonly called *slow waves*, waves over 13 Hz are called *fast waves*.

Although the electrical activity of the brain contains faster and slower waves than those of about 1–30 Hz, the frequency range clearly distinguished in the conventional EEG, these extremely fast and slow waves have not yet been shown to have clinical importance.

## 9.4 AMPLITUDE

*Amplitude* of EEG waves is measured in microvolts (μV). It is determined by measuring and comparing the total vertical distance of a wave (Fig. 9.1, Part 1) to the height of a calibration signal recorded at the same gain and filter settings (3.3.1). Thus, if the height of an EEG wave measures 14 mm and a calibration signal of 50 μV measures 7 mm, the amplitude of the wave is 100 μV. If the sensitivity of an amplifier is known to be 7 μV/mm (3.4.2), a wave of 7 mm can be inferred to have an amplitude of 50 μV without direct comparison with a calibration pulse. Amplitude should not be expressed in terms of the height of the pen deflection because this varies with the amplifier settings.

In clinical EEG, amplitude is often not reported in terms of microvolts but described loosely as *low* (under 20 μV), *medium or moderate* (20–50 μV), or *high* (over 50 μV). However, these terms often are used to describe amplitude of certain waves relative to that of other waves in the same record. For instance, a wave of 60 μV cannot be said to be of high amplitude if it occurs on a background of 40–50 μV.

An important abnormality is *asymmetry* of amplitude of the activity that is recorded simultaneously from corresponding parts of the two sides of the head. Even slight differences of amplitude may be of clinical importance (23.2) if they persist; this is true especially of the adult EEG, with the exception of the alpha rhythm (11.1).

Differences of amplitude are sometimes caused by factors outside the brain, especially by unequal spacing and impedance of the recording electrodes; the technician should therefore verify correct electrode placements (2.3) and impedances (2.2) before accepting that abnormal amplitude is genuine.

## 9.5 DISTRIBUTION

*Distribution* refers to the occurrence of electrical activity recorded by electrodes positioned over different parts of the head. EEG patterns may appear over large areas on both sides of the head, over one side only, or in a restricted, small area.

**9.5.1** *Widespread, diffuse or generalized* distribution refers to activity which occurs at the same time over most or all of the head. Generalized activity may have a clear maximum within its field of distribution, recognized by the highest amplitude in referential recordings and by phase reversal in bipolar recordings from that area (4.1).

**9.5.2** *Lateralized* distribution refers to activity which appears only or mostly on one side of the head. Lateralized activity is abnormal and suggests a cerebral abnormality either on the side where abnormal activity is present or on the side where normal activity is absent. Some normal patterns may appear on one side of the head at one time and then occur on the other side a few seconds or minutes later without being abnormal (9.7).

**9.5.3** *Focal* activity is that which is restricted to one or a few electrodes over an area of the head. Some of the neighboring electrodes may pick up the same activity with lower amplitude. This restricted distribution must be distinguished from a wide or generalized distribution which may have a maximum in one area. This distinction is important especially with regard to abnormal slow waves and to sharp waves. Criteria which sometimes help in this distinction are that *focal slow waves* often have a lower frequency at the area of maximum amplitude whereas generalized slow waves do not. *Focal sharp waves* with a tendency to spread can often be distinguished from generalized sharp waves with a local maximum of amplitude by their greater persistence at the focus.

Activity arising from a single unilateral focus is always abnormal. Activity from a midline focus or from two foci located symmetrically in the two hemispheres may be part of a normal pattern.

## 9.6 PHASE RELATION

*Phase* refers to the timing and polarity of components of waves in one or more channels. Waves of different frequency may occur in different channels so that the troughs and peaks occur at the same time; these waves are said to be *in phase*. If they do not coincide in this manner, they are said to be *out of phase*. The phase difference may be expressed in terms of phase angle. For instance, peaks pointing in opposite directions are said to be 180° out of phase. Such a *'phase reversal'* is the major indicator of the origin of EEG potentials in bipolar recordings (4.1.1). In a single channel, phase refers to the time relationship between different components of a rhythm; for instance, the peak of a sine wave is said to 'lead' the preceding crossing of the zero line by 90° and to 'lag' behind the next following peak by 360°.

## 9.7 TIMING

*Timing* of waves in different areas of the head may be similar or different. The terms *'simultaneous'* and *'synchronous'* are used to indicate that two events occurred at the same time. These terms are usually used with the same meaning, but 'synchronous' is sometimes used to denote precise coincidence while 'simultaneous' may be used more broadly to indicate the coincidence that is recognizable only imprecisely within the limits of the relatively slow recording speed of the EEG. The eye can hardly distinguish a horizontal difference of less than 1 mm between corresponding points on two waves even in neighboring channels. A horizontal distance of only 1 mm corresponds to a time difference of 33 msec at the conventional EEG recording speed. The resolution of time relations deteriorates if more distant channels are compared and if the writing units are not perfectly aligned; because of the curvilinear movement of the pens, synchronous excursions of different amplitude seem to have occurred at different times (3.6.1).

Waves which occur at the same time on both sides of the head are called *'bilaterally synchronous'* or *'bisynchronous'*. These terms consider mainly the relationship between the two sides but not necessarily that on the same side; thus, bilaterally synchronous waves may be out of phase in the same hemisphere. In some instances, waves are delayed against each other by the same amount in successive channels which record activity from electrodes placed from the front to the back of the head, giving the impression that these waves spread from front to back. For instance, this type of delay can be seen in triphasic waves of metabolic encephalopathies (19.2.6).

Waves which occur in different channels without constant time relation to each other are called *'asynchronous'*. This usually implies that the waves are present in different areas at the same time even though they do not fall in phase with each or do not have the same frequency. If waves occur in one area at one time and in other areas at another time, they are usually said to be *'independent'*; for instance, spikes in both temporal lobes may occur bisynchronously or independently; each case has different implications regarding a possible triggering mechanism.

## 9.8 PERSISTENCE

*Persistence* describes how often a wave or pattern occurs during a recording. Some waves occur only occasionally or intermittently, either in the form of a single wave or trains of waves; other waves are present through most or all of the recording. The persistence of waves can be estimated by measuring the proportion of time during which these waves appear. This is called the *index*. For instance, a delta index of 20% means that delta activity was present during one-fifth of a recording. Because the clinical importance of EEG patterns often depends not only on their persistence but also on their amplitude, the persistence and amplitude are often described together in terms of their *quantity, amount or prominence*. The term 'abundance', previously used to describe this combination of persistence and amplitude, is now obsolete.

Single waves and complexes may occur with a high, moderate or low persistence or incidence; the persistence of these events is best expressed as their average number in one second or one minute. They may occur periodically or at irregular intervals. Irregular and infrequent occurrence is sometimes called *'sporadic'*. The terms 'random' and 'diffuse' should not be used to describe persistence of EEG patterns.

## 9.9 REACTIVITY

*Reactivity* refers to changes which can be produced in some normal and abnormal patterns by various maneuvers. Some patterns are induced or increased, diminished or blocked by opening or closing the eyes, hyperventilation, photic or sensory stimuli, changes in levels of alertness, movements or other maneuvers. A common example is the blocking of alpha rhythm by eye opening or other alerting procedures (11.1.6). Abnormal slow waves in toxic and metabolic encephalopathies are often diminished by alerting and enhanced by hyperventilation and drowsiness whereas abnormal slow waves seen in cases of structural lesions usually show little reactivity.

## REFERENCES


Chatrian, G.E., Bergamini, L., Dondey, M., Klass, D.W., Lennox-Buchthal, M. and Petersén, I. (1974) A glossary of terms most commonly used by clinical electroencephalographers. Electroenceph. clin. Neurophysiol. 37: 538–548.

Gastaut, H. (1975) Section I. The significance of the EEG and of ictal and interictal discharges with respect to epilepsy. In: Rémond, A. (Ed.), Handbook of Electroenceph. clin. Neurophysiol., Vol. 13A, pp. 3–6.

Girton, D., Benson, K.L. and Kamiya, J. (1973) Observation of very slow potential oscillations in human scalp recordings. Electroenceph. clin. Neurophysiol. 35: 561–568.

Hall, R.A., Yaeger, C. and Yarbrough, R.B. (1967) Observations on high frequency electroencephalograms. Electroenceph. clin. Neurophysiol. 22: 262–265.

Kooi, K.A. (1966) Voltage-time characteristics of spikes and other rapid electroencephalographic transients: Semantic and morphological considerations. Neurology 16: 59–66.

# The normal EEG from premature age to the age of 19 years

# 10

SUMMARY

The development of the EEG from the newborn to the adult is not smooth. Milestones are summarized in Tables 10.1 and 10.2. The most abrupt changes occur between the early premature age and the first three months of life. The EEG of the premature baby depends less on the gestational age, i.e. the time between the onset of the mother's last menstrual period and the date of birth, than on the conceptional age, i.e. the gestational age plus the time since birth. The premature baby develops new EEG patterns and modifies the acquired ones within fairly narrow ranges of conceptional age. One may distinguish patterns characterizing the periods of the conceptional ages between

(10.1) *24 and 27 weeks*;

(10.2) *28 and 31 weeks*;

(10.3) *32 and 35 weeks*;

(10.4) *36 and 40 weeks*.

(10.5) *At the conceptional age of nine months*, the premature baby has developed EEG patterns similar to those of the full-term newborn.

(10.6) *After the first three months* of life, the neonatal patterns are replaced by patterns which show different rhythms in different areas. This differentiation, and the frequency of the rhythms, increase fairly rapidly during the first year of life.

(10.7) *During childhood and teenage*, the EEG develops rather steadily towards that of the adult with the exception of a few patterns which appear transiently during the childhood and teenage years.

(10.8) *EEG abnormalities* are less sharply defined below the age of 20 years. Patterns that are abnormal in adults may be normal at younger ages; synchrony, distribution and relation to sleep stages must be taken into consideration when deciding whether a waveform is normal or abnormal.

## 10.1 PREMATURE INFANTS OF 24 TO 27 WEEKS OF CONCEPTIONAL AGE

Wakefulness and sleep cannot yet be distinguished by EEG or behavior. Only one EEG pattern occurs (Pattern 1). It is *discontinuous*, i.e. it consists of periods of no

TABLE 10.1

Development of EEG patterns in premature and full-term infants

chronological age 0 — 4 weeks

conceptional age 24 — 28 — 32 — 36 — 40 — 44 weeks

| State | 24 weeks | 32 weeks | 36 weeks | Transition | 40 weeks |
|---|---|---|---|---|---|
| *Awake* | | | *Pattern 3*<br>Diffuse low voltage irregular activity | → | *Pattern 3*<br>('activité moyenne')<br>Diffuse low voltage irregular theta and delta |
| *Active sleep*<br>(later REM sleep)<br>1. Irregular breathing<br>2. Frequent eye and limb movements<br>3. No tonic neck EMG | | *Pattern 2*<br>Continuous slow waves, 1–2 Hz | | continuous theta and delta → | *Pattern 2*<br>Mixed low voltage irregular and 2–4 Hz slow waves |
| *Quiet sleep*<br>(later non-REM sleep)<br>1. Regular breathing<br>2. No eye and limb movement<br>3. Tonic neck EMG | *Pattern 1*<br>('Discontinuous')<br>a. Bursts ≤20 sec, delta ≥ theta ≥ alpha | | | 1–2 sec, 4–6 Hz; 1–2 Hz → | *Pattern 1*<br>('tracé alternant')<br>a. Bursts of 4–5 sec, 1–3 Hz |
| | b. Pauses: No activity ≤3 min | | | shorter pauses; low voltage may appear → | b. Low voltage activity, 4–5 sec |
| | | | | | *Pattern 4*<br>Continuous high amplitude slow waves |

Frontal sharp transients and sporadic spikes (dashed from 24 weeks, solid from about 33 to 40 weeks, dashed thereafter)

Delta brushes: 10–20 Hz on 0.3–1 Hz (dashed from about 28 weeks, solid from about 30 to 37 weeks, dashed to 40 weeks) activity for up to 3 minutes; these periods are separated from each other by bursts of activity lasting up to 20 seconds. The bursts usually appear over both hemispheres simultaneously, but individual waves in the bursts are not bilaterally synchronous. The waves are often rhythmical and fall in the delta, theta and alpha frequency range; delta waves have the highest amplitude. Sharp transients in the frontal regions and sporadic spikes in any location may occur in normal premature infants up to shortly after 40 weeks of age, although spikes and sharp waves are abnormal if they occur repetitively, unilaterally, with a consistent focus of origin, or during the pauses of the discontinuous pattern.

## 10.2 PREMATURE INFANTS OF 28 TO 31 WEEKS OF CONCEPTIONAL AGE

The EEG continues to show a single pattern of discontinuous activity (Pattern 1). The bursts of activity now last 1–2 seconds and consist mainly of rhythmical 4–6 Hz waves. These waves become bisynchronous at about 28 to 29 weeks and therefore may not be seen in bipolar recordings between electrodes on corresponding areas of the two hemispheres. Waves in the delta frequency range often re-appear in the bursts at the age of 30 weeks. Fast waves of 10–20 Hz, superimposed on slow waves of 0.3–1 Hz, begin to appear and can be seen until shortly before the age of 40 weeks. They are called 'delta brushes', 'ripples of prematurity' and many other names (Fig. 10.1).

## 10.3 PREMATURE INFANTS OF 32 TO 35 WEEKS OF CONCEPTIONAL AGE

Two EEG patterns may be present at different times. They correspond to the different levels of wakefulness and sleep which can first be distinguished between

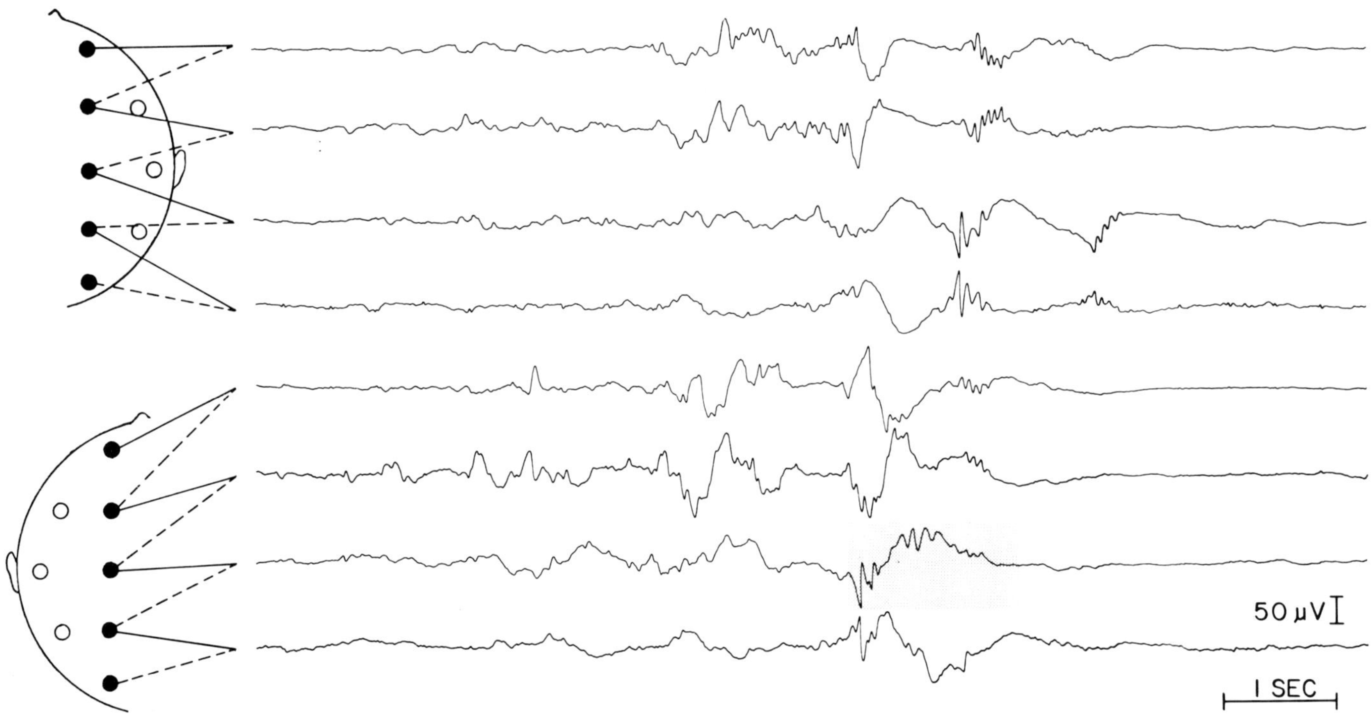


Fig. 10.1. Pattern of discontinuous activity of quiet sleep in a normal premature baby of a conceptional age of 34 weeks, recorded 5 days after birth. Delta brush is marked by shading.

the ages of 28 and 35 weeks although the correlation between these patterns and sleep stages is weak initially. Quiet sleep is characterized by regular breathing without other movements; active sleep is associated with irregular breathing and with eye and limb movements. Electromyographic recordings from electrodes below the chin (4.3.4) show tonic muscle activity during quiet sleep and loss of this activity during active sleep. The corresponding two patterns at this age are as follows:

*Pattern 1.* This pattern of discontinuous activity now shows bursts of slow waves of 1–2 Hz, mainly over the posterior head, and is usually associated with quiet sleep (Fig. 10.1).

*Pattern 2.* A new pattern of continuous slow waves of mainly 1–2 Hz appears often during wakefulness and active sleep. The slow waves appear in a wide distribution in the occipital, temporal and central regions. They are fairly rhythmical and may be synchronous on the two sides (Fig. 10.2).

### 10.4 PREMATURE INFANTS OF 36 TO 40 WEEKS OF CONCEPTIONAL AGE

The two earlier patterns are slightly modified and a third pattern emerges.

*Patterrn 1.* The pattern of discontinuous activity now has shorter pauses. Traces of low amplitude slow waves may appear between the bursts of slow waves. As before, this pattern is associated with quiet sleep.

*Pattern 2.* Continuous irregular slow waves of theta and delta frequency appear in wakefulness and active sleep. Delta brushes now occur less often in active sleep than in quiet sleep.

*Pattern 3.* A new pattern of diffuse irregular continuous slow waves of relatively low amplitude of less than 50 $\mu$V appears as an alternative to Pattern 2 during wakefulness and active sleep.

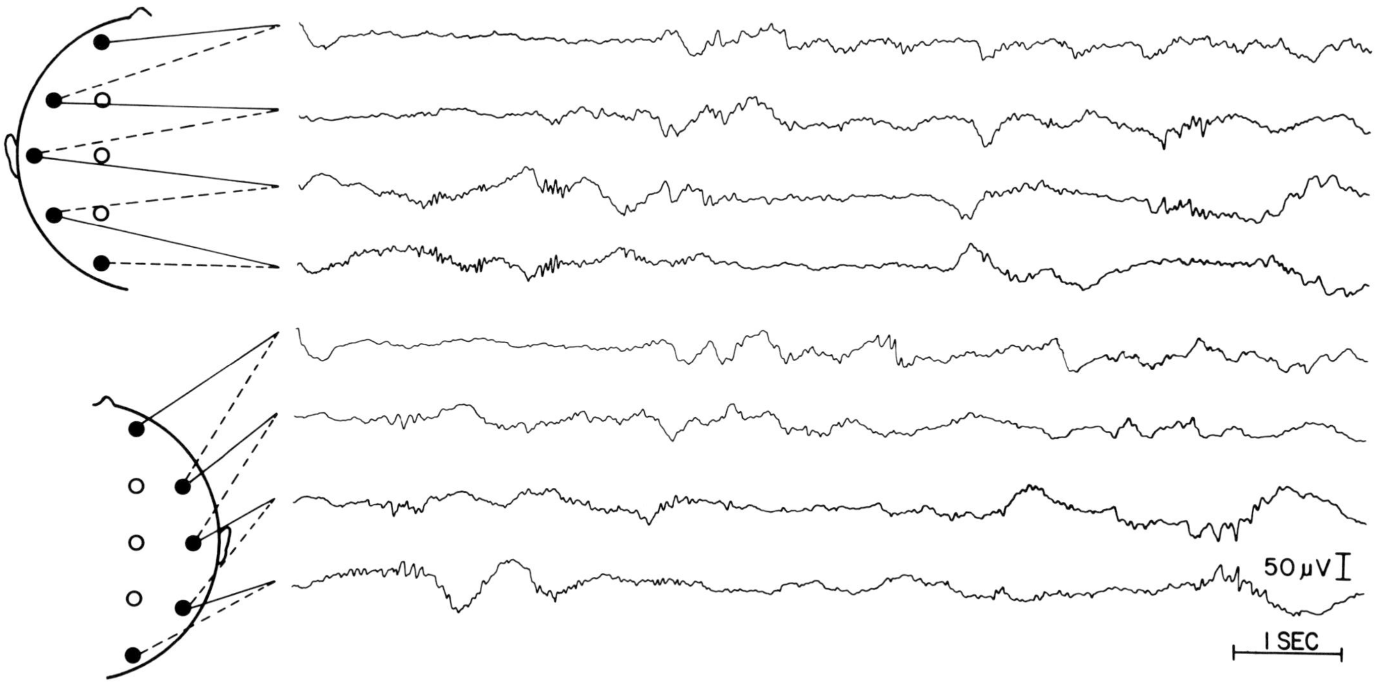


Fig. 10.2. Pattern of continuous slow waves of active sleep in a normal premature baby of a conceptional age of 35 weeks, recorded 3 days after birth.

## 10.5 INFANTS FROM FULL TERM TO 3 MONTHS OF AGE

The EEG may show up to four different patterns at different times. Three of them are slight modifications of the premature patterns; a newly acquired fourth pattern appears during wakefulness and active sleep.

*Pattern 1.* The 'tracé alternant' or alternating trace (Fig. 10.3) is a modification of the discontinuous pattern and appears during quiet sleep. Bursts of high amplitude waves of 1–3 Hz occur simultaneously on both sides of the head and last 4–5 seconds. They alternate with periods of low amplitude activity of similar duration. Frontal spikes appear during the bursts. This pattern disappears 3–4 weeks after term.

*Pattern 2.* This pattern, associated with active sleep, consists of continuous low amplitude mixed slow waves with superimposed larger delta waves which are either intermittent or continuous (Fig. 10.4).

*Pattern 3.* 'Acitivité moyenne' or medium activity (Fig. 10.5) is the most common pattern seen in wakefulness and active sleep at this age. It consists of continuous and fairly rhythmical waves mainly of 4–8 Hz of relatively low amplitude of less than 50 $\mu$V.

*Pattern 4.* A new pattern associated with quiet sleep consists of continuous slow waves of 0.5–2 Hz and of fairly high amplitude, maximal occipitally; ripples of 18–25 Hz may be superimposed (Fig. 10.6).

Drowsiness cannot be identified with certainty in the newborn. Transitions between active and quiet sleep are very rapid. In contrast to sleep in later life, sleep in infants up to the age of 3 months begins with the active phase. The newborn has sleep cycles which last 45–60 minutes and consist of about 25 minutes of active sleep and 20 minutes of quiet sleep. Such rhythmical alternations between active and quiet sleep cannot be clearly distinguished in the premature infant.

Tactile or auditory stimulation during sleep can produce one of several

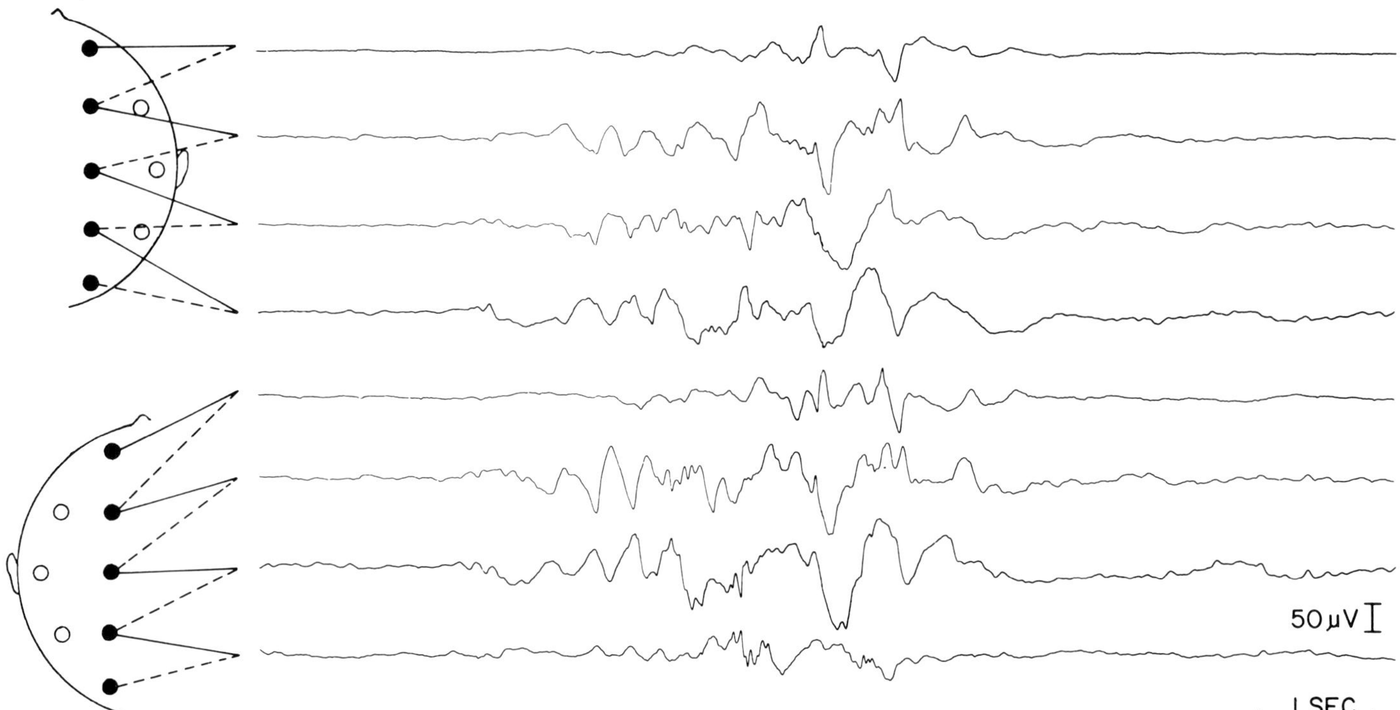


Fig. 10.3. Pattern of quiet sleep ('tracé alternant') in a normal full-term infant, 4 days old.

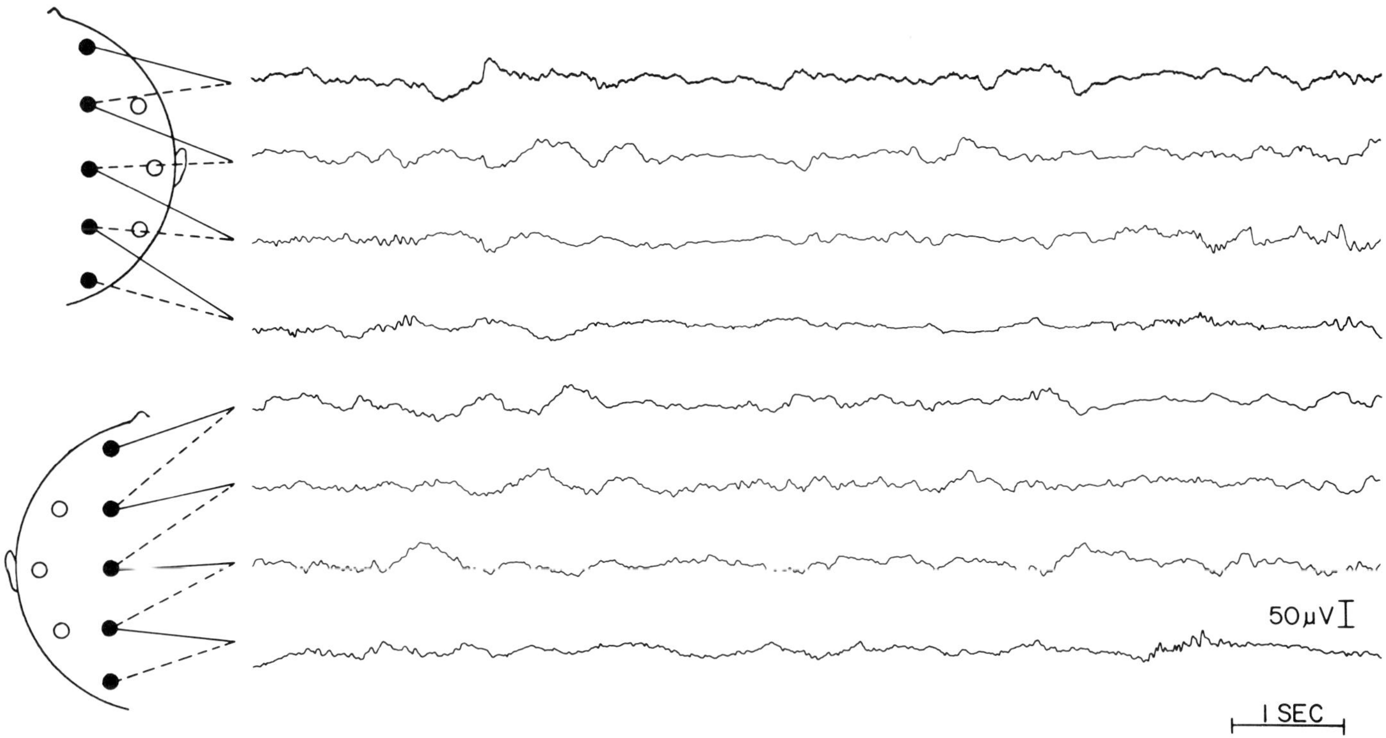


Fig. 10.4. Pattern of low voltage irregular slow waves, including larger delta waves, during active sleep in a normal full-term infant, 10 days old.

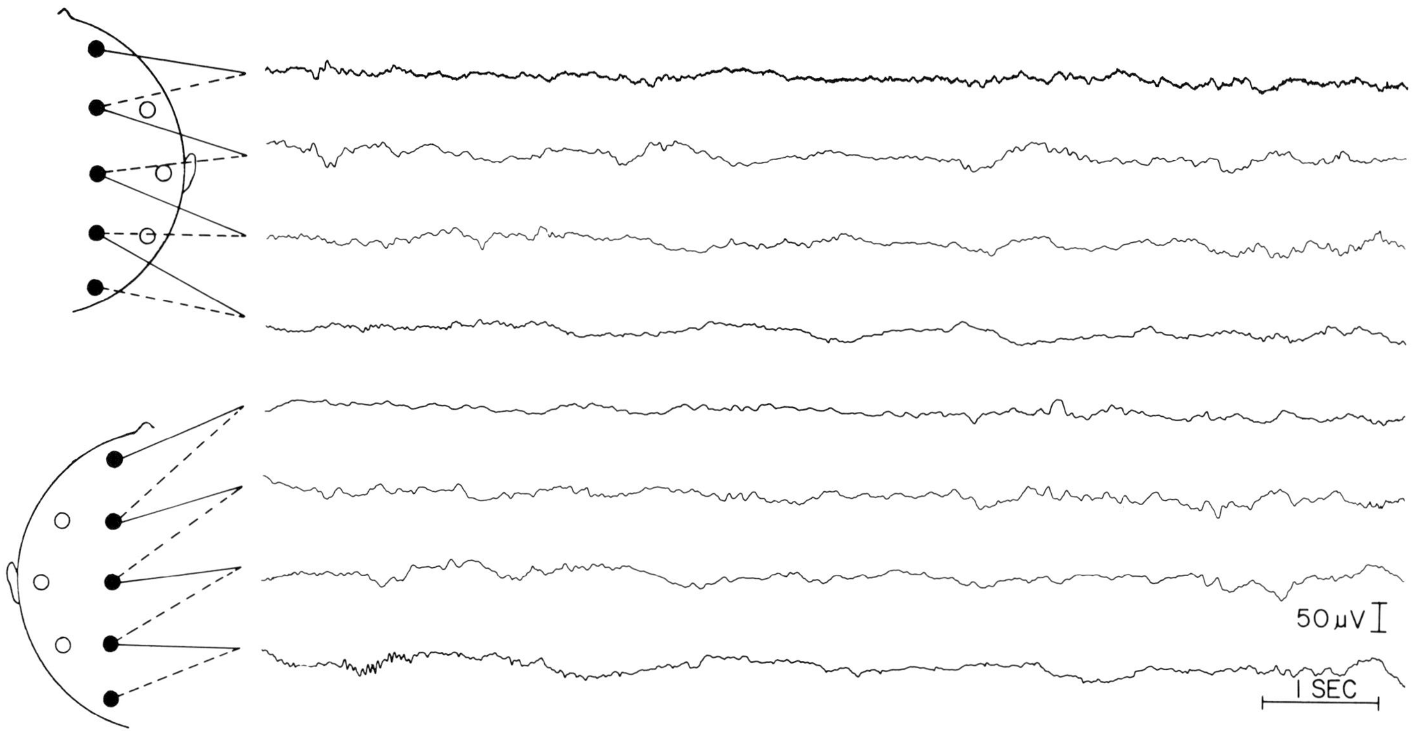


Fig. 10.5. Pattern of low voltage irregular theta and delta waves ('activité moyenne') in a wakeful normal full-term infant, 10 days old.

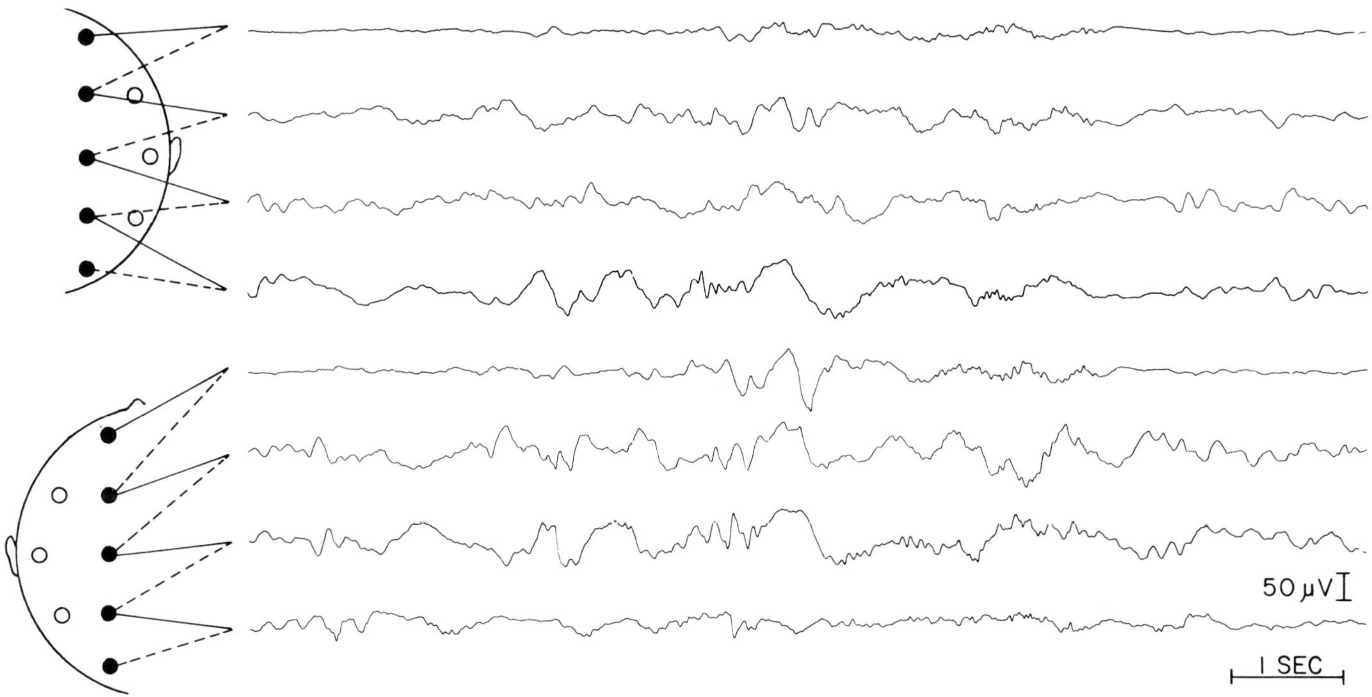


Fig. 10.6. Pattern of continuous high amplitude slow waves of quiet sleep in a normal full-term infant, 4 days old.

nonspecific reactions in the EEG: (a) a negative vertex spike up to 100 $\mu$V; (b) generalized flattening; (c) bursts of generalized slow waves; (d) bursts followed by flattening; (e) change in sleep stage, especially from tracé alternant to diffusely slow or low voltage pattern. In addition, more specific responses may be elicited during wakefulness and sleep in the form of visual evoked potentials in response to single flashes (5.2; 7.6.1; 14.3.1); photic driving in infants is obtained only rarely and only with low flash rates.

Some patterns which are abnormal in adults must be accepted as normal in infants. For example, sporadic nonfocal spikes in any part of the head, frontal sharp transients, and anterior slow waves are normal in neonates; transient asymmetry of patterns during wakefulness and sleep is not abnormal. Rhythmical activity of alpha frequency may be seen in the parietal or central areas during sleep. Normal sleep records may show rapid occipital rhythms of low amplitude; poorly defined spindles at the vertex and sharp waves in the central areas are precursors of more mature sleep activity. However, synchrony between bursts of the discontinuous sleep pattern increases and is nearly perfect at the conceptional age of 40 weeks.

## 10.6 INFANTS OF 3 TO 12 MONTHS OF AGE

Important changes appear in the EEG during wakefulness, drowsiness and sleep.

**10.6.1** *Wakefulness* is characterized by patterns which begin to show regional differences and to react to stimulation.

*Background activity* consists of rhythmical and arrhythmical slow waves in the delta and theta frequency range. These waves are generalized, and often more prominent over the occipital areas. They may appear synchronously over wide areas

Table 10.2
The EEG from the age of 1 month to adult age

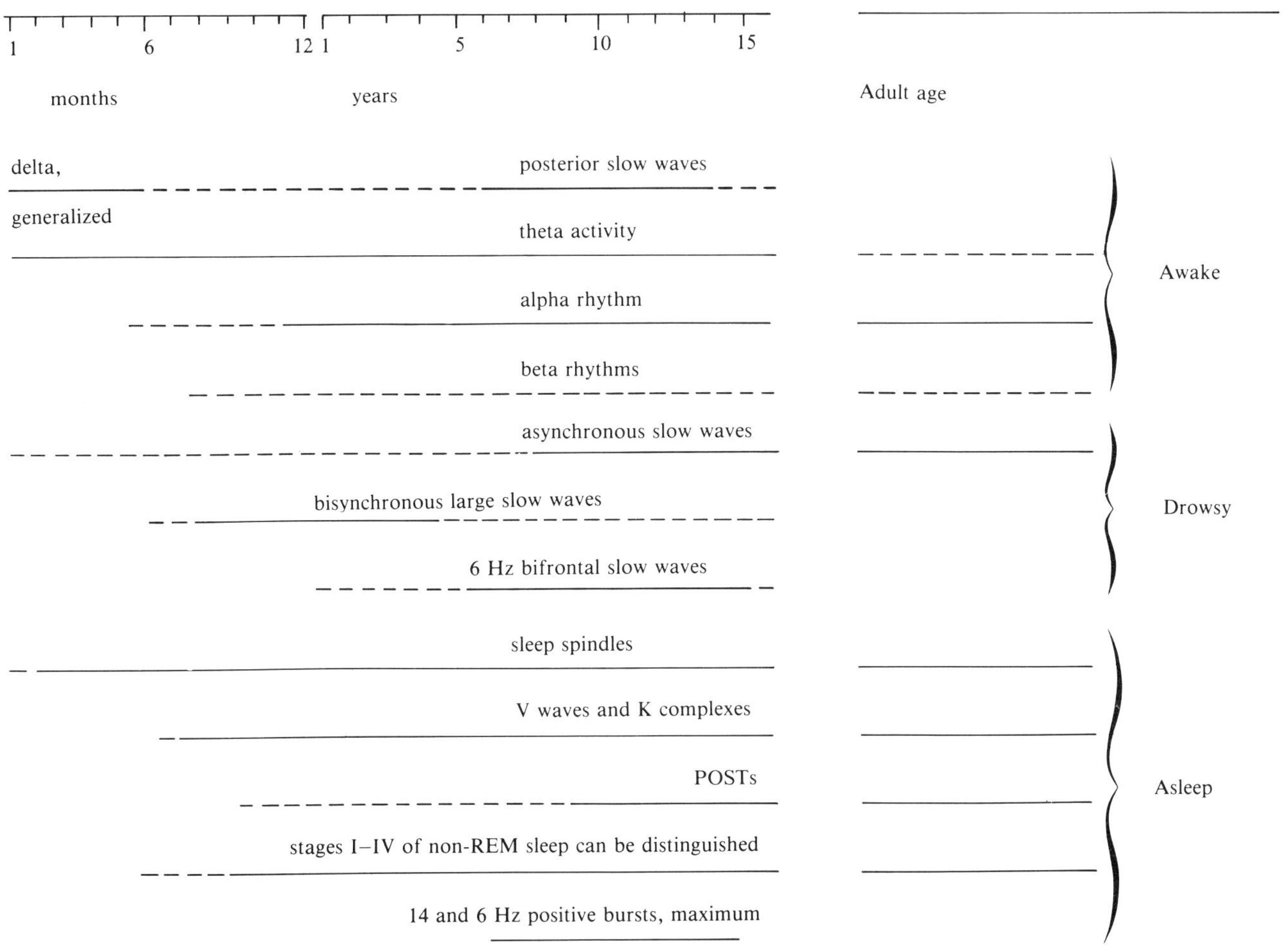

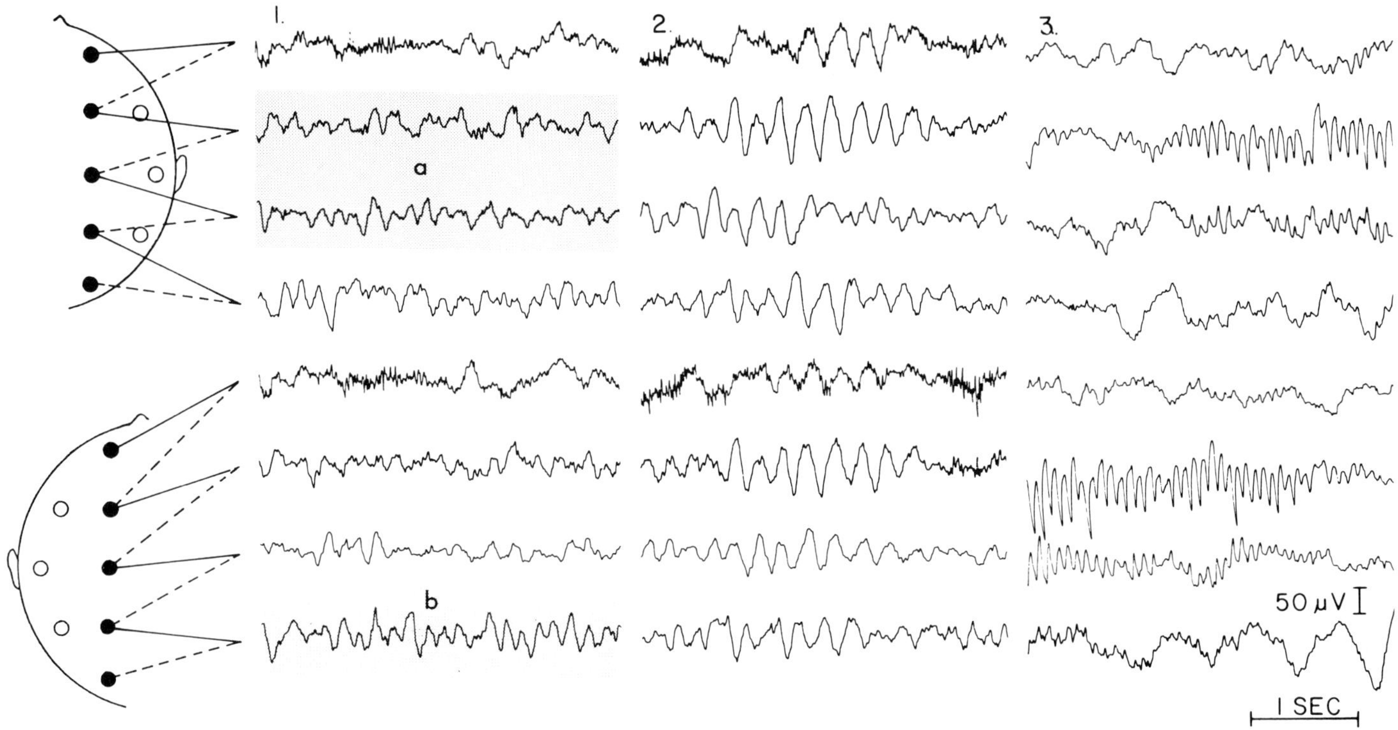


Fig. 10.7. Patterns of wakefulness (1), drowsiness (2) and sleep (3) in a normal 8 month old infant. 1. During wakefulness, rhythmical theta waves of 4–5 Hz in the central regions (a) can be distinguished from a rhythm of 6 Hz in the occipital areas (b); 2. Drowsiness is associated with high amplitude bisynchronous waves of 3–4 Hz; 3. During sleep, prominent spindles appear in the central regions, slightly asynchronous on the two sides; they are superimposed on generalized slow waves of under 2 Hz.

of both hemispheres. Delta waves become more rhythmical and diminish considerably during the first year. Before the age of 5 months, rhythmical occipital activity develops from the diffuse theta activity which is most prominent over the central and posterior regions (Fig. 10.7, Part 1). The absence of rhythmical theta activity after 5 months of age is considered abnormal.

*Occipital rhythms* which can be clearly distinguished from the background first appear at the age of about 3 months. These rhythms have frequencies of 3–4 Hz and are reduced in amplitude by eye opening. They become more regular and increase in frequency to about 5 Hz at 5 months of age and to 6–8 Hz at the end of the first year of life (Fig. 10.7, Part 1). The amplitude decreases from 50–100 $\mu$V to 50–75 $\mu$V at 12 months.

**10.6.2** *Drowsiness* up to the age of 6–8 months is associated with a smooth transition from patterns of wakefulness to those of sleep; the EEG shows a generalized and progressive increase of amplitude and a decrease of frequency to 2–3 Hz. At about this time, a specific pattern of drowsiness appears which consists of rhythmical and bi-synchronous 3–5 Hz waves of high amplitude of 75–200 $\mu$V (Fig. 10.7, Part 2). These waves begin rather abruptly in a wide distribution, sometimes with anterior, temporal or posterior predominance, and occur intermittently or continuously for up to several minutes at the beginning and at the end of sleep. This pattern vanishes gradually, usually before the age of 12 years. The rhythmical slow waves lose amplitude and become asynchronous and are thus transformed into the adult pattern of drowsiness. The childhood pattern of drowsiness has been called 'hypnagogic hypersynchrony', a name now considered objectionable because of its unproven implications. A few infants do not show this pattern of drowsiness but instead show occipital or widespread rhythmical and asynchronous 4–5 Hz waves of low to medium amplitude; this pattern more closely resembles the adult patterns of drowsiness.

**10.6.3** *Sleep* activity shows several major changes during the first year of life: (1) Active sleep develops into a sleep stage characterized by rapid eye movements (REM); the two infantile EEG patterns previously seen during active sleep are transformed into electrical patterns which gradually come to resemble the low amplitude patterns of the adult REM stage of sleep (12.2.6). (2) REM sleep, at first occupying about one-half of the total sleep time, decreases to about 40% of total sleep time at the age of 3–5 months, and to about 30% in the second half of the first year. (3) The alternating trace pattern and the continuous slow wave pattern of quiet sleep disappear 3–4 weeks after term and are replaced by sleep patterns which contain elements resembling those of adults (12.1). At the age of about 6 months, the EEG begins to show features similar to those which distinguish the adult non-REM sleep stages I–IV (12.2). (4) After the age of 3 months, sleep no longer begins with the active phase: infants now fall directly into non-REM sleep and go into REM sleep 40–50 minutes later.

*Sleep stages* in this age group are characterized by the following combinations of EEG patterns and behavioral characteristics.

*REM sleep* can generally be distinguished from non-REM sleep by EEG patterns, by the occurrence of eye and limb movements, and by irregular breathing. However, in infants and young children the behavioral manifestations of REM sleep are not very tightly correlated with the EEG pattern of REM sleep. For example, irregular breathing, characteristic of REM sleep in adults, occurs also in non-REM sleep in infants. Furthermore, the EEG patterns of REM sleep in infants consist of delta and theta waves which gradually change towards the pattern of low amplitude diffuse asynchronous slow waves characteristic of the adult EEG during REM sleep. In contrast to adults, normal infants may have sharp waves in the occipital regions during REM sleep.

*Non-REM sleep* is usually associated with regular breathing, absence of movements and presence of tonic neck muscle activity. Non-REM sleep can be divided into four stages characterized by EEG patterns similar to those of adults (12.2). These patterns begin to become distinguishable in the second half of the first year after the elements of these patterns are established.

The most important elements of sleep activity acquired during the first year of life are sleep spindles, vertex sharp transients and K complexes.

*Sleep spindles* consist of sinusoidal 12–15 Hz waves which develop in the central regions during the first few weeks of life and are usually well established by the age of 6–8 weeks (Fig. 10.7, Part 3). They continue to expand in distribution and become more prominent until they occur in bursts of at least 10 seconds or nearly continuously throughout non-REM sleep at the age of 2–6 months. After that time, the duration of spindle bursts decreases. An absence of sleep spindles between the ages of 3 and 6 months is probably abnormal. Spindle bursts are commonly asynchronous over the two hemispheres until the age of 6–8 months in normal infants; continuously asynchronous spindles after 1 year of age are probably abnormal. Spindle bursts are fairly asymmetrical in normal infants, but a marked and persistent reduction on one side raises the suspicion of a unilateral depression of activity.

*Vertex sharp transients (V waves) and K complexes* can be distinguished in rudimentary form in some infants during the neonatal period. They re-appear or appear for the first time at the age of 5–6 months. *V waves* have negative polarity, an amplitude of up to 250 $\mu$V, a wide distribution about the vertex, and a duration of usually less than 200 msec. V waves in the neonatal period tend to be smaller, longer lasting and more asymmetrical than later. In infants and young children, V waves often appear in the form of shorts bursts (Fig. 10.8, Part 3a). *K complexes* consist of a wave which is similar to a V wave but often of longer duration and preceded or followed by a positive wave; this diphasic wave is frequently followed by a sleep spindle. K complexes appear at deeper sleep stages than V waves. Both may appear without apparent stimulus or in response to sudden stimuli of any sensory modality (11.5).

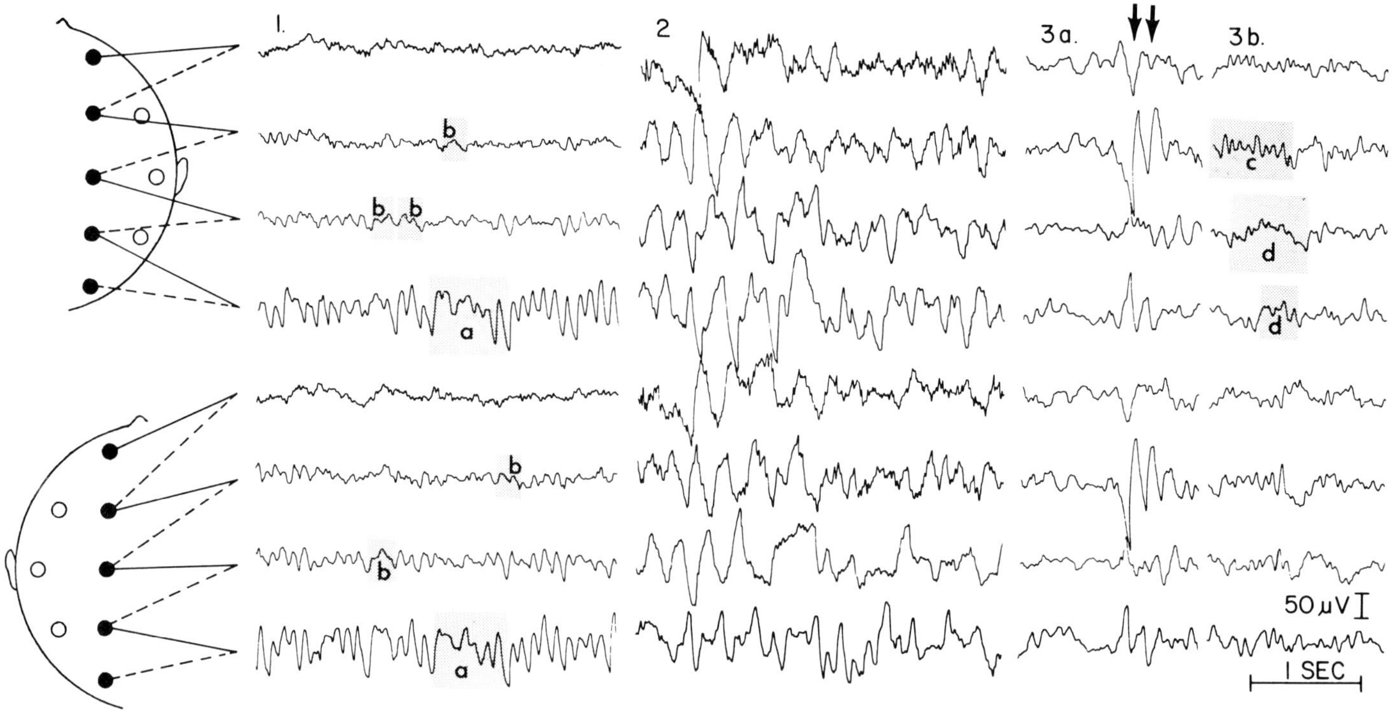


Fig. 10.8. Patterns of wakefulness (1), drowsiness (2) and sleep (3) in a normal boy of 12 years. 1. Wakefulness is associated with well developed occipital alpha rhythm of 9–10 Hz superimposed on bilaterally synchronous intermittent slow waves of 1–2 Hz (a), and with central theta waves (b); 2. Drowsiness is characterized by generalized bilaterally synchronous slow waves of 2–4 Hz of high amplitude; 3. Sleep is associated with repetitive V waves (arrows) in 3a, and with sleep spindles (c) and slow waves (d) in 3b.

The EEG during resting wakefulness can now be recorded more reliably and at greater length and shows differentiation of patterns towards those seen in adults. The waking record becomes the major indicator of structural lesions and metabolic abnormalities of the brain; the sleep EEG becomes useful for the activation of epileptiform activity. Hyperventilation and photic stimulation during wakefulness can be used as test conditions which may add information to that of the spontaneous EEG.

**10.7.1** *Resting wakefulness* is often associated with a mixture of alpha rhythm and slow waves of theta frequency.

*Alpha rhythm* develops from the rhythmical background activity in the occipital regions (Fig. 10.8, Part 1). It consists of sinusoidal waves of 8–13 Hz which occur over the posterior head regions and may extend forward to the central regions and beyond, often further than in the adult (11.1.4). Alpha rhythm appears during relaxed wakefulness, usually while the eyes are closed. It is blocked or clearly attenuated by eye opening, attention, and by mental effort. Alpha rhythm slows in frequency and then disappears in drowsiness. The frequency of the alpha rhythm increases gradually with age and becomes less variable in a given person. It reaches the range of 9–11 Hz between childhood and adolescence. Most normal children have well developed alpha rhythm at the age of 8 years. The amplitude of alpha rhythm increases up to the age of 10–12 years. As in adults (11.1.5), alpha rhythm is often of lower amplitude on the left side than on the right. However, the normal alpha asymmetry may be greater in children than in adults, reaching a ratio of 1:2 in some normal children. In contrast to adults (11.8), bilateral low amplitude or absence of alpha rhythm after the age of about 8 years is not normal in children.

*Slow waves* decrease in prominence with age. Theta waves are more prominent than alpha waves up to the age to 4 years. Between 5 and 6 years, the amounts of alpha and theta activity are about equal. After this age, alpha waves are normally more prominent than theta waves. Rhythmical theta waves during teenage years are usually most prominent in the temporal and posterior head regions (Fig. 10.8, Part 1). Intermittent slow waves of 1–3 Hz and of medium to high amplitude appear bisynchronously in the occipital regions of some teenagers (Fig. 10.8, Part 1). As in adults, rhythmical, bisynchronous, occipital slow waves of about half the frequency of alpha rhythm may alternate or mix with alpha rhythm to form slow alpha variants (11.1.7). Unlike adults, some normal teenagers show intermittent or briefly repetitive posterior slow waves of medium or high amplitude which transiently replace alpha rhythm.

*Beta rhythm* occurs only rarely in children and adolescents; when present, it is similar to that of the adult (11.2). As in the adult, neither the presence nor the absence of beta rhythm is abnormal, but persistent asymmetry, unilateral or focal distribution of beta rhythm is abnormal.

*Mu rhythm* may begin in childhood or adolescence and is similar to that in the adult (11.3).

**10.7.2** *Drowsiness* may be associated with one of two patterns.

*Bilaterally synchronous 3–5 Hz waves* of high amplitude, which began to occur in drowsiness during the first year of life (10.6.2), continue to be present during drowsiness in most children up to the age of 4 years. In some children this pattern may persist up to the age of 12 years (Fig. 10.8, Part 2).

*Rhythmical 6 Hz waves* of medium amplitude appear bisynchronously in the frontal regions during drowsiness in many children mainly between the ages of 5 and 16 years but are not normally seen after that age.

**10.7.3** *Sleep activity* shows maturation of stages and development of some new patterns.

*The sleep stages I–IV of non-REM* sleep and the *stage of REM sleep* become more similar to those of adults (12.2) and can be distinguished more easily from each other. Sleep cycles also mature. The proportion of time spent in REM sleep gradually drops from about 30% of the total sleep time at 1–2 years to the adult fraction of about 25%.

*Positive occipital sharp transients of sleep (POSTs)* similar to those of adults (12.1.2) begin to appear in light sleep during childhood or teenage.

*Fourteen and 6 Hz positive bursts* are frequently seen during drowsiness and sleep in children and adolescents and are more common at these ages than in adults. They are most likely a normal phenomenon (19.4.2).

## 10.8 MAJOR ABNORMALITIES

**10.8.1** *Spikes and sharp waves* are seen in normal EEGs of infants up to about 3 weeks of age. They appear in the frontal regions on both sides, either simultaneously or independently. However, they should have no discrete or consistent focus of origin. Spikes and sharp waves which are clearly focal and repetitive or which appear during the pauses of the alternating trace are abnormal. All spikes and sharp waves after the age of 3 months are abnormal except for V waves, positive sharp transients of sleep, 14 and 6 Hz positive bursts and a few other rare patterns of questionable clinical significance (19.4). Sharp waves and spikes have been reported in small portions of large populations of apparently normal children over the age of 3 months but cannot be accepted as normal EEG findings even if they are not accompanied by obvious clinical abnormalities.

**10.8.2** *Slow waves* are normal components of the EEG through teenage. They are abnormal only if they are (a) of focal or lateral distribution, or persistently and significantly asymmetrical; (b) clearly in excess of normal patterns for a given age, such as theta waves which are more prominent than alpha waves after the age of 6 years; (c) organized in the form of discrete trains of bilaterally synchronous sinusoidal slow waves of high amplitude unexplained by drowsiness or hyperventilation.

**10.8.3** *Abnormal amplitude* includes low amplitude in general and asymmetry of amplitude on the two sides of the head.

*Low amplitude* of all activity during an entire recording is abnormal between the age of 3 months and adulthood. Electrocerebral inactivity is diagnosed as in adults when special recordings techniques show no cerebral activity over 2 $\mu$V (5.4).

*Asymmetrical amplitude* is common in the normal EEG of infants. For instance, sleep spindles and V waves may be consistently asymmetrical for some time after their onset; these asymmetries are not abnormal unless other rhythms are also asymmetrical during the entire recording. Transient asymmetries, for instance those of the alternating trace of newborns, are not uncommon and not abnormal especially if the asymmetry is not consistent but fluctuates between the two sides in the same recording. The asymmetry of patterns which can be accepted as normal is greater in children and adolescents than in adults.

## REFERENCES

Corbin, H.P.F. and Bickford, R.G. (1955) Studies of the electroencephalogram of normal children: Comparison of visual and automatic frequency analyses. Electroenceph. clin. Neurophysiol. 7: 15–28.

Dreyfus-Brisac, C. and Curzi-Dascalova, L. (1975) Section II. The EEG during the first year of life. In: Rémond, A. (Ed.), Handbook of Electroenceph. clin. Neurophysiol., Vol. 6B, Elsevier, Amsterdam, pp. 24–30.

Dreyfus-Brisac, C. and Minkowski, A. (1968) Electroencephalographic maturation and low birth weight.

In: Kellaway, P. and Petersén, I. (Eds.), Clinical Electroencephalography of Children. Stockholm, Almqvist and Wiksell, pp. 49–60.
Dreyfus-Brisac, C. and Monod, N. (1975) Section I. The electroencephalogram of full-term new borns and premature infants. In: Rémond, A. (Ed.), Handbook of Electroenceph. clin. Neurophysiol., Vol. 6B, Elsevier, Amsterdam, pp. 6–23.
Engel, C.H. (1975) Abnormal Electroencephalograms in the Neonatal Period. Thomas, Springfield.
Goldie, L., Svedsen-Rhodes, U., Easton, J. and Roberton, N.R.C. (1971) The development of innate sleep rhythms in short gestation infants. Develop. Med. Child Neurol. 13: 40–50.
Hagne, I. (1968) Development of the waking EEG in normal infants during the first year of life. In: Kellaway, P. and Petersén, I. (Eds.), Clinical Electroencephalography of Children, Almqvist and Wiksel, Stockholm, pp. 97–118.
Hagne, I., Persson, J., Magnusson, R. and Petersén, I. (1973) Spectral analysis via fast Fourier transform of waking EEG in normal infants. In: Kellaway, P. and Petersén, I. (Eds.), Automation of Clinical Electroencephalography, Raven Press, New York, pp. 103–143.
Lenard, H.G. (1970) The development of sleep spindles in the EEG during the first two years of life. Neuropadiatrie 1: 264–276.
Lindsley, D.B. (1939) A longitudinal study of the occipital alpha rhythm in normal children: Frequency and amplitude standards. J. Genet. Psychol. 55: 197–213.
Lombroso, C.T. (1979) Quantified electrographic scales on 10 pre-term healthy newborns followed up to 40–43 weeks of conceptional age by serial polygraphic recordings. Electroenceph. clin. Neurophysiol. 46: 460–474.
Matousek, M. and Petersén, I. (1973) Frequency analysis of the EEG in normal children and adolescents. In: Kellaway, P. and Petersén, I. (Eds.), Automation of Clinical Electroencephalography, Raven Press, New York, pp. 75–102.
Matoušek, M. and Petersén, I. (1973) Automatic evaluation of EEG background activity by means of age-dependent EEG quotients. Electroenceph. clin. Neurophysiol. 35: 603–612.
Metcalf, D.R. (1970) EEG sleep spindle ontogenesis. Neuropaediatrie 1: 428–433.
Monod, N., Pajot, N. and Guidasci, S. (1972) The neonatal EEG: Statistical studies and prognostic value in full-term and pre-term babies. Electroenceph. clin. Neurophysiol. 32: 529–544.
Nolte, R. and Haas, G. (1978) A polygraphic study of bioelectrical brain maturation in preterm infants. Develop. Med. Child Neurol. 20: 167–182.
Parmalee, A.H. (1974) Ontogeny of sleep patterns and associated periodicities in infants. Pre- and postnatal development of the human brain. Mod. Probl. Pediat. 13: 298–311.
Parmalee, A.H., Akiyama, Y., Schultz, M.A., Wenner, W.H., Schulte, F.J. and Stern, E. (1968) The electroencephalogram in active and quiet sleep in infants. In: Kellaway, P. and Petersén, I. (Eds.), Clinical Electroencephalography of Children, Almqvist and Wiksell, Stockholm, pp. 77–88.
Parmalee, A.H., Schulte, F.J., Akiyama, Y., Wenner, W.H., Schultz, M.A. and Stern, E. (1968) Matu-

ration of EEG activity during sleep in premature infants. Electroenceph. clin. Neurophysiol. 24: 319–329.

Petersén, I., Eeg-Olofsson, O. and Selldén, U. (1968) Paroxysmal activity of normal children. In: Kellaway, P. and Petersén, I. (Eds.), Clinical Electroencephalography of Children. Almqvist and Wiksell, Stockholm, pp. 167–187.

Petersén, I. and Eeg-Olofsson, O. (1970) The development of the electroencephalogram in normal children from the age of 1 through 15 years. Nonparoxysmal activity. Neuropadiatrie 2: 247–304.

Petersén, I., Selldén, U. and Eeg-Olofsson, O. (1975) Section III. The evolution of the EEG in normal children and adolescents from 1 to 21 years. in: Rémond, A. (Ed.), Handbook of Electroenceph. clin. Neurophysiol., Vol. 6B, Elsevier, Amsterdam, pp. 31–68.

Samson-Dollfus, D., Forthomme, J. and Capron, E. (1964) EEG of the human infant during sleep and wakefulness during the first year of life. Normal patterns and their maturational changes; abnormal patterns and their prognostic significance. In: Kellaway, P. and Petersén, I. (Eds.) Neurological and Electroencephalographic Correlative Studies in Infancy, Grune and Stratton, New York, pp. 208–229.

Samson-Dollfus, D. and Goldberg, P. (1979) Electroencephalographic quantification by time domain analysis in normal 7–15 year-old children. Electroenceph. clin. Neurophysiol. 46: 147–154.

Slater, G.E. and Torres, F. (1979) Frequency-amplitude gradient. A new parameter for interpreting pediatric sleep EEGs. Arch. Neurol. 36: 465–470.

Smith, J.R. (1941) The frequency growth of the human alpha rhythms during normal infancy and childhood. J. Psychol. 11: 177–198.

Watanabe, K. and Iwase, K. (1972) Spindle-like fast rhythms in the EEGs of low-birthweight infants. Develop. Mec. Child Neurol. 14: 373–381.

# 11 The normal EEG of wakeful resting adults of 20–60 years of age

SUMMARY

The normal EEG of the wakeful adult at rest may show various types of activity alone or in combination:

(11.1) *Alpha rhythm* is most common and consists of sinusoidal 8–13 Hz waves maximal over the posterior head region which are blocked by eye opening, attention and sudden arousal and which disappear in drowsiness and sleep.

(11.2) *Beta rhythms* are less common and consist of waves over 13 Hz which appear either in a wide distribution, or limited to the frontal or posterior head regions.

(11.3) *Mu rhythm*,

(11.4) *Lambda waves*,

(11.5) *Vertex sharp transients*,

(11.6) *Kappa rhythm*,

(11.7) *Intermittent posterior theta rhythm* all are rarer than alpha and beta rhythms.

(11.8) *Low voltage activity* may be the only pattern of the EEG in some normal adults.

(11.9) *Abnormalities* are spikes and sharp waves, more than a minimum of slow waves, asymmetrical or very low amplitude activity, or specific deviations from normal patterns.

## 11.1 ALPHA RHYTHM

Alpha rhythm is defined by its frequency, its distribution and its reactivity (Fig. 11.1, Parts 1–5).

**11.1.1** The *wave form* is regular and often, but not always, sinusoidal. Alpha waves may have sharp points at the top or bottom. Single alpha waves with sharp peaks may be distinguished from abnormal sharp waves by the similarity to other, repetitive alpha waves in the same recording.

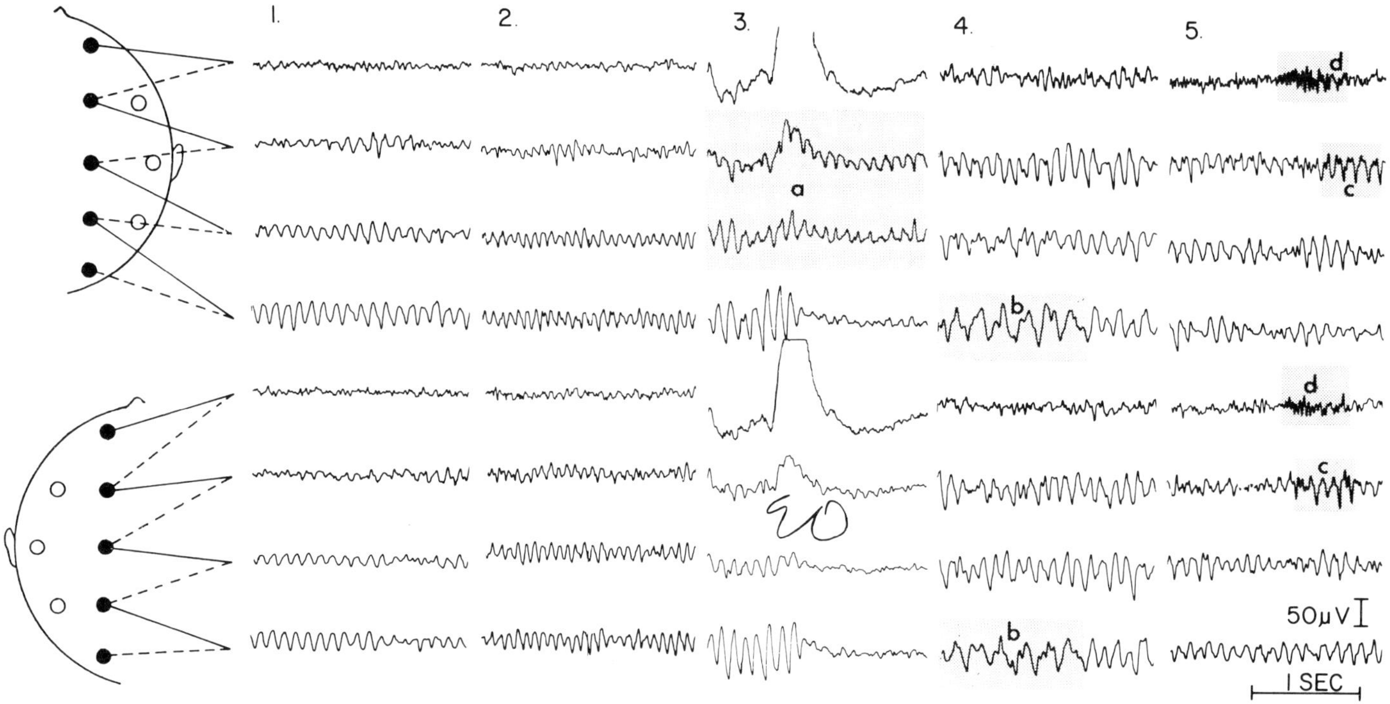


Fig. 11.1. Normal patterns of wakefulness in adults. 1. Alpha rhythm of 9 Hz in the posterior head regions and minimal beta activity in the frontal regions; 2. Alpha rhythm of 12–13 Hz extending from the posterior to the central regions; 3. Alpha rhythm of 9–10 Hz in the posterior head regions is present at the beginning of this part and is blocked by eye opening (E/O); a central mu rhythm on the right side persists after eye opening (a); 4. Slow alpha variant of 4–5 Hz, maximal in the occipital regions (b), alternates with alpha rhythm of about 9 Hz in a wider distribution in the posterior head regions; beta rhythm is present in the frontal regions; 5. Alpha rhythm of 8–9 Hz posteriorly, mu rhythm of similar frequency fronto-centrally (c), and beta rhythm frontally (d).

**11.1.2** The *frequency* ranges from 8 to 13 Hz in different subjects. It is fairly constant in a given subject but may decrease by 1 Hz or more with drowsiness and increase momentarily after eye closure. Because of this constancy, alpha rhythm within the normal frequency range may be found to be abnormally slow or fast when compared with other recordings in the same subject.

The frequency of alpha rhythm in the two hemispheres should be the same at any moment; even a slight difference is suspicious of abnormality if it persists, and a persistent difference of over 1 Hz at any time is definitely abnormal. The hemisphere with the lower frequency is likely to be abnormal.

Old persons may have an occipital background rhythm indistinguishable from alpha rhythm except for a frequency slightly below 8 Hz; these rhythms are nevertheless often called alpha rhythm even though they may be abnormal (13.1.1).

**11.1.3** The *phase relation* of alpha rhythm over different parts of the brain may vary. Individual alpha waves are often not synchronous in different areas in normal EEGs, even though alpha rhythm normally appears and disappears simultaneously in the two hemispheres.

**11.1.4** The *distribution* of alpha rhythm is posterior: Alpha rhythm has the greatest amplitude and is most persistent in the occipital and parietal areas. It often extends into the temporal areas and sometimes into the central areas, especially in young subjects. Alpha rhythm may appear in recordings from a frontal electrode referred to an electrode on the ear, the mastoid or other posterior placements because these reference electrodes pick up alpha rhythm in posterior locations (4.1.2; Fig. 11.2). Rhythms of alpha frequency which appear only or mainly in the frontal regions in an adult are abnormal (25.3.1). So are focal or lateralized alpha wave paroxysms in newborns (19.3.5).

**11.1.5** The *amplitude* of alpha rhythm. often waxes and wanes. While the amplitude may differ on the two sides at different times, an estimate of the average amplitude of alpha rhythm during a recording may show it to be symmetrical on the two sides. However, even persistent asymmetries of alpha rhythm are not necessarily abnormal. A higher amplitude of alpha rhythm on the right side is fairly common, but the amplitude on the left side should be no less than two thirds that on the right side (Fig. 11.1). Some normal subjects have alpha rhythm of slightly higher amplitude on the left side. The normal asymmetry of alpha rhythm does not seem to depend on whether a subject is right-handed or left-handed. Abnormal asymmetries can be seen in many conditions (23.7.1).

The amplitude and persistence of alpha rhythm decreases with age from its maximum in childhood (10.7.1). Because of the wide variation of alpha rhythm between normal adults, low amplitude, rare occurrence, or even complete absence of alpha rhythm on both sides (11.8) is not abnormal. Therefore, no clinical significance can be attached to distinctions which have been made between dominant and rare alpha rhythms, or between 'plus' or persistent ('P-type'), reactive ('R-type') and 'minus' or minimal ('M-type') alpha rhythms. Only if alpha rhythm changes significantly between sequential recordings from the same subject (24.1.2; 24.1.4) can one suspect the development of an abnormality (24.7).

**11.1.6** The *reactivity* of alpha rhythm can be tested with various maneuvers. Alpha rhythm is blocked by eye opening (Fig. 11.1, Part 3), sudden alerting, attention to visual and other stimuli, and mental concentration. The degree of reactivity varies in different subjects and in the same subject at different times. Alpha rhythm may be blocked completely for many seconds or its amplitude may be attenuated only briefly. However, the complete absence of any reduction suggests an abnormality (25.2.2). Unilateral blocking of alpha rhythm is definitely abnormal (25.2.1).

Alpha rhythm also attenuates when alertness decreases to the level of drowsiness (12.2.2). This attenuation may be associated with a decrease of frequency and is often gradual and intermittent. Drowsiness can also produce a normal variation of alpha blocking, namely *paradoxical alpha rhythm* which appears on eye opening as the result of partial alerting to that level of relaxed wakefulness which is usually associated with alpha rhythm: this alpha rhythm may disappear with eye closure if drowsiness returns (Fig. 11.2, Top). Subjects showing paradoxical alpha rhythm can be demonstrated to have normally reacting alpha rhythm if eye opening leads to complete alerting which is not associated with alpha rhythm and followed by alpha rhythm on eye closure (Fig. 11.2, Bottom).

The effect of eye opening should be studied in every routine clinical EEG recording (a) to study the reactivity and symmetry of alpha blocking, (b) to demonstrate the artifacts produced by eye opening, eye closing and eye movements and to distinguish them from frontal slow waves, (c) to bring out rhythms hidden by alpha rhythm, (d) to test the reactivity of other EEG activity, (e) to precipitate abnormal reactions to eye opening and eye closing, for instance paroxysmal discharges.

**11.1.7** *Alpha variants* are normal rhythms which resemble alpha rhythm in distribution and reactivity but differ from it by having slower or faster frequency.

*Slow alpha variants* are rhythms of 3.5–6 Hz, usually of 4–5 Hz or half the frequency of the alpha rhythm appearing in the same record (Fig. 11.1, Part 4). They appear over the posterior head, usually alternate or intermix with alpha rhythm of the usual frequency, and block like alpha rhythm. Slow alpha variants are rare but normal and should not be confused with the intermittent occipital slow waves seen in children (10.7.1) and adults (11.7.2).

*Fast alpha variants* are described with beta rhythms (11.2).

**11.1.8** The *physiological significance* of the alpha rhythm remains unknown. The

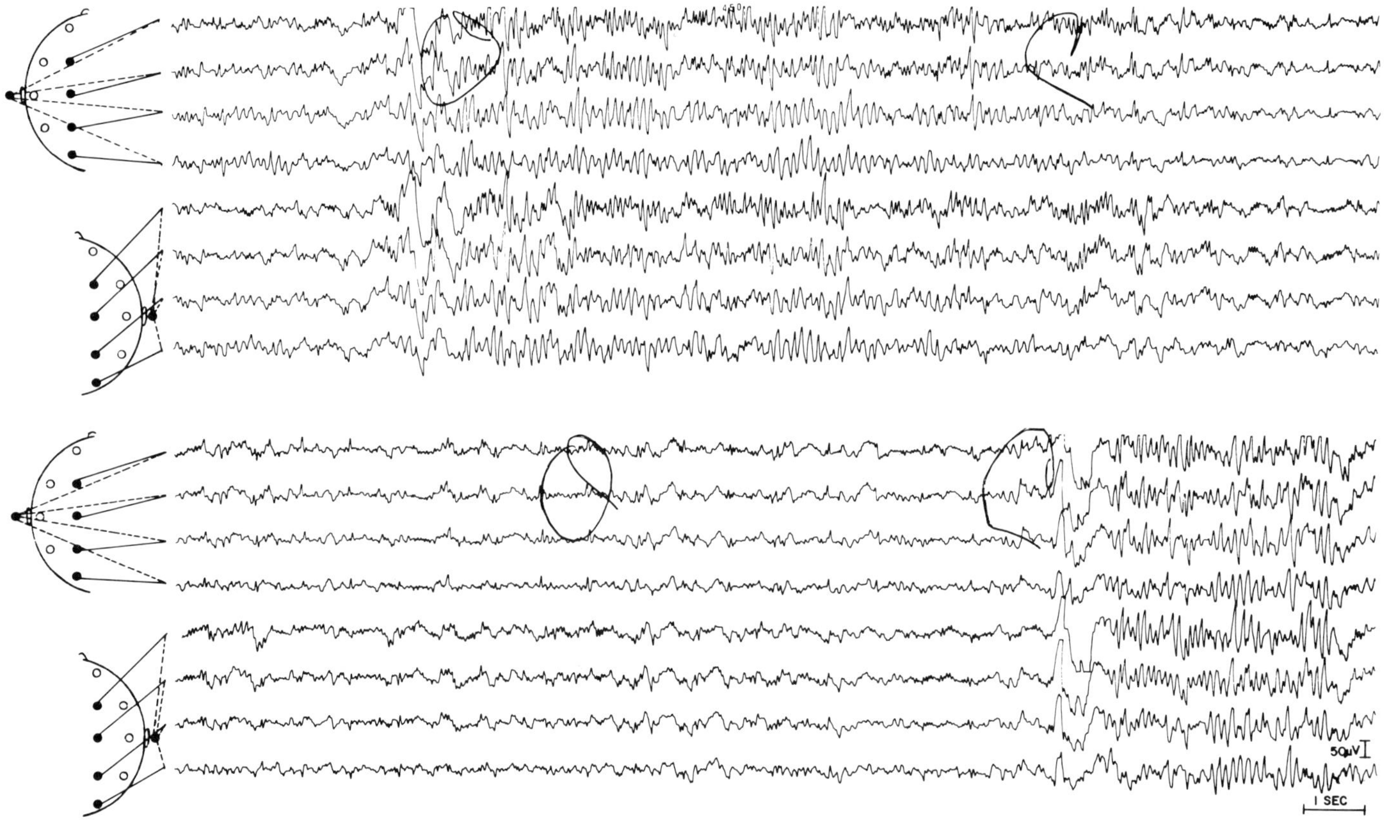


Fig. 11.2. Paradoxical alpha rhythm (top) and normal return of alpha rhythm (bottom) in a normal drowsy teenager. *Top*: Alpha rhythm appears on eye opening (O) and disappears soon after eye closure (C); activity characteristic of drowsiness is present before and after the period of eye opening; *Bottom*: Alpha rhythm appears after eye closure (C); activity before eye opening (O) and until shortly before eye closing is characteristic of drowsiness; the bottom part was recorded about 1 minute after the top part.

posterior distribution, the blocking by eye opening and other characteristics of alpha rhythm have suggested that it is related to the visual system and possibly represents an idling rhythm which appears in the absence of specific input to that system, perhaps as a result of a thalamic pacemaker (1.2).

## 11.2 BETA RHYTHMS

Unlike alpha rhythm, beta rhythms are defined only by frequency, but they can be subdivided by distribution and reactivity.

**11.2.1** The *frequency* of beta rhythms is over 13 Hz. Although any rhythmical activity above that frequency is called beta rhythm, beta rhythms of over 30 Hz have usually very low amplitude and are difficult to record with conventional EEG techniques (3.5.2).

**11.2.2** The *distribution* and reactivity of beta rhythms varies. Three types can be distinguished. All of them disappear in drowsiness and sleep, but the first two types usually persist longer than does alpha rhythm.

*Frontal beta rhythm* is the most common type. It often extends into the central regions (Fig. 11.1, Part 5). In some instances, this type of beta rhythm is blocked by movement, the intention to move, and tactile stimulation. The blocking effect is greater in the hemisphere contralateral to the moved or stimulated side.

*Widespread beta rhythm* can be recorded over most areas of the head, usually at the same time (Fig. 11.3, Part 1). It is not blocked by any stimulus.

*Posterior beta rhythm* or *fast alpha variant* has a frequency of usually up to 14–20 Hz, intermixes or alternates with alpha rhythm or replaces it (Fig. 11.3, Part 2). This beta rhythm is blocked by maneuvers which block alpha rhythm.

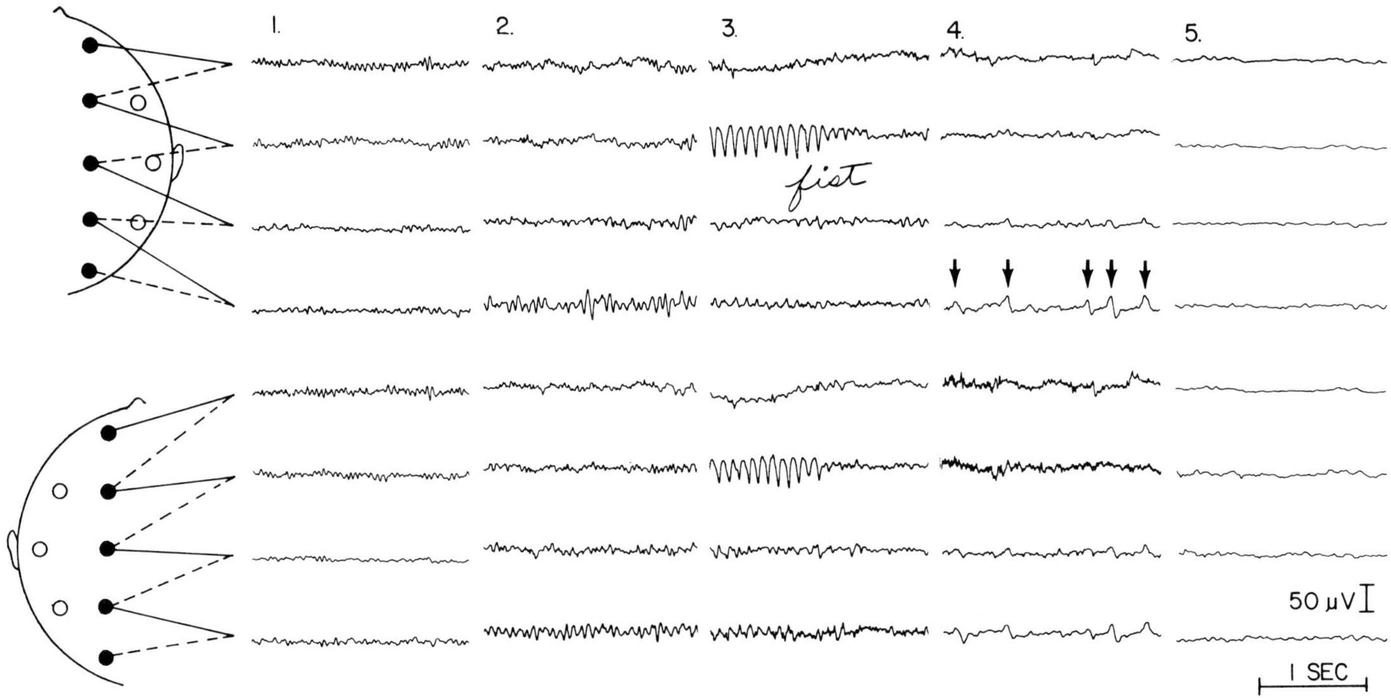


Fig. 11.3. Normal patterns of wakefulness in adults. 1. Generalized beta rhythm of a low amplitude or 'low voltage fast activity'; 2. Fast alpha variant of about 15 Hz in the posterior head regions and faster beta rhythm elsewhere; 3. Fronto-central mu rhythm, blocked by making a fist; posterior alpha rhythm is blocked by eye opening during this recording; 4. Lambda waves (arrows) in the occipital areas, triggered by visual scanning of a picture; 5. Low voltage pattern; subject was alert and had eyes closed during the recording.

**11.2.3** The *amplitude* of beta activity is usually lower than that of alpha rhythm in the same record, but amplitude and persistence of beta rhythm may be abnormally high (24.8). Amplitude and distribution of all normal beta rhythms is symmetrical: Asymmetry, unilateral or focal appearance of beta rhythm is abnormal (19.3.6; 23.7.2).

**11.2.4** The *persistence* of beta rhythms in the EEG of individuals and the incidence of beta rhythms in the general population increase with age. Since alpha activity tends to decrease during adult life (11.1.5), the ratio of beta to alpha activity increases with age (13.2). However, these age-dependent changes do not have definite clinical implications for a single subject. Only in a general manner does the presence of beta activity in an older person signal better cerebral function than does its absence.

The persistence and amplitude of beta activity may be excessive and then suggest an abnormality (24.8).

**11.2.5** The *physiological significance* of beta rhythms is not clear. The blocking mechanism of frontal beta rhythm suggests a relationship between this type of beta rhythm and sensorimotor functions of the underlying cortex; a similar relationship may be postulated for mu rhythm (11.3). Posterior beta rhythm probably has the same significance as alpha rhythm (11.1.8); it is of no clinical importance.

## 11.3 MU RHYTHM

Older names for this rhythm which should no longer be used are 'wicket', 'comb' or 'arceau' rhythm. Mu rhythm, seen in less than 10% of EEGs and most commonly in younger adults, consists of arch-shaped waves at 7–11 Hz which appear in trains of usually up to a few seconds over the central or centro-parietal regions (Fig. 11.3, Part 3). These trains often appear at different times on the two sides of the head. They are better seen in bipolar than in referential recordings. Mu waves intermix or alternate with beta activity (Fig. 11.1, Part 5) and then often have half the frequency of the beta waves. Because mu rhythm has a frequency similar to that of alpha rhythm, it usually is best recognized when alpha rhythm is blocked by eye opening (Fig. 11.1, Part 3). The appearance of mu rhythm is said to be facilitated while a subject scans visual images.

Like frontal beta rhythm, mu rhythm is often blocked by voluntary, reflex or passive movement, by the intention to move, or by tactile stimuli (Fig. 11.3, Part 3). The effect is greatest over the hemisphere opposite the side of the movement or stimulation. If alpha rhythm is present while mu reactivity is tested, alpha rhythm may be blocked along with mu rhythm if the test alerts the subject. Paradoxical mu rhythm is mu rhythm which is induced by contralateral movement or touch after mu rhythm has dropped out in drowsy subjects. The same events which induce paradoxical mu rhythm may also alert the subject, and paradoxical alpha rhythm may be induced at the same time.

Because mu rhythm is normally intermittent and asynchronous, an EEG is not abnormal if it shows only a few trains of mu rhythm on one side, or only a moderate difference in the incidence of mu rhythm on the two sides. However, frequent trains of mu rhythm appearing only on one side, or a consistent asymmetry of amplitude or frequency of mu rhythm suggests an abnormality on the side of the lower amplitude or frequency.

The physiological significance of mu rhythm may be related to somatosensory processes associated with movement. This is suggested by the distribution of mu rhythm, by the blocking effect of sensory stimuli and of passive movement, and by the onset of the mu blocking before actual and intended movement. Mu rhythm, like alpha rhythm, may represent the idling of a sensory system not processing specific input from thalamic nuclei.

## 11.4 LAMBDA WAVES

Sharp transients of sawtooth shape and of positive polarity occur in the occipital regions of some subjects when they look at images containing visual detail (Fig. 11.3, Part 4). Lambda waves are therefore rarely encountered in routine clinical EEGs. Neither the presence nor the absence of lambda waves is abnormal, but a marked asymmetry suggests an abnormality on the side of lower amplitude. Lambda waves resemble visual evoked potentials elicited by intermittent flash stimuli in many regards including distribution, wave form and latent period between the change of visual input and the wave peak. Each lambda wave is preceded by a scanning eye movement, sometimes recognizable as an eye movement artifact in frontal derivations. It is therefore likely that lambda waves partly represent visual evoked potentials. However, they persist to some extent after eye movements in the dark and probably also reflect other events, perhaps processes related to eye movement or to the blocking of visual input during changes of gaze.

## 11.5 VERTEX SHARP TRANSIENTS (V WAVES)

Sharp transients of negative polarity at the vertex are a common element of normal sleep activity (12.1.3). They occur very rarely in wakeful adults and then seem to follow sudden loud noise or other unexpected stimuli. The amplitude of V waves which occur during wakefulness is usually much lower than that of V waves occurring during sleep. V waves may form part of a generalized response to startling stimuli; such a response may also include eye blinks and scalp movements. Even though these three components occur at a similar interval after the stimulus, V waves are not due to eye or scalp movement.

V waves probably represent a late component of evoked potentials which is nonspecific insofar as it does not depend on the modality of the sensory stimulus and appears in a larger region of the cortex than the relatively small specific sensory area. Because of its wider distribution, this response part is more likely to be recorded in the EEG than the earlier parts of sensory responses which are restricted to the specific sensory pathways and cortical receiving areas and usually need enhancement by computer averaging to be seen clearly (7.6).

## 11.6 KAPPA RHYTHM

This rhythm consists of bursts of very low amplitude waves of alpha or theta frequency which have been recorded in a few instances in the temporal regions of subjects engaged in mental activity and are rarely, if ever, seen in routine clinical recordings. It is not clear whether these waves represent electrocerebral activity in the temporal lobes generated by mental effort or whether they are due to fine rhythmical eye movements associated with eyelid flutter.

## 11.7 NORMAL POSTERIOR THETA RHYTHMS

Two very rare patterns of rhythmical theta activity can be distinguished in some normal EEGs. Their distribution and reactivity resembles that of alpha rhythms. They are the only exceptions to the rule that synchronous and repetitive theta waves in the EEG of wakeful resting adults are abnormal (11.9.2).

**11.7.1** *Slow alpha variant* has been described (11.1.7).

**11.7.2** *Rhythmical slow waves of about 4–5 Hz* appear intermittently in the occipital and temporal areas in probably less than one percent of normal adults. Even though the distribution of these rhythms differs slightly from that of alpha waves, they are blocked by eye opening and alerting and disappear in drowsiness and sleep. The incidence of this pattern decreases during adult life.

## 11.8 THE LOW VOLTAGE EEG

Some EEGs show no activity over 20 $\mu$V in recordings from any part of the head (Fig. 11.3, Part 5). At a high gain, a wide range of frequencies can be distinguished, including beta, theta and some delta waves, and sometimes posterior alpha waves (Fig. 11.4). The term 'low voltage fast EEG', which has sometimes been used to describe this pattern, is therefore not appropriate. Waves of higher amplitude can sometimes be induced by hyperventilation, photic stimulation and sleep.

Low voltage EEGs are not seen in normal children, but they become more common with advancing age. They are sometimes seen in tense subjects who show normal amplitude when relaxed. However, low voltage EEGs may be abnormal reflecting bilateral reduction of amplitude which can be recognized only if a prior record from the same subject shows normal amplitude. Very low voltage, i.e. no activity over 10 $\mu$V, is more likely to be abnormal (24.2.2).

Low voltage EEGs must be clearly distinguished from recordings showing electrocerebral inactivity, i.e. absence of cerebral activity of over 2 $\mu$V (5.4).

## 11.9 MAJOR ABNORMALITIES

**11.9.1** *Spikes and sharp waves* are abnormal except for (a) vertex sharp transients (11.5); (b) lambda waves which can easily be recognized by their shape and distri-

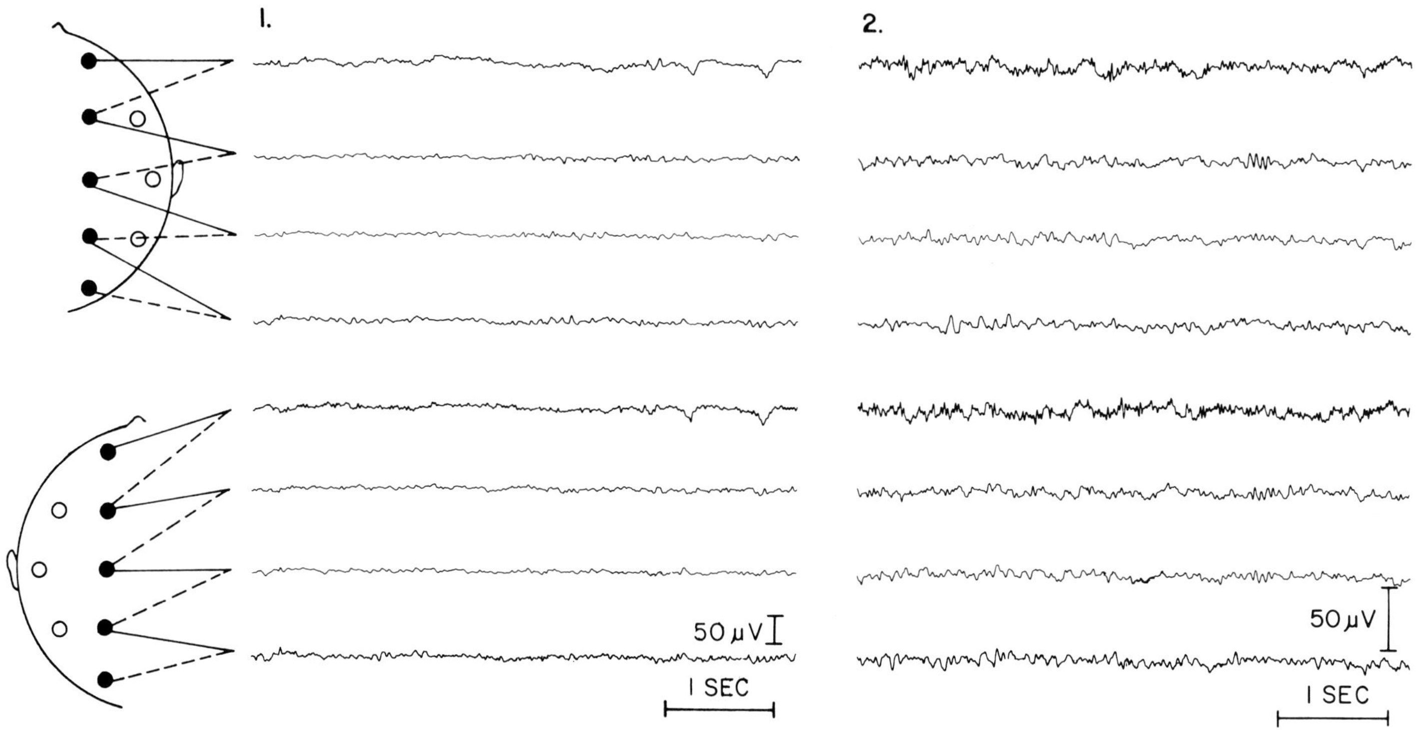


Fig. 11.4. Low voltage pattern in a normal adult. 1. Recording at the usual sensitivity shows an EEG without distinctive features; 2. Continuation at a higher sensitivity shows a mixture of a wide range of frequencies.

bution and by the specific precipitating mechanisms (11.4); (c) most 6 Hz spike-and-slow-wave complexes (19.4.1).

**11.9.2** *Slow waves* of less than 8 Hz should be absent or very rare. They can be accepted as normal only if they are single, of theta frequency, without focal, regional or lateral predominance, asynchronous and not much higher in amplitude than the background. Slow waves are abnormal if they are repetitive or frequent, of delta frequency, of focal, regional or lateral distribution, bilaterally synchronous or of clearly higher amplitude than the background. A rare exception are the bilaterally synchronous theta rhythms in the posterior head regions of a few adults (11.7).

**11.9.3** *Low amplitude* generally can best be diagnosed as being abnormal if the amplitude can be shown to be decreased in comparison with a preceding or subsequent record from the same subject. Moderately low amplitude observed in a single recording, although strictly an abnormal EEG feature, is often not associated with clinical abnormalities (24.2.2). However, a single recording of very low amplitude often indicates an abnormality, and complete absence of electrocerebral activity always does so (24.6). *Asymmetries* are abnormal except for the specified asymmetries of alpha rhythm (11.1.5).

**11.9.4** *Deviations from normal patterns* such as changes of the frequency or reactivity of alpha rhythm and the occurrence of alpha frequency patterns in coma and seizures may indicate important abnormalities (25).

## REFERENCES


Adrian, E.D. and Matthews, B.H.C. (1934) The Berger rhythm: Potential changes from the occipital lobes in man. Brain 57: 355–385.

Adrian, E.D. and Yamagiwa, K. (1935) The origin of the Berger rhythm. Brain 58: 323–351.

Aird, R.B. and Gastaut, Y. (1959) Occipital and posterior electroencephalographic rhythms. Electroenceph. clin. Neurophysiol. 11: 637–656.

Barlow, J.S. and Ciganek, L. (1969) Lambda responses in relation to visual evoked responses in man. Electroenceph. clin. Neurophysiol. 26: 183–192.

Chapman, R.M., Armington, J.C. and Bragdon, H.R. (1962) A quantitative survey of kappa and alpha EEG activity. Electroenceph. clin. Neurophysiol. 14: 858–868.

Chatrian, G.E., Petersen, M.C. and Lazarte, J.A. (1959) The blocking of the rolandic wicket rhythm and some central changes related to movement. Electroenceph. clin. Neurophysiol. 11: 497–510.

Chatrian, G.E. and Lairy, G.C., eds. (1976) Part A. The EEG of the waking adult. In: Rémond, A. (Ed.), Handbook of Electroenceph. clin. Neurophysiol., Vol. 6A, Elsevier, Amsterdam.

Fourment, A., Calvet, J. and Bancaud, J. (1976) Electrocorticography of waves associated with eye movements in man during wakefulness. Electroenceph. clin. Neurophysiol. 40: 457–469.

Garoutte, B. and Aird, R.B. (1958) Studies on the cortical pacemaker: Synchrony and asynchrony of bilaterally recorded alpha and beta activity. Electroenceph. clin. Neurophysiol. 10: 259–268.

Gibbs, F.A. and Gibbs, E.L. (1951) Atlas of electroencephalography, Vol. 1: Methodology and Controls, 2nd Ed., Addison-Wesley Publishing Co., Reading.

Gloor, P. (1969) Hans Berger on the electroencephalogram of man. The fourteen original reports on the human electroencephalogram. Electroenceph. clin. Neurophysiol., Suppl. 28.

Goodwin, J.E. (1947) The significance of alpha variants in the EEG, and their relationship to an epileptiform syndrome. Amer. J. Psychiat. 104: 369–379.

Green, J. (1957) Some observations on lambda waves and peripheral stimulation. Electroenceph. clin. Neurophysiol. 9: 691–704.

Harlan, W.L., White, P.T. and Bickford, R.G. (1958) Electric activity produced by eye flutter simulating frontal electroencephalographic rhythms. Electroenceph. clin. Neurophysiol. 10: 164–169.

Hoovey, Z.B., Heinemann, U. and Creutzfeldt, O.D. (1972) Inter-hemispheric 'synchrony' of alpha waves. Electroenceph. clin. Neurophysiol. 32: 337–347.

Hughes, J.R. and Cayaffa, J.J. (1977) The EEG in patients at different ages without organic cerebral disease. Electroenceph. clin. Neurophysiol. 42: 776–784.

Johnsson, L.C. and Ulett, G.A. (1959) Quantitative study of pattern and stability of resting electroencephalographic activity in a young adult group. Electroenceph. clin. Neurophysiol. 11: 233–249.

Koshino, Y. and Niedermeyer, E. (1975) Enhancement of rolandic mu-rhythm by pattern vision. Electroenceph. clin. Neurophysiol. 38: 535–538.

Kuhlman, W.N. (1978) Functional topography of the human mu rhythm. Electroenceph. clin. Neurophysiol. 44: 83–93.
Lehmann, D. (1971) Multichannel topography of human alpha EEG fields. Electroenceph. clin. Neurophysiol. 31: 439–449.
Leissner, P., Lindholm, L.-E. and Petersén, I. (1970) Alpha amplitude dependence on skull thickness as measured by ultrasound technique. Electroenceph. clin. Neurophysiol. 29: 392–399.
Lippold, O. (1973) The Origin of the Alpha Rhythm. Churchill Livingstone, Edinburgh and London.
Liske, E., Hughes, H.M. and Stowe, D.E. (1967) Cross-correlation of human alpha activity: Normative data. Electroenceph. clin. Neurophysiol. 22: 429–436.
Matoušek, M., Volavka, J. Roubíček, J. and Roth, Z. (1967) EEG frequency analysis related to age in normal adults. Electroenceph. clin. Neurophysiol. 23: 162–167.
Perez-Borja, C., Chatrian, G.E., Tyce, F.A. and Rivers, M.H. (1962) Electrographic patterns of the occipital lobe in man: A topographic study based on use of implanted electrodes. Electroenceph. clin. Neurophysiol. 14: 171–182.
Pfurtscheller, G., Maresch, H. and Schuy, S. (1977) Inter- and intrahemispheric differences in the peak frequency of rhythmic activity within the alpha band. Electroenceph. clin. Neurophysiol. 42: 77–83.
Schoppenhorst, M., Brauer, F., Freund, G. and Kubicki, S. (1980) The significance of coherence estimates in determining central alpha and mu activities. Electroenceph. clin. Neurophysiol. 48: 25–33.
Scott, D.F., Groethuysen, U.C. and Bickford, R.G. (1967) Lambda responses in the human electroencephalogram. Neurology 17: 770–778.

# The normal sleep EEG of adults over 20 years

# 12

Summary

The sleep EEG of adults shows less variation of patterns between individuals than does the waking EEG.

(12.1) The *elements* of the sleep EEG differ from those of the waking EEG and consist of slow waves, sleep spindles, positive occipital sharp transients of sleep (POSTs), vertex sharp transients (V waves) and K complexes. Eye movements and muscle activity may be picked up incidentally from routine electrode placements but are often recorded intentionally with special electrode placements.

(12.2) *Sleep stages* are distinguished by EEG patterns consisting of different combinations of electrographic elements. These patterns serve to distinguish *stages I–IV of slow wave sleep*, representing progressively deeper levels of dreamless sleep, and the *stage of rapid eye movement (REM) sleep*, which has characteristics of both very light and very deep sleep and is associated with dreaming.

(12.3) *Sleep cycles* are characteristic sequences of sleep stages. Cycles are best studied in all-night sleep recordings. Heart beat, respiration and other parameters are often included in such recordings.

(12.4) *Major abnormalities* which can be found in sleep recordings are spikes and sharp waves, REM periods at the onset of sleep ('sleep onset REM periods'), and sleep disorders characterized by disturbances of sleep cycles and of respiration.

## 12.1 ELEMENTS OF NORMAL SLEEP ACTIVITY

**12.1.1** *Slow waves* occur in a wide distribution and are often more prominent posteriorly than anteriorly. In lighter stages of non-REM sleep they are generally less persistent, more asynchronous, of lower amplitude and faster frequency (Fig. 12.1, Parts 2 and 3) than in deeper stages (Fig. 12.2, Parts 1 and 2).

**12.1.2** *Positive occipital sharp transients* (POSTs) are monophasic, triangular waves in the occipital regions (Fig. 12.1, Parts 2 and 3; Fig. 12.2, Part 1). Because they have positive electrical polarity, they produce upgoing pen deflections in channels connected to the occipital electrodes through input 2 (3.4.1). POSTs occur intermittently and apparently spontaneously, either simultaneously or independently, on the two sides of the head. They usually recur irregularly at intervals of over 1 second, but they may repeat up to 4–6 times a second. Their amplitude is moderate in most cases, but may be high. Intermittent independent POSTs of high amplitude may resemble focal epileptiform discharges but should not be confused with them.

POSTs have also been called 'lambdoid waves' because they resemble lambda waves in shape and distribution (11.4); like lambda waves, they depend on normal central visual acuity. However, because the mechanisms responsible for generating the two types of waves are not known, the term 'lambdoid' should not be used.

**12.1.3** *Vertex sharp transients (V waves)* are bilaterally synchronous waves which have a maximum of amplitude at the vertex and often extend into frontal, temporal and parietal areas (Fig. 12.1, Part 3). V waves have negative electrical polarity and therefore cause upgoing pen deflections in channels connected to an electrode closer to the vertex through input 1 and to a more distant electrode through input 2, whereas they cause a downgoing pen deflection in channels connected to electrodes near the vertex through input 2 and to more distant electrodes through input 1 (3.4.1; 4.1). V waves are symmetrical on average even though their amplitude on either side may fluctuate transiently. They are single and often recur at irregular intervals, rarely more often than two times a second. They sometimes appear in response to a sensory stimulus (11.5).

**12.1.4** *Sleep spindles* have a frequency of 11–15 Hz, usually 12–14 Hz, and last up to a few seconds (Fig. 12.1, Part 3, Fig. 12.2, Part 1). They have a wide distribution, often with a maximum over the central regions. They appear simultaneously and symmetrically over the two sides.

**12.1.5** *K complexes* resemble V waves in distribution, reaction to sensory stimuli and polarity of the major component, but they are usually longer and less sharp than V waves and are often preceded or followed by a positive wave; this biphasic or triphasic wave is often followed by a sleep spindle (Fig. 12.2, Part 1).

## 12.2 SLEEP STAGES

**12.2.1** *Stage W* or wakefulness at the transition to drowsiness may show some slowing and greater prominence of alpha rhythm (Fig. 12.2, Part 1). Beta rhythms may be present and continue into stage I of sleep; they are especially prominent when sleep is induced by sedatives. Movement and muscle artifacts may obscure the EEG at the transition to sleep.

**12.2.2** *Sleep stage I* begins with the disappearance of alpha rhythm and the appearance of slow waves of 2–7 Hz (Fig. 12.1, Part 2). At the early part of this stage, most persons show low amplitude activity of mixed frequencies, but some have medium amplitude slow wave bursts immediately after the disappearance of alpha rhythm. Alpha waves may recur briefly; this is the time when paradoxical alpha rhythm appears on slight alerting (11.1.6). Muscle activity diminishes. Slow eye movements may occur and last for several seconds. Slow waves during this light stage of sleep may be difficult to distinguish from abnormal generalized slow waves occurring during wakefulness, especially in persons who have little or no alpha rhythm during wakefulness and who have slow wave bursts at the beginning of drowsiness. However, the slow waves of drowsiness can usually be identified by their appearance preceding deeper sleep stages.

In deeper parts of stage I, slow waves are of medium amplitude and may form irregularly spaced bursts. V waves may occur in response to alerting stimuli or apparently spontaneously in this stage and in stage II. At the end of stage I, POSTs appear in many subjects.

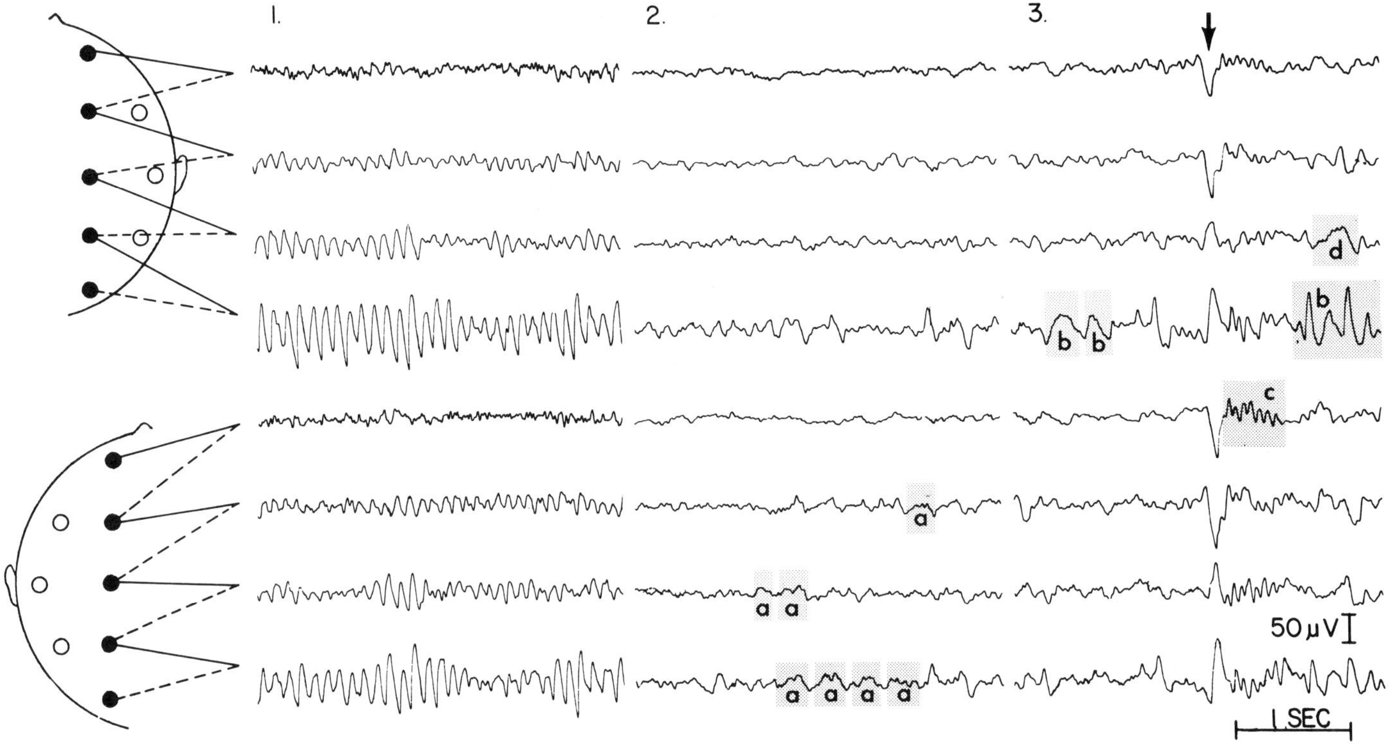


Fig. 12.1. Normal patterns of wakefulness and light sleep in an adult. 1. Stage W (wakefulness) with alpha rhythm and frontal beta rhythm; 2. Stage I (drowsiness) with irregular slow waves at 3–7 Hz (a); 3. Stage II (light sleep) with a V wave (arrow), POSTs (b), sleep spindles (c), and slow waves of 2–7 Hz (d).

**12.2.3** *Stage II* is characterized by the presence of sleep spindles of at least half a second in duration, K complexes or both (Fig. 12.1, Part 3). Slow waves of 2–7 Hz continue to be seen and are often bilaterally synchronous; slow waves of less than 2 Hz are absent or not prominent. POSTs often persist in stage II.

**12.2.4** *Stage III* is characterized by the presence of a moderate amount of very slow waves of high amplitude: 20–50% of the recording time is occupied by waves of 2 Hz or less of over 75 $\mu$V (Fig. 12.2, Part 1). K complexes are often present. Sleep spindles may be present or absent. POSTs can usually be distinguished.

**12.2.5** *Stage IV* is characterized by more slow wave activity than is present in stage III. Over 50% of the recording time is occupied by waves of 2 Hz or less and over 75 $\mu$V. K complexes blend with slow waves. Spindles and POSTs may be seen but are rare (Fig. 12.2, Part 2).

**12.2.6** *Stage REM* is characterized by low voltage EEG patterns, rapid eye movements, and generally reduced muscle activity; it is associated with dreaming. Although the EEG and some behavioral changes suggest that sleep is lighter during this stage, the threshold for arousal by auditory stimuli is increased, suggesting a deeper stage of sleep. These conflicting findings have prompted the use of the term 'paradoxical sleep'.

The *EEG* during REM sleep shows asynchronous low voltage waves of mixed frequency (Fig. 12.2, Part 3). It may resemble the pattern of stage I sleep except that it contains no V waves but may contain waves of sawtooth shape at the central and frontal regions. Alpha waves of 1–2 Hz less than the frequency of the alpha rhythm during wakefulness may be present.

*Rapid eye movements* are often picked up with routine prefrontal electrode placements but are more reliably monitored with recording electrodes placed near the

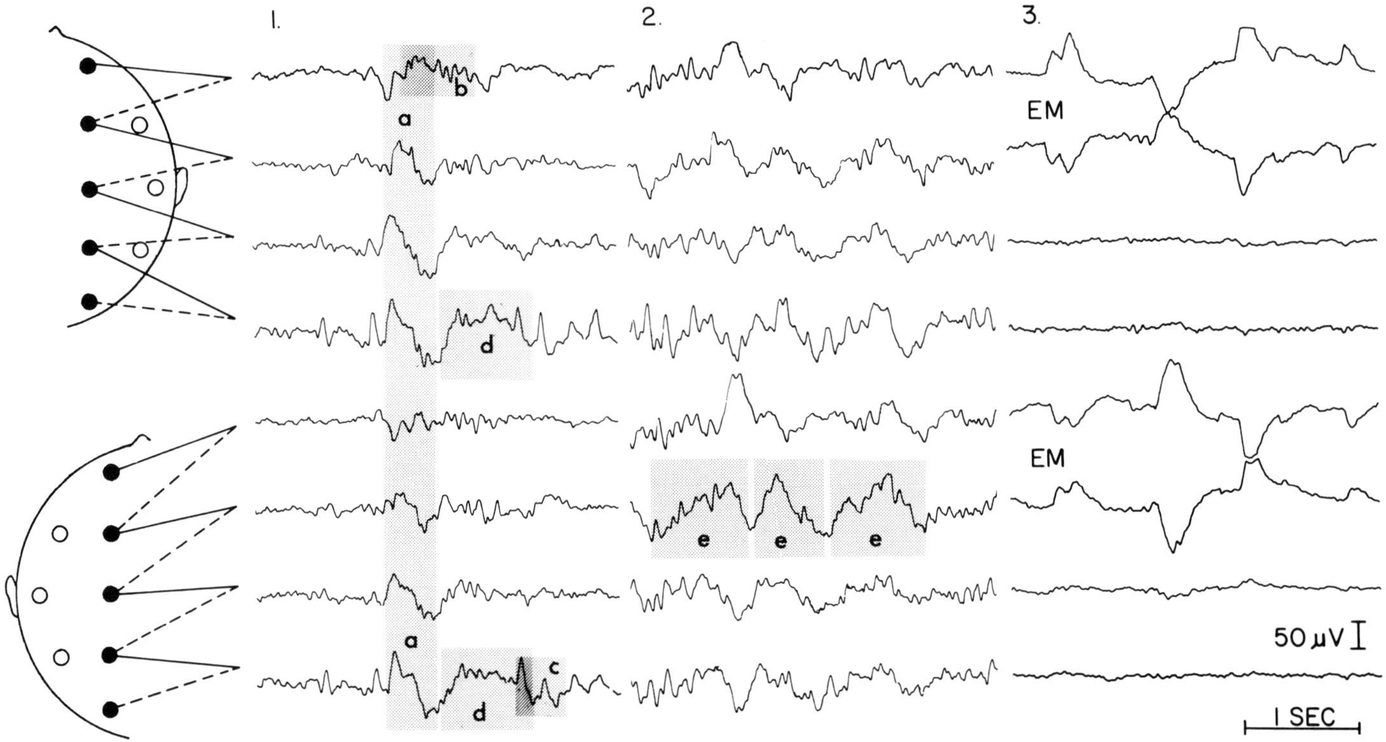


Fig. 12.2. Normal patterns of deep sleep and REM sleep in an adult. 1. Stage III (deep sleep) with a K complex (a), sleep spindle (b), POSTs (c), and slow waves of less than 2 Hz (d); 2. Stage IV (very deep sleep) with slow waves of less than 2 Hz and over 75 $\mu$V during over 50% of the recording (e); 3. Stage REM (rapid eye movement sleep) with eye movements indicated by eye movement monitors (EM) used during this part of the recording.

eyes (4.3.1). Such recordings show irregular deflections with extremely fast initial components due to rapid lateral changes of eye position (Fig. 12.2, Part 3).

*Changes of muscle tone and other activity* are sometimes monitored. Muscle tone can be recorded with EEG electrodes placed on neck muscles below the chin (4.3.4) and reaches its lowest level during the REM stage of sleep. However, paroxysms of muscle activity may appear in such recordings and often are associated with vigorous bursts of REM and brief twitches of face and limb muscles. Blood pressure and heart rate increase, breathing becomes faster and irregular, and gastrointestinal movement ceases; males have erections during almost every REM period.

## 12.3 SLEEP CYCLES

Normal nightly sleep is organized in characteristic sequences of sleep stages (Fig. 12.3). The first cycle begins with stage I and proceeds through increasingly deeper

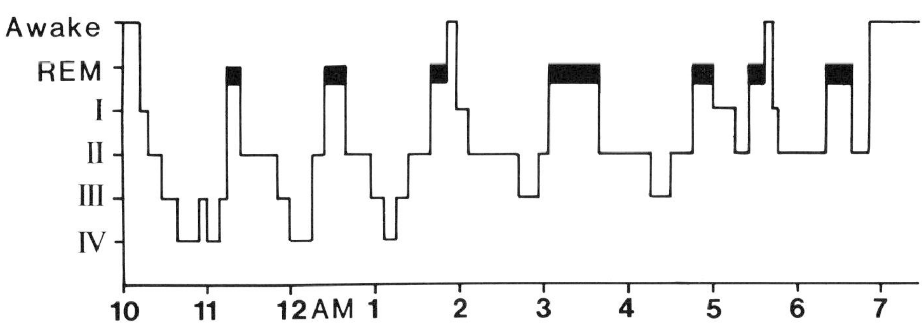


Fig. 12.3. Diagram of sleep cycles during an all-night sleep recording in a normal young adult. Sleep stages are plotted against time of the night.

stages of non-REM sleep to REM sleep. This resets the depth of sleep to a much lighter level and is followed by another cycle of gradual descent through non-REM sleep to REM sleep. Normally, people go through about 5–7 such cycles during a night. The first cycle is the shortest, but later cycles do not vary much in length and last about 80–120 minutes. REM sleep normally occurs only at the end of each cycle and thus first appears 70–90 minutes after the onset of sleep.

Several features of sleep vary with age. Although total sleep time is fairly constant through adulthood, the number and duration of the individual sleep stages changes. A normal young adult spends about 30–50% of sleep time in stage II, 20–40% in stages III and IV, and 5–10% in stage I. The percentage of stages III and IV decreases with age so that greater amounts of sleep time are spent in lighter stages. The proportion of REM sleep decreases slightly from about 25% in young adults to about 20% in the fifth decade.

To chart sleep stages, an all-night sleep recording is scored during successive periods of usually 20 or 30 seconds. The sleep stage prevailing during these periods is plotted as a function of time from the onset of sleep. To identify the sleep stages accurately, eye movements and muscle activity are recorded in addition to the EEG (5.3). A thorough study of sleep cycles requires that recordings be made during more than one night to overcome the distorting 'first night effect' which is due to the subject's unfamiliarity with the environment of the sleep laboratory and the recording procedures.

## 12.4 MAJOR ABNORMALITIES

Epileptiform activity, short latency to sleep onset, REM periods at sleep onset and other sleep disorders are often looked for in sleep recordings made as part of a routine EEG during the day. Such recordings are satisfactory for the detection of short sleep latency and may activate epileptiform activity, but all-night sleep recordings are more reliable for the study of sleep disorders.

**12.4.1** *Spikes and sharp waves* appear during sleep in many patients with convulsive disorders. Therefore sleep is often used as an activation procedure in the diagnosis of epilepsy (14.2.1). Spikes and sharp waves must be carefully distinguished from positive occipital sharp transients (12.1.2) and vertex sharp transients (12.1.3).

**12.4.2** *Short latency to sleep onset* of an average of less than 5 minutes can be found in patients with narcolepsy and other disorders (25.4.3) when they are given the opportunity to fall asleep during the day ('multiple sleep latency test').

**12.4.3** *Sleep onset REM periods* are characteristically seen in patients with narcolepsy and may occur in patients with sleep apnea (25.4.3). Daytime naps are not reliable indicators of this disorganization of the first sleep cycle because naps occasionally begin with REM sleep in persons without sleep disorders, and may begin without REM periods in some patients with narcolepsy and in many patients with sleep apnea.

**12.4.4** *Disorders of sleep cycles* such as abnormal length, number and distribution of sleep stages occur in various conditions (25.4.5). To diagnose these conditions, it is often necessary to record extracerebral physiological activity in addition to the EEG (4.3). For example, respiratory body movement and air flow must be monitored to study sleep apnea, characterized by frequent and long periods without breathing which can be the cause of undiagnosed daytime symptoms.

## REFERENCES


Brazier, M.A.B. and Finesinger, J.E. (1945) Action of barbiturates on the cerebral cortex. Arch. Neurol. Psychiat. 53: 51–58.

Daly, D.D. and Yoss, R.E. (1957) Electroencephalogram in narcolepsy. Electroenceph. clin. Neurophysiol. 9: 109–120.

Decoster, R. and Foret, J. (1979) Sleep onset and first cycle of sleep in human subjects: Change with time of day. Electroenceph. clin. Neurophysiol. 46: 531–537.

Dement, W. and Kleitman, N. (1957) Cyclic variations in EEG during sleep and their relation to eye movements, body mobility, and dreaming. Electroenceph. clin. Neurophysiol. 9: 673–690.

Dement, W., Rechtschaffen, A. and Gulevich, G. (1966) The nature of the narcoleptic sleep attack. Neurology 16: 18–33.

Dement, W.C. (1976) Daytime sleepiness and sleep 'attacks'. In: Guilleminault, D., Dement, W.C. and Passouant, P. (Eds.), Narcolepsy, Spectrum, New York, pp. 17–42.

Hishikawa, Y. and Kaneko, Z. (1965) Electroencephalographic study on narcolepsy. Electroenceph. clin. Neurophysiol. 18: 249–259.

Kales, A. and Kales, J.D. (1974) Sleep disorders. Recent findings in the diagnosis and treatment of disturbed sleep. New Engl. J. Med. 290: 487–499.

Lavie, P., Gadoth, N., Gordon, C.R., Goldhammer, G. and Bechar, M. (1979) Sleep patterns in Kleine-Levin syndrome. Electroenceph. clin. Neurophysiol. 47: 369–371.

Loomis, A.L., Harvey, E.N. and Hobart, G.A. (1938) Disturbance patterns in sleep. J. Neurophysiol. 1: 413–430.

Mitler, M.M., van den Hoed, J., Carskadon, M.A., Richardson, G., Park, R., Guilleminault, C. and Dement, W.C. (1979) REM sleep episodes during the multiple sleep latency test in narcoleptic patients. Electroenceph. clin. Neurophysiol. 46: 479–481.

Moses, J.M., Hord, D.J., Lubin, A., Johnson, L.C. and Naitoh, P. (1975) Dynamics of nap sleep during a 40 hour period. Electroenceph. clin. Neurophysiol. 39: 627–633.

Rechtschaffen, R., Wolpert, E.A., Dement, W.C., Mitchell, S.A. and Fisher, C. (1963) Nocturnal sleep of narcoleptics. Electroenceph. clin. Neurophysiol. 15: 599–609.

Rechtschaffen, A. and Kales, A. (1968) A Manual of Standardized Terminology, Techniques and Scoring System for Sleep Stages of Human Subjects. PHS, U.S. Government Printing Office, Washington, D.C.

Richardson, G.S., Carskadon, M.A., Flagg, W., van den Hoed, J., Dement, W.C. and Mitler, M.M. (1978) Excessive daytime sleepiness in man: Multiple sleep latency measurement in narcoleptic and control subjects. Electroenceph. clin. Neurophysiol 45: 621–627.

Roth, M., Shaw, J. and Green, J. (1956) The form, voltage distribution and physiological significance of

the K-complex. Electroenceph. clin. Neurophysiol. 8: 385–402.
Vignaendra, V., Matthews, R.L. and Chatrian, G.E. (1974) Positive occipital sharp transients of sleep: Relationships to nocturnal sleep cycle in man. Electroenceph. clin. Neurophysiol. 37: 239–246.
Williams, R.L., Karacan, I. and Hursch, C.J. (1974) Electroencephalography (EEG) of Human Sleep. Wiley, New York.

# The normal EEG of adults over 60 years of age

# 13

SUMMARY

The normal EEG of adults over 60 years of age is similar to that of younger adults with a few exceptions.

(13.1) *Alpha rhythm* may be slower, less persistent and less reactive.

(13.2) *Beta rhythm* is often more prominent.

(13.3) *Sporadic generalized slow waves* may be slightly more common than in younger adults.

(13.4) *Intermittent temporal slow waves* appear in some apparently normal subjects, especially on the left side.

(13.5) *Sleep* is less deep and more often interrupted by wakefulness.

(13.6) *Major abnormalities* at this age are also similar to those of younger adults except that a wider range of slow waves is acceptable as normal in old age. Asymmetrical or extremely low amplitude, and spikes and sharp waves remain abnormal as before.

## 13.1 ALPHA RHYTHM

Alpha rhythm decreases in frequency, prominence and reactivity.

**13.1.1** The *frequency* of alpha rhythm drops from mean values of about 10–11 Hz in groups of young adults to means of about 9 Hz in persons over 60 years and of 8–9 Hz in centenarians. This progression to slower rates can be seen in recordings from the same individual made at different ages.

The frequency of alpha rhythm may fall below 8 Hz in old persons; although such rhythms are outside the defined lower frequency limit of alpha rhythm, they are commonly, however imprecisely, called 'alpha rhythm' as long as they retain the distribution and reactivity of alpha rhythm. The significance of alpha frequencies below 8 Hz in elderly persons is not entirely clear. It was previously thought that a frequency as low as 7 Hz was not abnormal in persons between 60 and 70 years of age and that frequencies of 6–7 Hz could be normal in some persons over 70 years, but it is now often believed that such low rates are not found in mentally intact old persons.

**13.1.2** The *voltage and persistence* of alpha rhythm decrease with age. Low voltage patterns (11.8) become more common after age 60.

**13.1.3** The *reactivity* of alpha rhythm is decreased. In older persons, blocking is slower and of shorter duration than in younger people.

## 13.2 BETA RHYTHM

The incidence and amplitude of beta rhythms increase during middle life (11.2.4). Beta activity is found in at least half of the elderly, more commonly in women than in men. Fast activity tends to disappear in very old age. Its disappearance is probably not a normal phenomenon but generally correlates with the development of cerebral atrophy.

## 13.3 SPORADIC GENERALIZED SLOW WAVES

Sporadic generalized slow waves are not much more prominent between 60 and 75 years than in younger adults. After age 75, a slight increase of slow waves mainly in the theta range may represent normal, age-dependent EEG changes, but more continuous theta activity or the appearance of generalized delta waves represents an EEG abnormality. Abnormal generalized slow waves correlate more strongly than other age-related EEG changes with senile dementia. However, senile dementia may progress to considerable severity before the EEG shows any deviation from the normal range.

### 13.4 INTERMITTENT TEMPORAL SLOW WAVES

Intermittent temporal slow waves of elderly persons have several characteristic features. They appear in the form of single waves or of brief bursts of usually arrhythmical waves of theta, delta or both frequencies (Fig. 13.1). Some bursts contain sharp transients. Although these bursts have medium or high amplitude, they occur infrequently and remain separated from each other by normal background activity. They usually arise from the left anterior or middle temporal area. Similar slow waves of lower amplitude sometimes appear simultaneously or independently in the right temporal regions. Rarely do such slow waves occur predominantly in the right temporal areas.

Although these slow waves are probably the result not of normal aging but of degenerative or vascular cerebral changes, they are often found in otherwise normal old persons. These slow waves can usually be distinguished from an abnormal slow wave focus by their clearly intermittent occurrence between long periods of normal background activity and by their restricted distribution. In contrast, abnormal focal slow waves of comparable amplitude are much more likely to be continuous, to extend into neighboring areas, especially the frontal regions, and to be associated with generalized slow waves. The sharp transients occurring with some temporal slow wave bursts may resemble focal sharp waves (17.1.2), but their configuration usually varies more than that of sharp waves.

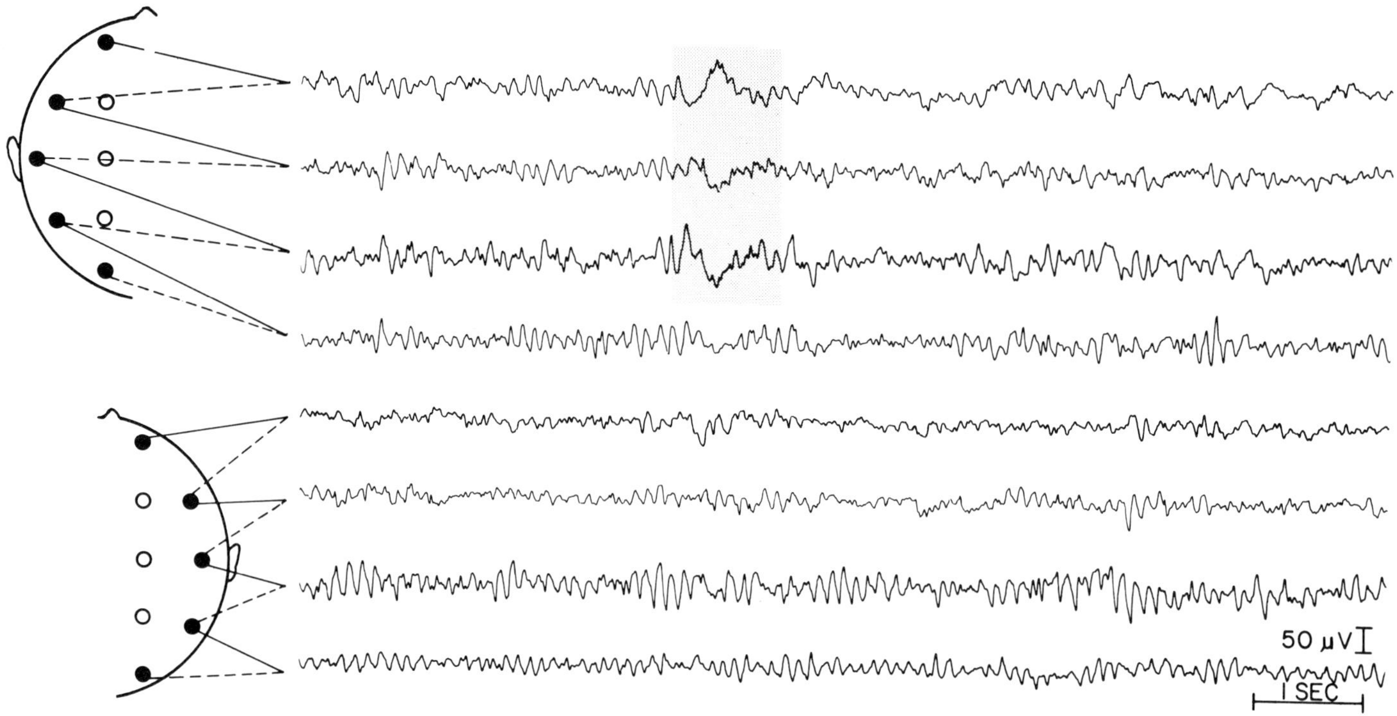


Fig. 13.1. Sporadic left temporal slow waves with sharp contours in 61-year-old subject without clinical abnormalities (shaded).

## 13.5 SLEEP

**13.5.1** *Sleep onset* may be associated with fairly prominent slow waves beginning abruptly as soon as alpha activity has dropped out. Some normal old persons show trains of bilaterally synchronous delta waves in drowsiness.

**13.5.2** *Sleep depth* is reduced. The proportion of time spent in stages III and IV decreases through adult life and reached a minimum of less than 10% in old age. The time spent awake between periods of sleep increases with age.

**13.5.3** *REM sleep* decreases to less than 20% of total sleep time at the ages of 70–80 years.

## 13.6 MAJOR ABNORMALITIES

**13.6.1** *Slow waves* in excess of those acceptable as normal at this age (13.3) indicate abnormality. Abnormal slow wave patterns at this age, in contrast to those of younger adults, consist more often of bilaterally synchronous trains of rhythmical delta waves and less often of focal slow waves.

**13.6.2** *Extremely low amplitude* and *asymmetry of amplitude* are abnormal; the standards are the same as for younger adults (11.9.3).

**13.6.3** *Spikes and sharp waves* are abnormal with the same exceptions as for younger adults during wakefulness (11.9.1) and sleep (12.4.1).

## REFERENCES


Agnew, H.W., Webb, W.W. and Williams, R.L. (1967) Sleep patterns in late middle age males: An EEG study. Electroenceph. clin. Neurophysiol. 23: 168–171.

Harner, R.N. (1975) EEG evaluation of the patient with dementia. In: Benson, D.F. and Blumer, D. (Eds.), Psychiatric Aspects of Neurological Disease, Grune and Stratton, New York and London, pp. 63–82.

Hubbard, O., Sunde, D. and Goldensohn, E.S. (1976) The EEG in centenarians. Electroenceph. clin. Neurophysiol. 40: 407–417.

Ingvar, D.H., Sjölund, B. and Ardö, A. (1976) Correlation between dominant EEG frequency, cerebral oxygen uptake and blood flow. Electroenceph. clin. Neurophysiol. 41: 268–276.

Marsh, G.R. and Thompson, L.V. (1977) Psychophysiology of aging. In: Handbook of the Psychology of Aging. In: Birren, J.E. and Schaie, K.W. (Eds.), Reinhold van Nostrand, New York, pp. 219–248.

Mundy-Castle, A.C., Hurst, L.A., Beerstecher, D.M. and Prinsloo, T. (1954) The electroencephalogram in the senile psychoses. Electroenceph. clin. Neurophysiol. 6: 245–252.

Obrist, W.D., Sokoloff, L., Lassen, N.A., Lane, M.H., Butler, R.N. and Feinberg, I. (1963) Relation of EEG to cerebral blood flow and metabolism in old age. Electroenceph. clin. Neurophysiol. 15: 610–619.

Obrist, W.D. (1976) Section V. Problems of aging. In: Rémond, A. (Ed.), Handbook of Electroenceph. clin. Neurophysiol., Vol. 6A, Elsevier, Amsterdam, pp. 275–292.

Otomo, E. and Tsubaki, T. (1966) Electroencephalography in subjects sixty years and over. Electroenceph. clin. Neurophysiol. 20: 77–82.

Silverman, A.J., Busse, E.W. and Barnes, R.H. (1955) Studies in the processes of aging: Electroencephalographic findings in 400 elderly subjects. Electroenceph. clin. Neurophysiol. 7: 67–74.

# 14 Activation procedures

SUMMARY

Activation procedures are used to induce, enhance or better define abnormal EEG patterns. These procedures also may induce normal patterns which are not seen in the spontaneous EEG.

(14.1) *Hyperventilation* is used routinely in most laboratories. The normal response consists of a buildup of generalized slow waves; this response is seen especially in persons who are young or in those who are hypoglycemic. Abnormal responses include spike-and-wave discharges, spikes, sharp waves, focal slow waves or enhancement of abnormal slow waves and of asymmetries.

(14.2) *Sleep* recordings are made after routine daytime waking records in many laboratories and are indicated especially in patients who are suspected of having epilepsy but show no epileptiform activity in the waking record; all-night sleep recordings are occasionally used for that purpose. Recordings after a period of *sleep deprivation* should be used in patients who give a history of having seizures after insufficient sleep.

(14.3) *Photic stimulation* with stroboscopic flashes of diffuse light is used in some laboratories. Normal responses are visual evoked potentials to intermittent flashes and photic driving to repetitive flashes. Photomyoclonic responses are unusual; photoconvulsive responses are abnormal.

(14.4) *Other stimuli* such as patterned light, startling noise, or musical sounds should be used during EEG recordings in those patients who are known to react to these stimuli with behavior suspected of representing seizure activity.

(14.5) *Pentylene tetrazol* and other convulsant drugs are used only rarely and for very narrowly defined reasons.

## 14.1 HYPERVENTILATION

Hyperventilation should be performed for 3–5 minutes in all routine recordings with the few exceptions described in 5.1.

**14.1.1** *Normal responses* consist of generalized slow waves which may begin soon

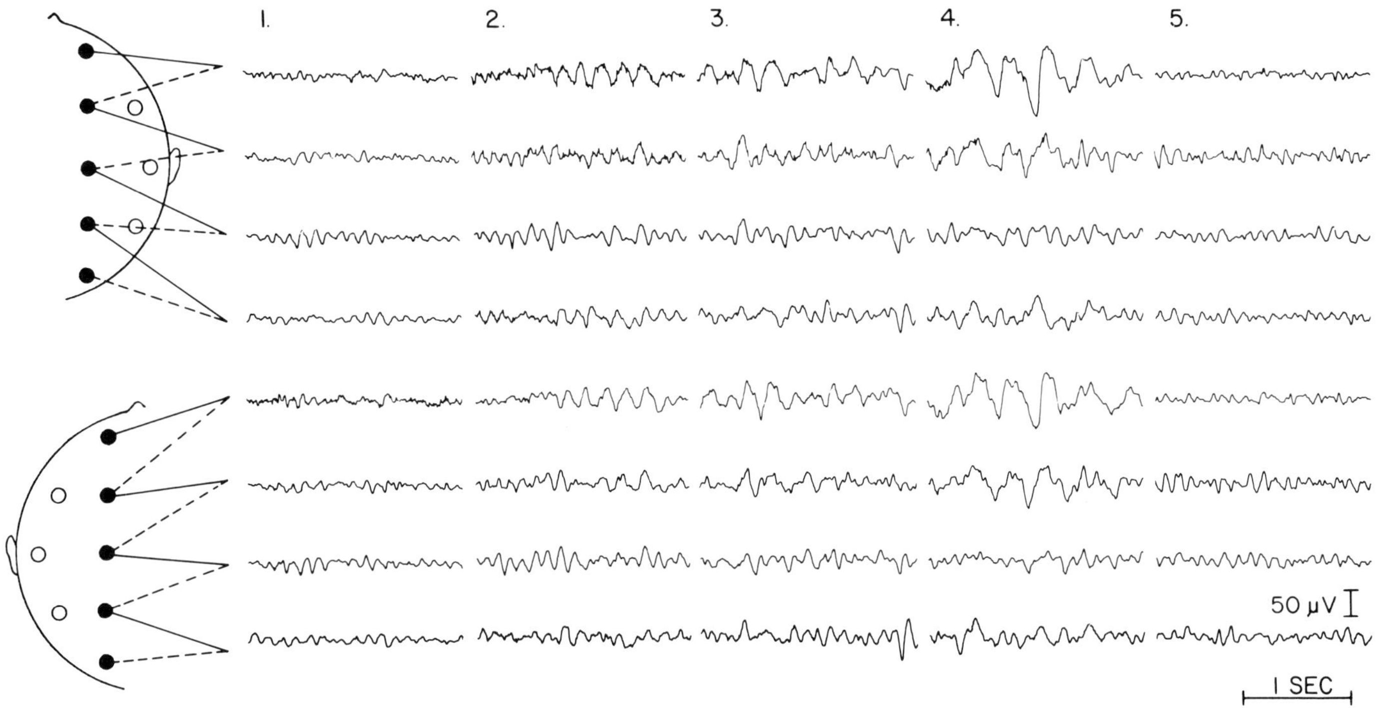


Fig. 14.1. Normal hyperventilation response in 45-year-old subject, 4–5 hours after the last meal. 1. Before hyperventilation: Normal EEG; 2. After 1 minute of hyperventilation: Rhythmical theta waves with frontal maximum; 3. After 2 minutes of hyperventilation: Theta and delta waves with frontal maximum; 4. After 3 minutes of hyperventilation: Fairly rhythmical delta waves, maximal frontally; 5. 1 minute after the end of hyperventilation: Return to initial EEG pattern.

after the onset of hyperventilation (Fig. 14.1). Initially, the slow waves are often intermittent and may appear in the form of bilaterally synchronous bursts containing waves with sharp contours. The slow waves sometimes start as, or often develop into, long trains of rhythmical, bisynchronous, generalized delta waves of high amplitude which may become continuous. Normal slow waves of hyperventilation are not focal or lateralized in distribution even though they may have a maximum in the frontal or occipital regions. The normal response ends within one minute after the patient stops hyperventilating. Hyperventilation is sometimes prolonged by sobbing or crying which develops in some patients during this procedure.

**14.1.2** *The incidence and intensity* of the hyperventilation response depend on age, blood sugar level and cerebral oxygen supply. Hyperventilation responses are most common and most extensive in children and teenagers. They diminish in young adults and are rare in old persons, presumably because of reduced respiratory effort, reduced gas exchange across alveolar membranes or reduced reactivity of cerebral blood vessels. Hyperventilation responses are more prominent in persons having low blood sugar or cerebral ischemia at the time of hyperventilation. This is probably due to the fact that hyperventilation produces its effects by constricting small cerebral blood vessels, thus reducing cerebral blood flow and the delivery of oxygen and glucose to the brain.

**14.1.3** *Abnormal responses* to hyperventilation can occur at any age. Subjective symptoms in a patient's history such as dizziness, numbness, tingling, transient blurring of vision, episodic changes of consciousness or awareness, or ringing in the ears often raise the clinician's suspicion of a convulsive disorder and prompt an EEG examination. The specific symptoms of the patient may be reproduced during hyperventilation. If the EEG at that time shows no epileptiform abnormalities, it is very unlikely that the symptoms are due to a seizure disorder. This is one of the most common and useful pieces of information which can be obtained from hyperventilation. The technician should therefore document whether hyperventilation reproduced any of the patient's symptoms (5.1), and the EEG reader should report the reproduction and state whether or not it was associated with EEG abnormalities (26.1.3).

*An extremely intense or abnormally prolonged hyperventilation response*, especially if occurring in a person after adolescence, raises the suspicion of low blood sugar or cerebral anoxia.

*Epileptiform discharges* may be induced or enhanced by hyperventilation in some cases. Spike-and-wave discharges of 3 Hz are particularly sensitive to hyperventilation and in many cases appear only during this procedure.

*Slow waves* in a wide distribution, if present in the spontaneous recording, may be enhanced during hyperventilation, but they may merge with the generalized slow waves of a normal hyperventilation response and are then difficult to recognize as abnormal. Hyperventilation is more likely to enhance rhythmical and generalized slow waves than arrhythmical and focal slow waves.

*Asymmetries* of background activity may be enhanced and become clearly significant during hyperventilation, or they may become less prominent and reduce the suspicion of an abnormality. Persistent asymmetries of the hyperventilation response itself are abnormal. It may be difficult to determine whether the underlying abnormality is on the side of higher or lower amplitude.

## 14.2 SLEEP

**14.2.1** *Sleep recordings* can help in the diagnosis of epilepsy (12.4.1). Although most epileptiform abnormalities can be found in waking records, recordings which contain a period of sleep can help to (1) detect these abnormalities in some patients who do not show them during wakefulness and (2) discover or delimit an epileptogenic focus in patients showing epileptiform activity without clear focal origin during wakefulness. Foci in the temporal lobes are especially likely to fire in sleep. An attempt should therefore be made to obtain a sleep recording, either spontaneous or drug-induced (5.1), (a) in all patients who are suspected of having a convulsive disorder and who do not show epileptiform discharges in the waking EEG, and (b) in patients whose clinical findings or waking EEG suggest a focal epileptiform abnormality but whose waking EEG does not clearly indicate a focus. Epileptiform activity may occur in any non-REM stage of sleep and is less likely to appear during REM sleep.

**14.2.2** *Sleep deprivation* of a day or more can induce epileptiform activity in recordings made during continued wakefulness or during sleep at the end of the deprivation period. This procedure may be effective in patients with convulsive disorders who do not show epileptiform activity in routine waking and sleep recordings. However, sleep deprivation is used rather rarely, partly because it is somewhat difficult to keep a patient without sleep for over a day, and partly because paroxysmal abnormalities have been induced by sleep deprivation in a few persons without convulsive disorders. However, sleep deprivation should be used in patients who have a history suggesting seizures occurring after insufficient sleep and who do not show epileptiform activity in routine waking and sleep recording.

## 14.3 PHOTIC STIMULATION

**14.3.1** *Normal cerebral responses* to stimulation with flashes of diffuse light (5.1) consist of visual evoked potentials produced by intermittent flashes, and of photic driving in response to repetitive flashes. These responses appear mainly in the oc-

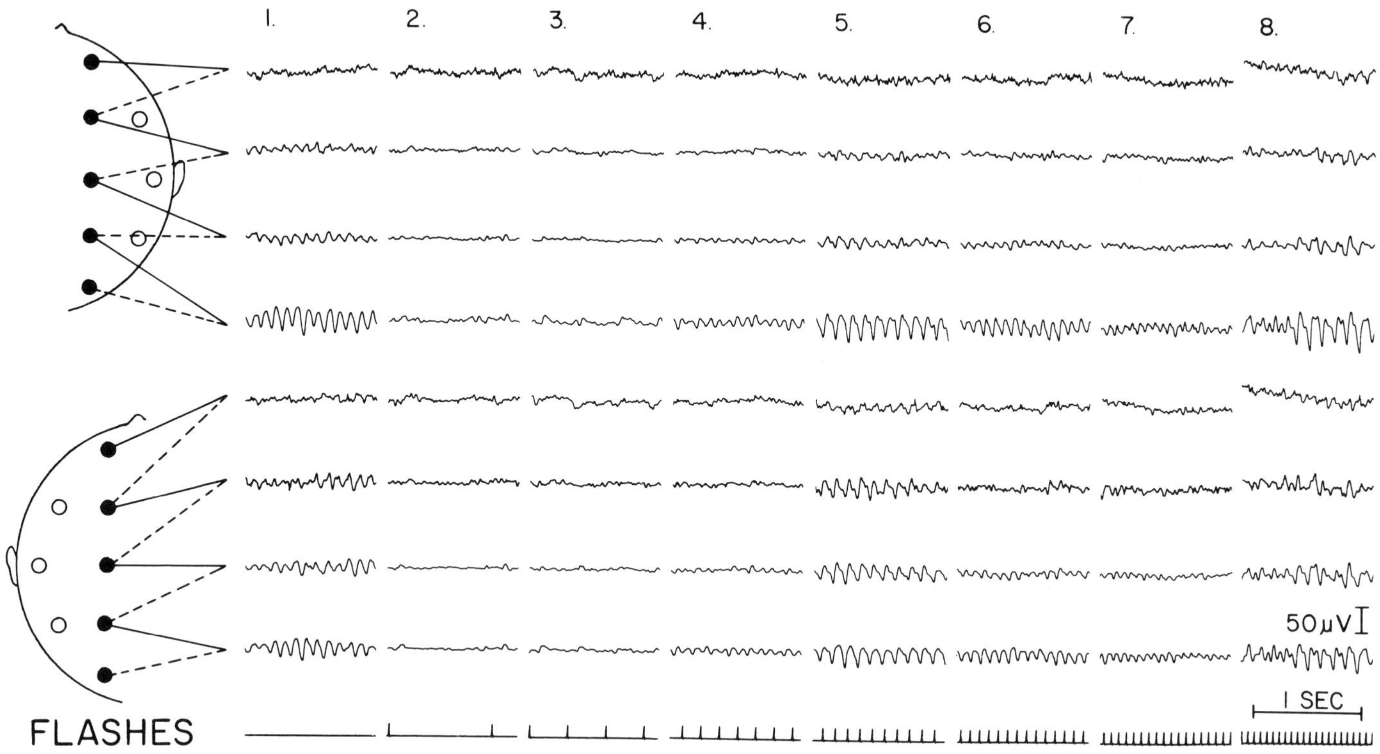


Fig. 14.2. Normal responses to photic stimulation in a 58-year-old subject with closed eyes. Flashes are indicated on the bottom line. 1. Before stimulation: Normal EEG with posterior alpha rhythm; 2. to 8. During photic stimulation at rates of 1, 3, 6, 9, 12, 15 and 18 Hz. Note that the posterior responses have the highest amplitude at a rate near that of the alpha rhythm (Part 5) and at twice that rate (Part 8).

cipital areas but may extend into the parietal, posterior temporal and even more anterior areas.

*Visual evoked potentials* recorded in the EEG usually consist of a monophasic wave of positive polarity with a peak appearing 50 to 150 msec after the flash. When extracted from the ongoing EEG by computer averaging techniques, the potential often shows additional smaller components (7.6.1).

*Photic driving* usually occurs at flash rates over 3 Hz (Fig. 14.2). At these rates, individual components of the visual evoked potential merge into rhythms which consist of some components having the frequency of the stimulus and of other components often having harmonic or subharmonic frequencies. The response may develop gradually and change in amplitude and configuration as the repetitive stimulation continues. The response on one side may differ from that on the other, both in wave form and in amplitude; these differences may vary with the stimulus rate. The largest responses are often obtained with stimulus frequencies at or near the frequency of the subject's alpha rhythm.

While the amplitude of photic driving, like that of alpha rhythm, is often higher on the right side, even a 2-fold difference of amplitude of photic driving on either side is not definitely abnormal. High frequency components of the response may be so prominent as to form spikes as part of a normal photic driving response.

*The incidence and prominence* of photic responses depends on the frequency, intensity, color and pattern of the stimulus, and on the alertness and attention of the subject. Flashes given while the eyes are closed often elicit a response of higher amplitude and different configuration than flashes given while the eyes are open. Responses may appear, change and disappear during continued stimulation. Many subjects show photic driving only at some stimulus frequencies, usually in the range of 8–15 Hz. Driving at high rates is rare in young infants and old persons. Driving cannot be elicited in newborns. Photic responses may be entirely absent in normal subjects even though they can be demonstrated in virtually all subjects of any age by computer averaging of evoked potentials (7.6.1).

**14.3.2** *Photomyoclonic or photomyogenic responses* consist of brief muscle contractions triggered in a few susceptible subjects by flashes given while the eyes are closed. The contractions involve mainly the eyelids but may extend into other muscles of the head, neck and body and lead to rather violent twitching. Although they are usually considered to be a normal phenomenon, they will be described together with the abnormal photoconvulsive responses (25.5.3).

**14.3.3** *Abnormalities of photic responses* consist of extreme variations of response amplitude, or of photoparoxysmal responses.

*Asymmetry of amplitude of photic responses* recorded on the two sides is likely to be abnormal if it consistently exceeds a ratio of 2:1. It may be associated with asymmetry of alpha rhythm in the same area. The question of whether the higher or the lower amplitude indicates the abnormal side can often be answered if the recording also contains unilateral slow waves or spikes and sharp waves indicating the abnormal side.

*A marked bilateral increase or decrease of amplitude*, established by comparison with a control recording obtained from the same subject under the same recording and stimulating conditions, raises the suspicion of an abnormality. However, a single recording showing the extremes of either very high amplitude or complete absence of responses is not abnormal.

*Photoconvulsive or photoparoxysmal responses* consist of spikes and other epileptiform activity (25.5.2). While normal photic responses may contain sharp waves and spikes which repeat at the stimulus rate, remain maximal in the posterior head regions and end with the cessation of stimulation, photoconvulsive responses usually show no clear relationship to the stimulus frequency, often involve the entire head and may outlast the end of stimulation.

## 14.4 OTHER STIMULI

Other activation procedures may be used in cases where episodic symptoms or signs suggest a convulsive disorder triggered by known stimuli and where a diagnosis is wanting. These procedures should be used with caution and with the intention of inducing EEG abnormalities while avoiding precipitation of a seizure. The benefits of the diagnostic information obtainable by activation of EEG discharges must be weighed against the risk of inducing a seizure. Great care should be taken to precisely reproduce the triggering conditions which are suspected to bring on seizures in the patient under study. Many of these triggering conditions consist of very specific visual, auditory or other sensory stimuli.

**14.4.1** *Pattern sensitivity* is characterized by paroxysmal discharges, similar to photoconvulsive responses, which can be induced in the EEG while a patient looks at an image containing visual detail. The triggering mechanism can be further analyzed in terms of visual content and manner of looking. A patient may be sensitive to stripes of a certain width, direction, brightness, contrast and color, but may be insensitive to other, slightly different, patterns. The pattern may be effective only when the patient keeps scanning it, when he switches from looking at the pattern to looking at a blank surface or vice versa, when he opens or closes his eyes while facing the pattern, etc. While the effective stimulus condition remains constant in some patients, responsiveness varies in others. Some patients have seizures while watching television. This may be due to one or more mechanisms, including the appearance of effective patterns. In some cases, television becomes an effective stimulus only when the television set malfunctions so as to produce a flickering stimulus.

**14.4.2** *Auditory stimuli* of several different kinds may trigger paroxysmal discharges in the EEG and seizures. In some patients, a sudden loud noise may be more effective than other startling stimuli. Other patients require more specific auditory stimuli such as a certain sound, a tune, a tune in a certain instrumentation, or a tune played by a certain orchestra ('musicogenic epilepsy'). Certain stimuli may have an emotional impact on the patient, and this may be at least as important for the triggering as the sensory quality of the stimulus. This is probably true of some rare triggering mechanisms such as the hearing of a particular word or sentence or the confrontation with the need to make a decision.

**14.4.3** *Reading* may induce paroxysms through one of two mechanisms.

*Primary reading epilepsy*, also called 'intrinsic' or 'perceptive', is characterized by paroxysmal abnormalities which appear only with reading. Paroxysms occur after a period of reading, have a maximum in the parieto-occipital regions, and are often associated with jaw jerking or clicking preceding a generalized seizure.

*Secondary reading epilepsy*, also called 'extrinsic' or 'sensorial', is characterized by paroxysmal discharges which appear not only with reading but also under other conditions. This form of reading epilepsy may be associated with pattern sensitivity, photoconvulsive and photomyoclonic responses, suggesting that the abnormal responses depend not on the deciphering of the written text but on the photic stimulation resulting from the scanning eye movements during reading.

**14.4.4** *Tactile stimulation* of certain parts of the body may induce or abolish paroxysmal EEG discharges and seizures in some patients.

### 14.5 PENTYLENE TETRAZOL, BEMEGRIDE AND OTHER CONVULSANT DRUGS

When given in sufficient doses, these drugs can induce generalized seizures in anyone. The addition of photic stimulation during administration of pentylene tetrazol ('photometrazol test') often brings out paroxysms and seizures at slightly lower drug doses. Because the effective doses for the production of seizures and of epileptiform EEG discharges under either condition are not clearly different for persons with and without epilepsy, convulsant drugs cannot be used to establish the diagnosis of epilepsy.

The use of convulsant drugs is indicated only in patients who have seizures which cannot be controlled medically and which are suspected of arising from a focus or an area of hyperexcitable brain tissue. Because these patients may benefit from surgical removal of the epileptogenic tissue, the use of convulsant drugs is justified to (a) determine the precise location of the abnormality; (b) reproduce a seizure typical for that patient and ascertain that it arises from a focus observed in the EEG; (c) exclude the existence of additional foci which could continue to produce seizures after removal of a focus seen in the spontaneous EEG or with other activation procedures (17.1.2). While graded intravenous injection of pentylenetetrazol can provide the answer to most of these questions, the technique of injecting pentylene tetrazol and short-acting barbiturates into each carotid artery may be used to study the triggering of seizure discharges by epileptogenic foci in each hemisphere separately. This technique is complicated and requires study of carotid blood flow through each hemisphere by cerebral angiography.

Because activation with convulsant drugs can induce generalized seizures, precaution must be taken to avoid injury to the patient, and diazepam or a short-acting barbiturate should be kept available for immediate injection.

## REFERENCES

Bickford, R.G., Whelan, J.L., Klass, D.W. and Corbin, K.B. (1956) Reading epilepsy: Clinical and electroencephalographic studies of a new syndrome. Trans. Amer. Neurol. Assn. 81: 100–102.

Binnie, C.D., Coles, P.A. and Margerison, J.H. (1969) The influence of end-tidal carbon dioxide tension on EEG changes during routine hyperventilation in different age groups. Electroenceph. clin. Neurophysiol. 27: 304–306.

Bostem, F. (1976) Section II. Hyperventilation. In: Rémond, A. (Ed.), Handbook of Electroenceph. clin. Neurophysiol., Vol. 3D, pp. 74–88.

Chatrian, G.E., Lettich, E., Miller, L.H. and Green, J.R. (1970) Pattern-sensitive epilepsy. Part 1. An electrographic study of its mechanisms. Epilepsia 11: 125–150.

Chatrian, G.E., Lettich, E., Miller, L.H., Green, J.R. and Kupfer, C. (1970) Pattern-sensitive epilepsy. Part 2. Clinical changes, tests of responsiveness and motor output, alterations of evoked potentials and therapeutic measures. Epilepsia 11: 151–162.

Coull, B.M. and Pedley, T.A. (1978) Intermittent photic stimulation. Clinical usefulness of non-convulsive responses. Electroenceph. clin. Neurophysiol. 44: 353–363.

Engel, J. (1974) Selective photoconvulsive responses to intermittent diffuse and patterned photic stimulation. Electroenceph. clin. Neurophysiol. 37: 283–292.

Gastaut, H. and Tassinari, C.A. (1966) Triggering mechanisms in epilepsy. The electroclinical point of view. Epilepsia 7: 85–138.

Gloor, P., Tsai, C. and Haddad, F. (1958) An assessment of the value of sleep-electroencephalography for the diagnosis of temporal lobe epilepsy. Electroenceph. clin. Neurophysiol. 10: 633–648.

Gloor, P. (1976) Section V. Intracarotid amobarbital and pentylenetetrazol activation. In: Rémond, A. (Ed.), Handbook of Electroenceph. clin. Neurophysiol., Vol. 3D, Elsevier, Amsterdam, pp. 121–151.

Gloor, R., Rasmussen, T., Altazurra, A. and Garretson, H. (1976) Role of the intracarotid amobarbital-pentylenetetrazol EEG test in the diagnosis and surgical treatment of patients with complex seizure problems. Epilepsia 17: 15–31.

Hishikawa, Y., Yamamoto, J., Furuya, E., Yamada, Y., Miyazaki, K. and Kaneko, Z. (1967) Photosensitive epilepsy: Relationships between the visual evoked responses and the epileptiform discharges induced by intermittent photic stimulation. Electroenceph. clin. Neurophysiol. 23: 320–334.

Jeavons, P.M., Harding, G.F.A., Panayiotopoulos, C.P. and Drasdo, N. (1972) The effect of geometric patterns combined with intermittent photic stimulation in photosensitive epilepsy. Electroenceph. clin. Neurophysiol. 33: 221–224.

Klass, D.W. and Fischer-Williams, M. (1976) Section I. Sensory stimulation, sleep and sleep deprivation. In: Rémond, A. (Ed.), Handbook of Electroenceph. clin. Neurophysiol., Vol. 3D, Elsevier, Amsterdam, pp. 5–73.

Maheshwari, M.C. and Jeavons, P.M. (1975) The clinical significance of occipital spikes as a sole response to intermittent photic stimulation. Electroenceph. clin. Neurophysiol. 39: 93–95.

Mattson, R.H., Pratt, K.L. and Calverley, J.R. (1965) Electroencephalograms of epileptics following sleep deprivation. Arch. Neurol. 13: 310–315.

Maulsby, R.L. and Markand, O.N. (1972) Use of activation procedures in routine EEG examinations. Spike and Wave, Special Issue, No. 5: 15–31.

Panayiotopoulos, C.P., Jeavons, P.M. and Harding, G.F.A. (1972) Occipital spikes and their relation to visual evoked responses in epilepsy, with particular reference to photosensitive epilepsy. Electroenceph. clin. Neurophysiol. 32: 179–190.

Panayiotopoulos, C.P. (1974) Effectiveness of photic stimulation on various eye-states in photosensitive epilepsy. J. neurol. Sci. 23: 165–173.

Paulson, O.B. and Sharbrough, F.W. (1974) Physiologic and pathophysiologic relationship between the electroencephalogram and the regional cerebral blood flow. Acta neurol. scand. 50: 194–220.

Pratt, K.L., Mattson, R.H., Weikers, N.J. and Williams, R. (1968) EEG activation of epileptics following sleep deprivation: A prospective study of 114 cases. Electroenceph. clin. Neurophysiol. 24: 11–15.

Rodin, E.A., Luby, E.D. and Gottlieb, J.S. (1962) The electroencephalogram during prolonged experimental sleep deprivation. Electroenceph. clin. Neurophysiol. 14: 544–551.

Rovit, R.L., Gloor, P. and Rasmussen, T. (1961) Intracarotid amobarbital in epileptic patients. Arch. Neurol. 5: 606–626.

Takahashi, T. and Tsukahara, Y. (1976) Influence of color on the photoconvulsive response. Electroenceph. clin. Neurophysiol. 41: 124–136.

Vignaendra, V., Thian Ghee, L., Chong Lee, L. and Siew Tin, C. (1976) Epileptic discharges triggered by blinking and eye closure. Electroenceph. clin. Neurophysiol. 40: 491–498.

White, J.C. (1970) A case of reading epilepsy with observations on the effect of sleep deprivation and fasting on EEG correlates. Electroenceph. clin. Neurophysiol. 28: 510–513.

Wilkins, A.J., Andermann, F. and Ives, J. (1975) Stripes, complex cells and seizures. An attempt to determine the locus and nature of the trigger mechanism in pattern-sensitive epilepsy. Brain 98: 365–380.

Wilkins, A.J., Darby, C.E., Binnie, C.D., Stafansson, S.B., Jeavons, P.M. and Harding, G.F.A. (1979) Television epilepsy. The role of pattern. Electroenceph. clin. Neurophysiol. 47: 163–171.

# Part C
# The abnormal EEG

# Abnormal EEG patterns, correlation with underlying cerebral lesions and neurological diseases

# 15

SUMMARY

(15.1) An EEG is usually called abnormal not because it lacks normal patterns but because it contains: A. Epileptiform activity, B. Slow waves, C. Abnormalities of amplitude, or D. Deviations from normal patterns. These abnormalities can be subdivided into a few basic abnormal EEG patterns.

(15.2) The basic abnormal EEG patterns correspond fairly well with a few kinds of cerebral lesions.

(15.3) However, the basic abnormal EEG patterns do not correlate directly with specific neurological diseases because similar cerebral lesions, and thus similar EEG patterns, may be produced by a great variety of neurological diseases. Moreover, many diseases may produce more than one abnormal pattern. The EEG therefore cannot make a clinical diagnosis but can help to select one of several possible diagnoses.

## 15.1 DEFINITION OF THE ABNORMAL EEG

An EEG is abnormal if it contains A. epileptiform activity, B. slow waves, C. amplitude abnormalities, or D. certain patterns resembling normal activity but deviating from it in frequency, reactivity, distribution or other features. In most abnormal EEGs, the abnormal patterns do not entirely replace normal activity: they appear only intermittently, only in some channels, or only superimposed on a normal background.

The most important EEG abnormalities can be divided into the following basic abnormal EEG patterns which are discussed in the subsequent chapters.

A. Epileptiform activity

1. Localized epileptiform activity
2. Generalized epileptiform activity

    3. Special epileptiform patterns
B. Slow waves
    1. Localized slow waves
    2. Generalized asynchronous slow waves
    3. Bilaterally synchronous slow waves
C. Amplitude abnormalities
    1. Localized amplitude changes: Asymmetries
    2. Generalized amplitude changes
D. Deviations from normal patterns.

## 15.2 CORRELATION BETWEEN ABNORMAL EEG PATTERNS, GENERAL CEREBRAL PATHOLOGY AND SPECIFIC NEUROLOGICAL DISEASES

Each of the basic abnormal EEG patterns listed above can be caused by one or a few types of cerebral abnormalities. The abnormalities are characterized by their irritative or destructive character and by their cortical, subcortical and epicortical location. The correlation between EEG patterns, cerebral pathology and specific diseases is summarized in a series of tables and discussed in the subsequent chapters. The four major categories of abnormal EEG patterns are the subject of Table 15.1 – Basic epileptiform patterns, 15.2 – Basic patterns of slow wave abnormalities, 15.3 – Basic patterns of abnormal amplitude and 25.1 – Deviations from normal patterns. The epileptiform patterns listed in Table 15.1 are further detailed in Tables 17.1, 18.1, 19.1, 19.2, 19.3 and 19.4; the patterns of abnormal amplitude listed in Table 15.3 are shown in more detail in Tables 23.1 and 24.1

**15.2.1** *Epileptiform activity* is outlined in Table 15.1. Local epileptiform activity is usually due to a focal irritative lesion of the cerebral cortex; in infants, such activity

TABLE 15.1
Basic epileptiform patterns: Pathological and clinical correlates

| Basic patterns | General pathological correlates | Examples of specific diseases |
|---|---|---|
| 1. *Local epileptiform activity* (Table 17.1) | (1) Chronic local cortical lesions | Cortical scars after strokes and injuries, tumors; with or without recurring partial seizures: symptomatic epilepsy |
| | (2) Acute local cortical lesions | Acute strokes, head injuries; with or without acute partial seizures |
| | (3) In young infants | |
| | (a) Widespread structural damage | Perinatal injury, anoxia, ischemia; with or without partial, uni- or bilateral seizures |
| | (b) Toxic, metabolic, electrolytic abnormalities | Hypoglycemia, pyridoxine deficiency, phenylketonuria; with or without seizures as above |
| | (4) Children without detectable lesion | Benign epilepsy of childhood with partial seizures |
| 2. *Generalized epileptiform activity* (Table 18.1) | (1) No detectable abnormality | Idiopathic epilepsy with primary generalized seizures |
| | (2) Diffuse cortical and subcortical disorders: | |
| | (a) Structural | |
| | (aa) Acute damage | Acute anoxia, head injury, encephalitis; with or without primary generalized seizures |
| | (bb) Chronic diseases | Postanoxic and posttraumatic generalized cerebral damage, myoclonus epilepsy; with or without primary generalized seizures |
| | (b) Toxic, metabolic, endocrine, electrolytic disorders | Hypoglycemia, renal encephalopathy, alcohol withdrawal; with or without primary generalized seizures during the disorder |
| 3. *Special epileptiform patterns* | | |
| 3.1 Infantile and juvenile patterns of multifocal and generalized spikes (Table 19.1) | Widespread structural or metabolic cerebral disease; patterns are more specific for age than for cause | Pre-, peri- and postnatal injury, cerebromacular degeneration, tuberous sclerosis, phenylketonuria, leukodystrophies; with or without partial or generalized seizures |
| 3.2 Periodic complexes (Table 19.2) | Acute or subacute, fairly widespread cerebral damage or metabolic derangements | Fresh cerebral infarcts, Jakob-Creutzfeldt disease, subacute sclerosing panencephalitis, barbiturate intoxication, herpes simplex encephalitis, metabolic encephalopathies; with or without myoclonus |
| 3.3 Ictal patterns without spikes and sharp waves (Table 19.3) | No common pathological correlate | Certain partial complex seizures, tonic seizures, neonatal seizures, absence seizures, epilepsia partialis continua |
| 3.4 Epileptiform patterns without known pathological correlates and without seizures (Table 19.4) | No detectable abnormality | No known diseases or seizures |

may be the result of widespread lesions or of toxic, metabolic or electrolytic abnormalities whereas some children have local spikes without any detectable cerebral lesions. Generalized epileptiform activity is either not associated with demonstrable lesions or associated with a variety of conditions which increase the excitability of subcortical centers, of wide parts of the cerebral cortex, or of both. Special epileptiform patterns have a great variety of pathological correlates.

**15.2.2** *Slow wave abnormalities* and their correlates are shown in Table 15.2.

TABLE 15.2
Basic patterns of slow wave abnormalities: Pathological and clinical correlates

| Basic patterns | General pathological correlates | Examples of specific diseases |
|---|---|---|
| 1. Local slow waves | (1) Local structural damage of | |
| | (a) Subcortical white matter | Strokes, tumors, abscesses |
| | (b) Thalamus | As above |
| | (2) Local disorders of cerebral blood flow or metabolism | Transient ischemic attacks, migraine, postictal condition |
| 2. Generalized asynchronous slow waves | (1) No detectable abnormality in some cases of mild or moderate slow waves | No known disease, in 10–15% of normal adults |
| | (2) Widespread structural damage including subcortical white matter | Widespread degenerative and cerebrovascular disease |
| | (3) Generalized disorders of cerebral function | Acute anoxia, syncope, coma, postictal condition |
| 3. Bilaterally synchronous slow waves | Deep midline grey matter involvement by | |
| | (1) Diffuse diseases damaging subcortical and cortical grey matter more than white matter | Presenile dementia, progressive supranuclear palsy |
| | (2) Local structural lesions which directly involve or compress, distort or render ischemic deep midline structures of the mesencephalon, diencephalon, mesial and orbital parts of frontal lobe | Tumors, strokes at or near the bottom of the anterior, middle or posterior fossa |
| | (3) Metabolic, toxic, and endocrine encephalopathies | Hepatic, renal, hypoparathyroid encephalopathies |

Local slow waves are often due to circumscribed damage of the white matter of the hemispheres with or without involvement of the cortex. Generalized asynchronous slow waves suggest a widespread disturbance of cerebral function, often due to greater involvement of subcortical white matter than of the cerebral cortex. Bisynchronous slow waves are often due to widespread involvement of subcortical and cortical grey matter or to local involvement of deep midline structures; this may be due to structural damage or to metabolic, toxic or endocrine disorders.

**15.2.3** *Amplitude changes* are described in Table 15.3. Local reductions of amplitude are often due either to superficial lesions which reduce the electrical potentials generated in the cortex or to material that is interposed between cortex

TABLE 15.3
Basic patterns of abnormal amplitude: Pathological and clinical correlates

| Basic patterns | General pathological correlates | Examples of specific diseases |
|---|---|---|
| 1. Local differences of amplitude (asymmetries) (Table 23.1) | (1) Locally decreased EEG production | |
| | (a) Structural cortical damage | Cortical infarct, contusion |
| | (b) Disorder of cortical function | Cortical transient ischemia, migraine |
| | (2) Local change of media between cortex and recording electrode | |
| | (a) Increase | Subdural hematoma, subgaleal hematoma |
| | (b) Decrease | Surgical skull defect |
| 2. Generalized changes of amplitude (Table 24.1) | (1) Generally decreased EEG production | |
| | (a) No detectable abnormality in some cases of mild or moderate reduction | No known disease, in 5–10% of normal adults |
| | (b) Structural diseases of cerebral cortex | Huntington's chorea, postanoxic encephalopathy |
| | (c) Disorders of cortical function | Hypothyroidism, acute anoxia, hypothermia, intoxications, anxiety, postictal |
| | (2) Bilateral increase of media between cortex and recording electrodes | Subdural hematoma |

and recording electrodes and interferes with the electrical conduction of cortical potentials to the recording electrodes; a local increase of amplitude often results from skull defects. Generalized reductions of amplitude are due either to a widespread decrease of the production of electrocortical potentials or to a generalized increase of the conducting media between cortex and recording electrodes.

**15.2.4** *Deviations from normal patterns* are listed in Table 25.1. These patterns resemble normal patterns but deviate from them in specific regards, for instance in frequency, reactivity or distribution; some of them correlate with particular cerebral abnormalities.

## 15.3 THE DIAGNOSTIC VALUE OF THE EEG

Each cerebral lesion can be caused by many different neurological diseases. Examples are listed in the right columns of the tables. It is obvious that not any one EEG pattern is specific for any one disease: each pattern can be caused by several diseases. The correlation between patterns and diseases is further weakened by several facts. (a) Many diseases cause more than one type of cerebral lesion and, therefore, more than one pattern. (b) Not all cases of a neurological disease cause an EEG abnormality; the EEG may be normal especially if the cerebral lesion is small, chronic or located deeply in the brain. A disease may also produce EEG abnormalities which are intermittent and so rare that they do not appear during the period of a routine EEG recording. (c) The EEG may be abnormal in some persons who show no other evidence for a disease; for instance, the EEG abnormality may precede or outlast all other signs of a disease.

Because each abnormal EEG pattern can be caused by more than one disease and because some diseases cause more than one abnormal EEG pattern, the EEG alone cannot be used to make a specific clinical diagnosis but can only suggest a set of possible diagnoses. Even so, the EEG can become a powerful diagnostic tool when it is applied to the specific clinical presentation of a case. Like other laboratory tests, the EEG can limit the differential diagnosis and thereby lead to the selection of the correct diagnosis. For example, in an alcoholic patient in coma who is suspected of having either a subdural hematoma or a hepatic encephalopathy, focal slow waves or depression of amplitude would clearly favor the former diagnosis and bisynchronous generalized triphasic waves the latter even though each of these diseases can cause many other EEG patterns and even though each of these EEG patterns occurs in many other diseases.

Even in cases where the clinical options are wider, the EEG may select some of them as being more likely. For instance, an elderly patient with increasing episodes of confusion may have spikes in the temporal lobe suggesting that he suffers from psychomotor seizures; he may show focal slow waves over a frontal area and suffer from a structural lesion such as a frontal lobe tumor; he may have an EEG of very low amplitude and suffer from Huntington's chorea, hypothyroidism, bilateral subdural hematomas or postanoxic encephalopathy; or he may have a normal EEG or an exaggeration of the EEG changes normally appearing with advancing age and suffer from presenile dementia.

In general, the EEG reflects changes of cerebral function more directly and reliably than it detects structural lesions, especially if the structural lesions are not discrete and localized near the surface of the hemispheres. As a result, the EEG has been found to be more useful in the differential diagnosis of some disorders than in that of others. The indication for ordering an EEG therefore depends on the diagnoses entertained in each case. The *diagnostic value* of an EEG is likely to be:

(a) *High* in sudden and rapidly progressive disorders of the hemispheres and of midline diencephalic and mesencephalic structures, for instance in: (1) Seizure disorders; (2) Toxic-metabolic encephalopathies; (3) Coma of undetermined cause;

(4) Suspected cerebral death; (5) Reduction of cerebral blood flow during carotid endarterectomy; (6) Encephalitis; (7) Jakob-Creutzfeldt disease, Huntington's chorea.

(b) *Moderate* in recent or progressive focal mass lesions of the hemispheres or of midline diencephalic and mesencephalic structures; although these lesions are usually more precisely localized by isotope and computerized tomographic brain scans, in some cases they may be recognized earlier or only by EEG. Examples are: (1) Brain tumor; (2) Strokes; (3) Head injury; (4) Chronic subdural hematoma; (5) Cerebral abscesses.

(c) *Low* in lesions below the hemispheres and not impinging upon midline diencephalic and mesencephalic structures, and in mild, old stationary or slowly progressive generalized disorders of the hemispheres, namely in: (1) Cerebellar diseases and lesions; (2) Brainstem lesions involving cranial nerves and long tracts but not the reticular core; (3) Psychiatric diseases; (4) Alzheimer's disease, Parkinson's disease, Wilson's disease, spinocerebellar degenerations; (5) Chronic headaches of undetermined cause.

Even though the diagnostic value of the EEG is generally low in certain diseases, the EEG may be of value in many cases of these diseases by excluding other diagnostic possibilities; for instance, although the EEG in Alzheimer's disease may show only mild generalized slow waves, the finding of such slow waves may help to rule out other possible causes of dementia such as a frontal tumor or hypothyroid encephalopathy. The EEG is often also useful in monitoring the progress of a patient's disease or the effect of treatment. This is true for a wide variety of acute and subacute disorders of cerebral structure and function. For instance, the EEG may help to demonstrate recovery from postanoxic coma, intoxications, metabolic encephalopathy or status epilepticus. It is very important to obtain a baseline recording early in the course of these disorders and before the beginning of any treatment.

# REFERENCES

Goldensohn, E.S. and Koehle, R. (1975) EEG Interpretation: Problems of Overreading. Futura, Mount Kisco.

Kiloh, L.G., McComas, A.J. and Osselton, J.W. (1972) Clinical Electroencephalography. Butterworths, London.

Kooi, K.A., Tucker, R.P. and Marshall, R.E. (1978) Fundamentals of Electroencephalography. Harper and Row, Hagerstown.

Laidlaw, J. and Stanton, J.B. (1966) The EEG in Clinical Practice. Livingstone, Edinburgh.

Rémond, A., ed. (1971–1978) Handbook of Electroencephalography and Clinical Neurophysiology, Elsevier, Amsterdam, Vols. 1–16.

Werner, S., Stockard, J.E. and Bickford, R.G. (1977) Atlas of Neonatal Electroencephalography. Raven Press, New York.

# 16 Classification of seizures

SUMMARY
This chapter differs from those which follow in that it does not deal with EEG patterns. To prepare the reader for the clinical correlates of epileptiform EEG patterns, this chapter gives definitions and classifications of clinical seizure disorders. These disorders have recently been re-classified in a system germane to EEG; a complete account is not yet readily available in current texts and is therefore given here.

(16.1) *Definitions*: *Seizures* are episodes of sudden disturbances of mental, motor, sensory or autonomic activity caused by a paroxysmal cerebral malfunction. *Convulsions* are seizures consisting of violent involuntary contractions of somatic muscles. *Seizure disorder and convulsive disorder* are terms describing the condition of patients who have had one or more seizures or convulsions. *Epilepsy* consists of seizures recurring as the result of a primary and fairly lasting cerebral abnormality; the cause may be known ('symptomatic epilepsy') or unknown ('idiopathic epilepsy' or 'cryptogenic epilepsy'). *Status epilepticus* is the recurrence of seizure episodes at intervals too short to allow recovery of the pre-seizure condition. *Epilepsia partialis continua* consists of repetitive seizure manifestations, usually rhythmical twitching of a limb, persisting for several days or weeks and not forming discrete seizure episodes.

(16.2) *The international classification of epileptic seizures* divides seizures by their clinical manifestations as shown in Table 16.1.

## 16.1 DEFINITIONS

**16.1.1** *Seizures*, in neurological terms, are episodes of sudden disturbances of consciousness, mental functions, motor, sensory and autonomic activity, caused by a paroxysmal malfunction of cerebral nerve cells. Seizures are discrete episodes lasting only one or a few minutes and involving either only a part of the brain or the entire brain. Most seizures show varying manifestations during their course. They may progress from one area of the body to the other, and they may produce one manifestation, for instance a sustained tonic contraction, before another manifestation, for instance a rhythmical, clonic contraction. Seizures are often followed by a transient paralysis of that function which had been hyperactive during the seizure ('Todd's paralysis'). Seizures occurring in the same person usually resemble each other closely. These characteristics in most instances clearly distinguish seizures from other conditions producing episodic loss of consciousness or change of behavior such as syncope, transient ischemic attacks and psychiatric disturbances.

**16.1.2** *Convulsions* are violent involuntary contractions of the body musculature. In neurology, the term is usually limited to contractions produced by cerebral seizure activity.

**16.1.3** *Seizure disorder* and *convulsive disorder* are terms used to describe the condition of patients who have had one or more seizures or convulsions.

**16.1.4** *Epilepsy* describes the condition of patients who have recurring seizures due to some lasting cerebral abnormality. Patients who have had only one seizure or who have recurrent seizures due to transient cerebral abnormalities or to abnormalities primarily outside the brain such as alcohol withdrawal, hypoglycemia or fever are not usually said to have epilepsy.

**16.1.5** *Status epilepticus* describes the recurrence of seizures at intervals too short to allow recovery of the condition which existed before the onset of the seizures. Usually more than two or three seizures occur and form cycles of discrete seizure episodes separated from each other by only brief pauses. The seizure episodes consist of constant or progressively changing manifestations, each episode usually resembling the others. This repetition of discrete episodes distinguishes status epilepticus from epilepsia partialis continua. However, the seizures may be indistinguishable from the intervals in status epilepticus consisting of seizures which lead only to reduced alertness or confusion.

**16.1.6** *Epilepsia partialis continua* is a continuous and rather stereotyped repetition of one, fairly constant, type of epileptic activity, usually rhythmical jerking of a limb or of part of a limb; alertness is usually reduced. This activity may last for weeks or months. Sometimes, it may be interrupted by discrete partial or generalized seizures or may become less violent or more restricted and even disappear intermittently.

**16.1.7** *Reflex epilepsy* denotes seizures triggered by sensory stimuli and other mechanisms specific for each patient (14.4; 25.5.2). Many patients with reflex epilepsy also have seizures which are not triggered by these mechanisms.

## 16.2a CLASSIFICATION OF SEIZURES – GENERAL

The International Classification of Epileptic Seizures is becoming widely accepted now (Table 16). Although not without shortcomings, this classification draws on recent insights into seizure mechanisms and gives a more complete framework than older classifications. Seizures are divided by their clinical manifestations into I. Partial, II. Generalized, III. Unilateral and IV. Unclassified seizures. *Partial seizures* involve only part of the cerebral hemisphere and produce symptoms in corresponding parts of the body or in some related mental functions. *Generalized seizures* involve the entire brain and produce bilateral motor symptoms usually with loss of consciousness. Both partial and generalized seizures can occur at all ages. In contrast, *unilateral seizures* are observed almost exclusively in newborn and very young infants. The manifestations of unilateral seizures are similar to those of

TABLE 16.1
International classification of epileptic seizures

- I. Partial seizures or seizures beginning locally
  - A. Partial seizures with elementary symptoms
    - 1. Partial seizures with motor symptoms
      - (i) Partial seizures with focal motor symptoms
      - (ii) Partial motor seizures with Jacksonian march (Jacksonian seizures)
      - (iii) Partial seizures with versive motor symptoms (adversive and contraversive seizures)
      - (iv) Partial seizures with postural motor symptoms
      - (v) Partial seizures with inhibitory motor symptoms
      - (vi) Partial seizures with aphasic symptoms
      - (vii) Partial seizures with phonatory symptoms (vocalization and speech arrest)
    - 2. Partial seizures with special sensory and somatosensory symptoms
      - (i) Partial seizures with somatosensory symptoms
      - (ii) Partial seizures with visual symptoms
      - (iii) Partial seizures with auditory symptoms
      - (iv) Partial seizures with olfactory symptoms
      - (v) Partial seizures with gustatory symptoms
      - (vi) Partial seizures with vertiginous symptoms
    - 3. Partial seizures with autonomic symptoms
    - 4. Partial seizures with compound elementary symptoms
  - B. Partial seizures with complex symptoms
    - 1. Partial seizures with impaired consciousness only
    - 2. Partial seizures with cognitive symptoms
      - (i) Partial seizures with dysmnesic symptoms (conscious amnesia, déjà vu, déjà vécu)
      - (ii) Partial seizures with ideational symptoms ('forced thinking', 'dreamy state')
    - 3. Partial seizures with affective symptoms
    - 4. Partial seizures with psychosensory symptoms
      - (i) Partial seizures with illusions (macropsia, metamorphopsia)
      - (ii) Partial seizures with hallucinations
    - 5. Partial seizures with psychomotor symptoms (automatisms)
    - 6. Partial seizures with compound complex symptoms
  - C. Partial seizures secondarily generalized

II. Generalized seizures (bilateral symmetrical seizures, or seizures without local onset)
1. Absences ('petit mal' seizures)
   (a) Simple absences (with impaired consciousness only)
   (b) Complex absences (with impaired consciousness and other phenomena)
      (i) Myoclonic absences
      (ii) Retropulsive absences
      (iii) Atonic absences
      (iv) Automatic absences
      (v) Autonomic absences
      (vi) Mixed absences
2. Bilateral massive epileptic myoclonus (myoclonic jerks)
3. Infantile spasms
4. Clonic seizures
5. Tonic seizures
6. Tonic-clonic seizures ('grand mal' seizures)
7. Atonic seizures
   (a) Brief atonic seizures (epileptic drop attacks)
   (b) Long atonic seizures (including atonic absences)
8. Akinetic seizures

III. Unilateral or predominantly unilateral seizures

IV. Unclassified seizures

generalized seizures except that they involve only one side of the body. *Unclassified* seizures is a category to be used only for cases without sufficient information to allow classification in one of the other groups.

The International Classification has eliminated many of the traditional names of common seizure types. The term 'focal seizures' is largely replaced by 'partial seizures' because many seizures with symptoms referrable to a cortical focus also involve subcortical structures. 'Temporal lobe seizures' is no longer used because many seizures with partial complex symptoms of the type seen in seizures originating from the temporal lobe involve other parts of the brain during the seizure, for instance frontal and association cortex, and nonspecific thalamic nuclei. 'Grand mal' is replaced by the more precise 'generalized tonic-clonic seizure', and 'petit mal', often misused to denote any minor seizure, is replaced by 'absence'.

## **16.2b** CLASSIFICATION OF SEIZURES – SPECIFIC

### I. *Partial seizures*

These seizures are restricted to part of the brain and produce symptoms in those body parts or mental functions which are represented in the cerebral areas involved by the seizure.

#### A. *Partial seizures with elementary symptoms*

These seizures produce focal motor, sensory, autonomic or mixed symptoms, usually without change of consciousness.

1. *Partial seizures with motor symptoms*:

(i) *Focal motor seizures* consist of sustained tonic contractions or intermittent clonic contractions, or of a sequence of tonic and clonic movements. They involve the face, one part of a limb, an entire limb or half of the body.

(ii) *Jacksonian seizures* are focal motor seizures which successively involve adjacent parts on one side of the body during a seizure. This march is due to the spread of the seizure activity over adjacent parts of the motor cortex.
(iii) *Versive seizures* cause turning of the body, usually in a direction away from the side of the seizure discharge. They are also called 'adversive' or 'contraversive' seizures.
(iv) *Postural seizures* consist of involuntary changes of body posture.
(v) *Inhibitory motor seizures* may cause a paroxysmal cessation of all muscle tone in a part of the body.
(vi) *Aphasic seizures* are characterized by expressive, receptive or global loss of language. They result from seizure activity in speech areas.
(vii) *Phonatory seizures* consist of vocalization or of speech arrest.

2. *Partial seizures with special sensory and somatosensory symptoms*:
(i) *Somatosensory seizures* produce sudden sensations such as tingling, heaviness, numbness or burning which, like motor symptoms, either remain in one part of the body or march over part, or all, of the side of the body opposite to the seizure discharge in the somatosensory area of the brain.
(ii) *Visual seizures* produce hallucinations of white or colored simple shapes, for instance stars and flashes.
(iii) *Auditory seizures* cause hallucinations of simple sounds.
(iv) *Olfactory seizures* produce hallucinations of odors; they often precede partial complex seizures.
(v) *Gustatory seizures* consist of hallucinations of taste.
(vi) *Vertiginous* seizures cause transient vertigo; unless associated with other seizure manifestations, these rare seizures may be difficult to distinguish from vertigo of other causes.

3. *Partial seizures with autonomic symptoms* are rarely seen in isolation, but autonomic symptoms are often part of other partial seizures. The seizure symptoms

consist of salivation, perspiration, changes in pupillary size, heart beat, respiration or skin color, sexual symptoms, urination, epigastric discomfort or increased gastrointestinal activity. Abdominal epilepsy is a rare cause of periumbilical pain and may be associated with symptoms of partial complex seizures, but this diagnosis requires strict exclusion of local abdominal abnormalities as a cause of the paroxysmal pain. The autonomic symptoms seem to depend on seizure discharges in the insula, the depth of the Sylvian fissure or the mesial frontal areas.

4. *Compound forms* of partial seizures with elementary symptoms consist of combinations of simple motor, sensory or autonomic symptoms.

B. *Partial seizures with complex symptoms*

These seizures have often been called 'temporal lobe seizures' because they usually arise from foci in the mesial and inferior part of the temporal lobe or adjacent parts of the frontal lobe. The complex symptoms generally consist of changes of the content of consciousness which reduce the ability of patients to interact with their surroundings; complete loss of consciousness is not a primary symptom. A variety of other mental symptoms can be seen. In general, patients have no recollection or only incomplete memory of events which occur during the seizure although they may remember simple symptoms at the onset of the seizure such as an awareness of a bad odor. Such olfactory hallucinations presumably arise from the uncus of the temporal lobe and are called 'uncinate fits'.

1. *Partial seizures with impaired consciousness only* are associated with a reduction of awareness which is manifested by confusion.

2. *Partial seizures with cognitive symptoms* may lead to disturbances of memory. Some patients feel and act as though in a dream ('dreamy state'). Other patients become conscious of a lack of memory while some feel that they have seen, heard, or lived through the same situation before ('déjà-vu', 'déjà-entendu', 'déjà-vécu') or that they are strangely unfamiliar with their situation ('jamais vu'). Idea-

tional symptoms include the appearance and persistence of an idea or a thought which is out of context and seems to be forced upon the mind ('forced thinking') during the seizure.

3. *Partial seizures with affective symptoms* may cause sudden, unprompted and seemingly inappropriate changes of affect. Most common is a display of fear. Less common are laughing and crying. Rage is not usually a primary seizure manifestation but may be induced as a reaction to restraining environmental factors. Patients with partial complex seizures are not capable of volitionally directed violent behavior; they may commit violent acts by accident, not by intention.

4. *Partial seizures with 'psychosensory symptoms'* consist of illusions or hallucinations. Illusions include disturbances of visual perception such as micropsia, macropsia and metamorphopsia, somesthetic and auditory illusions. Hallucinations are frequently visual or auditory. In contrast to the hallucinations of partial seizures with simple symptoms, the hallucinations of partial complex seizures consist of structured, recognizable objects and sounds. The patient may believe he is viewing entire scenes or hearing conversations or music; these hallucinations may, partly or entirely, consist of previous experiences.

5. *Partial seizures with 'psychomotor symptoms'* consist of repetitive movcmcnts which sccm purposcful in thcmsclvcs although thcy scrvc no obvious purpose in the actual situation; these movements may seem automatic ('automatism'). Simple movements may consist of scratching, patting, chewing, swallowing, mumbling and lip smacking. More highly organized symptoms include facial, gestural and verbal expressions.

6. *Compound forms* consist of combinations of several complex symptoms or of complex and simple symptoms, which appear together or in sequence during a seizure.

### C. *Partial seizures secondarily generalized*

These seizures begin like other partial seizures. They then evolve into a generalized seizure either suddenly or after gradually spreading to larger areas. Secondary generalized seizures are usually symmetrical and tonic-clonic, but may be asymmetrical and tonic or clonic. The partial onset of the generalized seizure may be remembered by the patient or observed by witnesses; it may, however, be too short to produce any clinical manifestations. A focal onset may be suggested by the EEG in some cases of apparently primary generalized seizures, but it remains an open question whether some, many or all apparently primary generalized seizures are really secondary generalizations from clinically and electroencephalographically undetected foci.

## II. *Generalized seizures*

These seizures involve the entire brain and produce bilateral and fairly symmetrical motor changes; autonomic manifestations may be pronounced. Most generalized seizures begin and remain associated with loss of consciousness. In general, any type of seizure may occur in children; infants do not usually have bilaterally synchronous and symmetrical seizures whereas adults rarely have generalized seizures other than bilateral massive epileptic myoclonus or tonic-clonic seizures.

### 1. *Absences ('petit mal' seizures)*

Absence attacks, formerly called 'petit mal' seizures, usually occur in childhood and rarely persist into adulthood. In most cases they are an idiopathic form of epilepsy and not associated with clinical or EEG abnormalities except during the attacks ('typical absences' or 'typical petit mal'). However, in some cases, absence attacks are associated with a wide variety of diseases acquired early in life and manifested by various EEG and clinical abnormalities which persist independent of attacks ('atypical absence' or 'petit mal variant').

(a) *Simple absence attacks* consist of impairment of consciousness without loss of muscle tone and posture. They often manifest as a momentary apparent inattentiveness, an empty stare, or an interruption of speech or motion. Usually the interrupted activity is promptly resumed after the attack and the patient has no memory of the lapse of awareness. Some patients retain a limited degree of awareness and continue simple repetitive movements. Attacks may go unnoticed unless they interrupt some motor activity or unless a lapse of awareness or memory can be demonstrated (5.1). Attacks are often triggered by hyperventilation and photic stimulation.

Absences may follow each other closely or continue without noticeable pause so that the patient remains confused or stuporous. This form of status epilepticus, sometimes called 'absence status' occurs usually in children. However, a similar condition may appear in patients over 60 years of age, especially in women, who have not previously had absence attacks (Fig. 18.4).

(b) *Complex absence attacks* are characterized by a combination of impaired consciousness and motor or autonomic changes.

(i) *Myoclonic absences* show rhythmical twitching, for instance fluttering of eyelids, head nodding or widespread limb twitching, usually at a frequency of 3 Hz.

(ii) *Retropulsive absences* are associated with a sudden increase of postural tone causing the patient to move backward.

(iii) *Atonic absences* are combined with a decrease of postural tone producing drop attacks similar to those occurring in brief atonic seizures.

(iv) *Automatic absences* are associated with seemingly automatic behavior, for instance rhythmical movements of mouth and hands, which may resemble partial complex seizures.

(v) *Autonomic absences* combine lapses of awareness with loss of bladder control, changes of heart rate, respiration, skin color, perspiration, gastro-intestinal symptoms, etc.

(vi) *Mixed forms* of absences may contain more than one of the components listed above.

2. *Bilateral massive epileptic myoclonus (myoclonic jerks)*

Bilateral massive epileptic myoclonus or myoclonic jerks are brief contractions which involve mainly flexor muscles on both sides of the body and may vary in distribution. The contractions may recur at irregular or regular intervals. In some cases, they are precipitated by photic stimulation. This type of generalized seizure is so brief that a loss of consciousness cannot usually be detected. Epileptic myoclonus, in contrast to nonepileptic myoclonic contractions, is associated with brief epileptiform activity in the EEG. Thus, epileptic myoclonus precipitated by photic stimuli differs from the more common photomyoclonic response (25.5.3).

3. *Infantile spasms*

Infantile spasms are brief sudden contractions mainly of flexor muscles of the limb girdle producing quick nodding or jack-knife movements of the body. The contractions may last for several seconds and they may recur irregularly for several minutes. Akinesia and reduced responsiveness follow the spasms in some instances and are the only seizure manifestation in others.

4. *Clonic seizures*

Clonic seizures consist of generalized rhythmical myoclonic movements which last for a minute or more and are associated with loss of consciousness. These seizures commonly occur as febrile seizures in childhood.

5. *Tonic seizures*

Tonic seizures consist of contractions of the axial musculature of the entire body and produce flexor positions. They last up to one minute and are associated with loss of consciousness.

6. *Tonic-clonic seizures ('grand mal' seizures)*

Tonic-clonic seizures, formerly called 'grand mal', are the most severe form of generalized seizures and are the most common type of generalized seizures in adults. They begin suddenly with loss of consciousness, sometimes preceded by a shrill cry. Few patients have vague premonitions up to a few hours or days before a seizure, but well-described symptoms preceding the loss of consciousness ('aura') raise the suspicion of a partial seizure with secondary generalization. During the initial tonic phase, most muscles of the body contract intensely, causing stiffening and occasional quivering of the entire body, respiratory arrest with cyanosis, increased heart rate and blood pressure, pupillary dilatation, and perspiration. After 10–20 seconds, the tonic muscle contraction gives way to rhythmic twitching which builds up to violent, generalized and bilaterally synchronous jerking movements of the entire body. This clonic phase may result in injury, tongue biting, irregular respiration and foaming at the mouth. The clonic phase stops in about 30 seconds and leaves the patient in deep coma from which he gradually recovers after passing through the stages of sleep, somnolence and confusion. Urinary and fecal incontinence may occur in this stage.

7. *Atonic seizures*

Atonic seizures consist of sudden loss of muscle tone. They may be associated with myoclonic jerks to form myoclonic-atonic seizures.

(a) *Brief atonic seizures or epileptic drop attacks* lead to sudden falls; the attacks usually last one or two seconds.

(b) *Long atonic seizures* cause patients to suddenly lose consciousness, fall to the floor and remain completely flaccid for one or several minutes.

8. *Akinetic seizures*

Akinetic seizures consist of cessation of movement without loss of tone or posture. Consciousness is impaired or lost.

## III. *Unilateral seizures*

Unilateral seizures occur almost exclusively in infants and very young children. Unilateral seizures have the motor features of generalized seizures except that impairment of consciousness and autonomic changes are less severe. Motor manifestations may change sides during seizures ('seesaw seizures') or involve different sides in successive seizures ('alternating seizures'). Many unilateral seizures begin at the same time in the entire side of the body; they are 'primary unilateral'. Other unilateral seizures begin in a part of the body and then extend to other parts or the entire half of the body; they may be 'secondary unilateral'. Primary unilateral seizures may be idiopathic, i.e. occur without apparent cerebral abnormality, or they may be associated with a wide variety of cerebral abnormalities. Secondary unilateral seizures usually indicate underlying local damage. Unilateral seizures can be divided into unilateral tonic-clonic, clonic and tonic seizures, unilateral infantile spasms, unilateral massive epileptic myoclonus, and unilateral atonic epileptiform seizures ('unilateral drop attacks', 'unilateral hemiplegia').

## IV. *Unclassified seizures*

It may be impossible to classify the seizures of a patient if sufficient information is not available or if his seizures are of a type not yet recognized. This category is not for seizures of undetermined etiology.

## REFERENCES

Currie, S., Heathfield, K.W.G., Henson, R.A. and Scott, D.F. (1971) Clinical course and prognosis of temporal lobe epilepsy. A survey of 666 patients. Brain 94: 173–190.

Daly, D.D. (1975) Ictal clinical manifestations of complex partial seizures. In: Penry, J.K. and Daly, D.D. (Eds.), Advances in Neurology, Vol. 11, Raven Press, New York, pp. 57–83.

Gastaut, H. (1970) Clinical and electroencephalographical classification of epileptic seizures. Epilepsia 11: 102–113.

Gastaut, H. and Broughton, R. (1972) Epileptic Seizures. Clinical and Electrographic Features, Diagnosis and Treatment. Thomas, Springfield.

Masland, R.L. (1974) The classification of the epilepsies. A historical review. In: Vinken, P.J. and Bruyn, G.W. (Eds.), Handbook of Clinical Neurology. North-Holland, Amsterdam, pp. 1–29.

# 17 Localized epileptiform patterns

SUMMARY

(17.1) *The patterns* of localized epileptiform activity consist of single or repetitive focal spikes, sharp waves and their combinations with slow waves. Paroxysms lasting less then a few seconds are called "interictal activity" because they generally appear between seizures. Longer bursts of epileptiform activity are called "ictal" or "seizure activity" and are often associated with seizures. The shape of ictal discharges usually differs from that of interictal discharges in the same person. Interictal localized activity is usually restricted to one or a few electrodes, while ictal activity may occupy wider areas or both hemispheres in some cases.

(17.2.1) *Clinical correlates* of localized epileptiform activity are partial seizures. The type of partial seizure depends on the location of the ictal discharges in the brain. Local discharges in motor and sensory areas generally cause partial seizures with elementary motor and sensory symptoms. Local discharges in the temporal areas are likely to cause partial seizures with complex symptoms. The correlation between the appearance of epileptiform discharges and clinical seizures is not perfect. Some patients suffer from seizures but show no epileptiform activity during the EEG recording, whereas a few patients show epileptiform activity without ever having had a seizure.

(17.2.2) *Causes* of focal epileptiform activity in adults are acute or chronic lesions which produce partial damage in a circumscribed cortical area. It is not known why some lesions cause epileptiform activity while other, similar, lesions do not. In infants and children, single or multiple foci may be the result of fairly widespread cortical damage; such foci tend to shift in distribution and have little localizing value. In some patients with focal epileptiform activity, no underlying structural lesion can be demonstrated.

(17.3) *Other EEG abnormalities* associated with focal epileptiform activity may suggest specific clinical correlates and causes.

(17.4) *Grading* of focal epileptiform activity reflects the degree and type of EEG abnormality.

(17.5) *Mechanisms* underlying focal epileptiform activity are thought to involve paroxysmal depolarizing shifts of the membrane potential of a group of cells synchronized by a few pacemaker neurons ('epileptic neurons', 'epileptic neuronal aggregate'). The depolarizing shifts are limited in time and space by hyperpolarizing mechanisms except during seizures when the depolarization becomes repetitive and may spread in area.

(17.6) *Specific disorders* causing focal epileptiform activity are mainly cerebral injuries, tumors and strokes, but also include a wide variety of degenerative, developmental, metabolic, and infectious diseases.

## 17.1 DESCRIPTION OF PATTERNS

**17.1.1** *Local epileptiform activity* consists of spikes and sharp waves which may combine with slow waves and appear at one or a few neighboring electrodes. Local epileptiform activity is divided into interictal and ictal activity (9.1). This distinction is based on the duration of the epileptiform activity. Interictal activity lasts less than a few seconds while ictal activity lasts longer than a few seconds, often up to 1 or 2 minutes.

Interictal and ictal activity often also differ in (1) wave shape and (2) distribution (Table 17.1).

(1) *The wave shape* of interictal activity consists of spikes or sharp waves which are sometimes followed by a slow wave; these discharges are usually intermittent but may repeat briefly with little or no variation of shape. In contrast, ictal activity consists of paroxysmal rhythmical waves which continue to change in shape, frequency and amplitude during the discharge. Ictal discharges often contain components other than spikes and sharp waves. The interictal activity of a patient usually consists of waveforms which differ from those of his ictal patterns. Although the shapes of interictal and ictal patterns differ between patients, most adult patients have only one or a few interictal and ictal patterns; infants and children show a much greater variety of patterns and often have several interictal and ictal patterns. Both interictal and ictal activity may occur in the same recording, but interictal activity is seen much more commonly.

(2) *The distribution* of interictal discharges is usually limited to one or a few electrodes over an area which is often called a 'spike focus', 'sharp wave focus' or 'epileptogenic focus'. Ictal discharges often have a wider distribution; they may

TABLE 17.1
Localized epileptiform activity

| Interictal epileptiform pattern | Ictal epileptiform pattern | Clinical seizure type | Underlying brain lesion |
|---|---|---|---|
| Intermittent focal spikes, sharp waves, spike-and-waves, rarely repetitive | Episodes of repetitive epileptiform activity, usually different from interictal patterns | Partial seizures | |
| A. *Located usually outside of temporal and fronto-temporal areas, in:*<br>1. Motor cortex<br>2. Sensory cortex<br>3. Insula, sylvian fissure, mesial frontal cortex<br>4. Cortex of more than one area | *Located usually in similar distribution as interictal patterns, but may occupy wider area*<br>Patterns include: Fast waves of increasing amplitude and decreasing frequency; paroxysmal theta, delta or alpha activity; no EEG change; | *Partial seizures with elementary symptoms* ('focal seizures')<br>1. With motor symptoms<br>2. With sensory symptoms<br>3. With autonomic symptoms<br>4. Compound forms | Often history or findings of fresh or old local cortical lesions |
| B. *Located usually in temporal or fronto-temporal areas* | *Located usually in similar distribution as interictal patterns but may occupy wider and bilateral areas*<br>Patterns include those in A. above; 4–6 Hz unilateral or bisynchronous waves; bilateral 14–20 Hz waves; flattening of EEG | *Partial seizures with complex symptoms* ('temporal lobe seizures')<br>1. With impaired consciousness<br>2. With cognitive symptoms<br>3. With affective symptoms<br>4. With illusions and hallucinations<br>5. With automatisms ('psychomotor seizures')<br>6. Compound forms | Often no history or clinical evidence for a lesion |
| C. *Followed by generalized epileptiform activity*<br>As in A. and B., occasionally followed by generalized epileptiform activity | *Ictal discharges* begin as above in A. and B., then involve the entire brain | *Partial seizures secondarily generalized*<br>Begin as above in A. and B., followed by generalized seizure | As above in A. and B. |

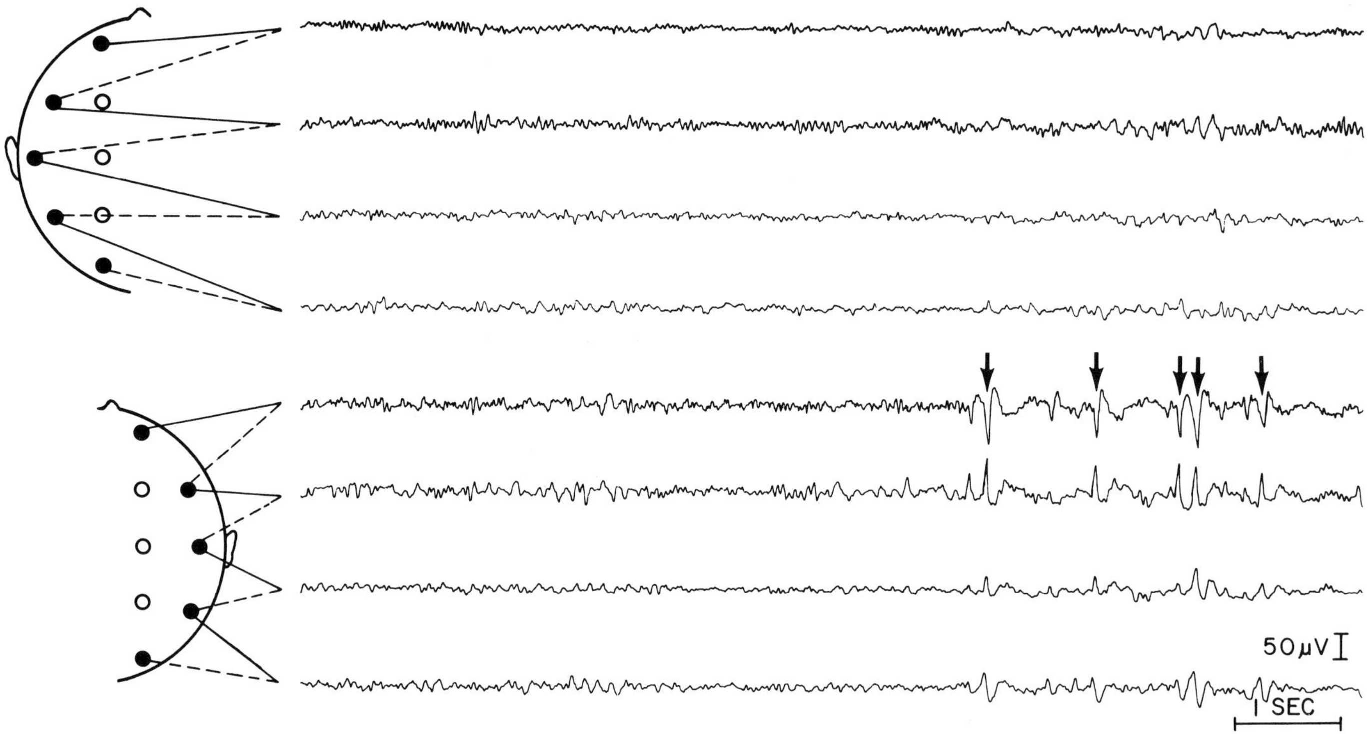


Fig. 17.1. Focal sharp waves in the right anterior temporal region (arrows). The patient is a 30-year-old man with a history of birth injury; for 15 years he has had partial seizures characterized by confusion and automatic behavior.

start at the focus of interictal activity and gradually extend to a larger area or they may initially appear in such a larger area which includes the focus of interictal activity.

It is important to realize that the terms 'ictal' and 'interictal' describe the EEG, not the patient. While interictal activity in most instances is not associated with clinical seizure manifestations and ictal activity is usually associated with such manifestations, some discharges having a short duration characteristic of interictal activity may be associated with clinical manifestations such as twitching. Conversely, some discharges having a long duration and other characteristics of ictal discharges may be unassociated with any detectable clinical manifestations, and are then called 'subclinical' or 'electrographic' ictal or seizure discharges.

**17.1.2** *Specific interictal patterns* consist of spikes or sharp waves (Figs. 17.1, 20.4) which may combine with slow waves to form spike-and-wave complexes or sharp-and-slow wave complexes (Figs. 17.3, 17.4). The major component of most spikes and sharp waves has negative electrical polarity and therefore causes upgoing pen deflections in channels connected to an electrode near the focus through input 1, and downgoing pen deflections in channels connected to such an electrode through input 2 (4.1). Focal epileptiform activity is usually intermittent and rarely repeats to form polyspikes and repetitive spike-and-wave or polyspike-and-wave complexes; the repetition of these elements is often irregular in contrast to that of most generalized epileptiform activity. Some types of focal epileptiform activity which repeat periodically are described under 'special epileptiform patterns' (19.2).

The location of foci remains fixed in many adults but may vary slightly in some. More than one focus may occur in the same patient and the shape of the discharges from each focus may be different. Pairs of foci are often located in corresponding parts of the hemispheres, especially in the temporal areas; they are often called 'mirror foci'. One focus may fire only when the other one fires suggesting that it is

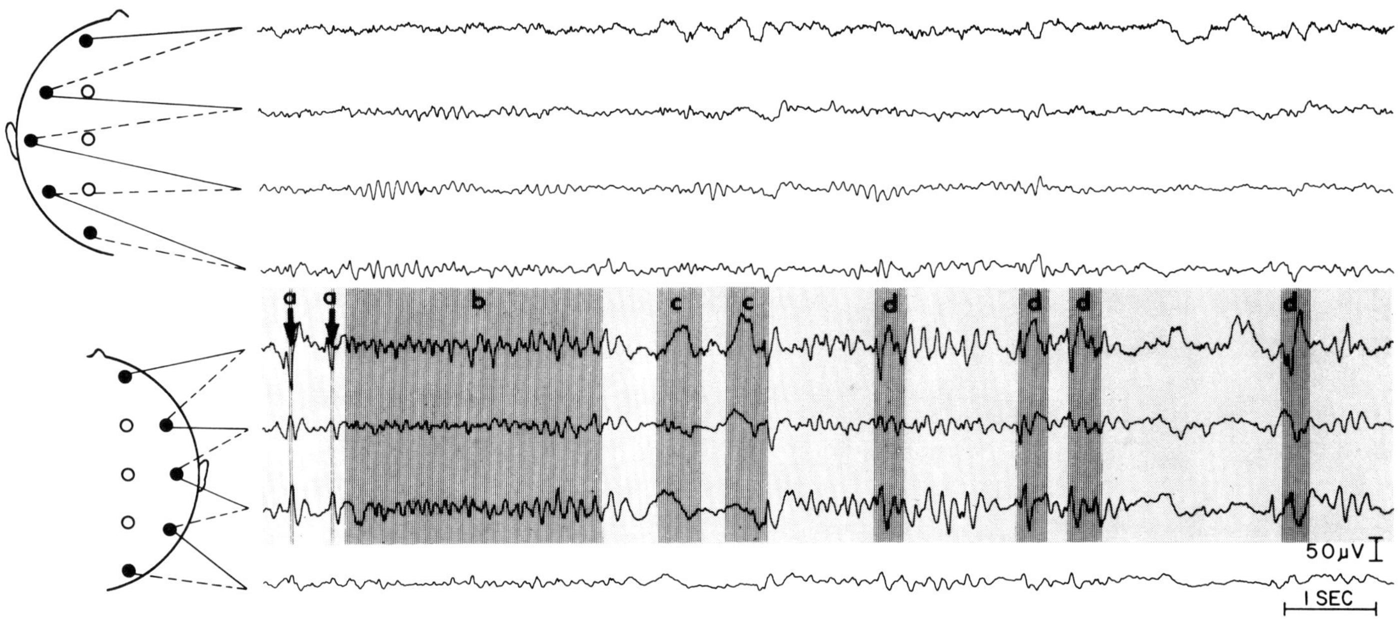


Fig. 17.2. Focal ictal discharge in the right anterior temporal region, consisting of initial intermittent spikes (a) followed by a rhythm of 10 Hz of increasing amplitude and decreasing frequency (b) which is interrupted by slow waves (c) and forms irregular spike-and-wave complexes (d). This short ictal discharge, occurring during light sleep, was not associated with any clinical manifestations. This 57-year-old man had a series of generalized convulsions three days before the EEG recording.

triggered by the other, or both foci may fire independently of each other. Multiple foci which shift location from moment to moment are common in infants (18.2.3) and young children (19.1.1). Foci in older children are slightly more stable in location but may change location between different recordings made at fairly short intervals (19.1.3). Slight shifts in the location of foci are more common up to the age of adolescence than during adulthood (17.6.6).

**17.1.3** *Specific ictal patterns* consist of repetitive waves which, in many instances, change configuration and distribution as the discharge progresses (Fig. 17.2). They often contain spikes or sharp waves mixed with slow waves and form a variety of patterns. Many ictal discharges are preceded by a disappearance of interictal epileptiform activity and begin with low amplitude rhythmical activity which increases in amplitude and decreases in frequency. Only some ictal discharges begin with spikes of the interictal type and only rarely do ictal discharges consist of a repetition of interictal discharges. Ictal discharges end abruptly or with a few intermittent bursts and may be followed by a depression of amplitude and then by slow waves in the distribution of the discharge.

Ictal discharges in adults are generally distinguished from those in children in that they are more uniform among different patients and show little variation in the same patient. Newborn and young infants in particular show a great variety of local ictal patterns. These patterns consist of repetitive spikes, sharp waves, complexes, paroxysmal slow waves or rhythmical waves in the alpha (19.3.5) and beta (19.3.6) frequency range (18.2.3, 25.3.2). The shape and distribution of the waves during one ictal discharge may differ considerably from those in another ictal discharge in the same patient. The discharges may involve an entire hemisphere from the start or after gradually extending from a focus; they may change from one side to the other and become bilateral, but are rarely symmetrical and synchronous.

Several types of ictal discharges can be distinguished (Table 17.1):

(1) A rhythm of small fast waves of about 10–12 Hz which increase in amplitude to form rhythmical spikes; this rhythm extends in distribution and then gradually decreases in frequency. The spikes may then be interrupted by intermittent slow waves to form regular or irregular spike-and-wave or polyspike-and-wave discharges (Fig. 17.2).

(2) Paroxysms of rhythmical focal waves of theta, delta or alpha frequency which undergo progressive changes of amplitude and frequency.

(3) Absence of ictal discharges or other changes in the EEG during episodes that are diagnosed as seizures on clinical grounds.

(4) Unilateral or bilaterally synchronous waves of 4–6 Hz or of slightly higher or lower frequency which often have sharp contours and may appear in one or both temporal or frontotemporal areas, often building up from local fast activity which increases in amplitude and decreases in frequency.

(5) Bilateral fast waves of 14–20 Hz appearing paroxysmally.

(6) A paroxysmal decrease of amplitude or complete flattening which may be the only ictal manifestation.

Ictal discharges of the first three types, restricted to one hemisphere, are commonly seen in patients who have interictal foci outside the temporal and frontotemporal areas and who suffer from partial seizures with simple symptoms. Ictal patterns of any of the types described, especially those involving both hemispheres, are usually seen in patients who have interictal foci in the frontal and frontotemporal areas and who usually suffer from partial seizures with complex symptoms.

## 17.2 CLINICAL SIGNIFICANCE OF FOCAL EPILEPTIFORM ACTIVITY

**17.2.1** *Association with seizures.* Many patients who show local epileptiform activity in their EEG have a history of partial or generalized seizures, and many patients with such a history show local epileptiform EEG activity. However, a few patients showing epileptiform activity in their EEG never had a seizure, and many patients with a history of seizures do not show epileptiform activity in an EEG recording. This fairly loose correlation between epileptiform activity and clinical seizures holds true especially for interictal epileptiform activity which is much more commonly recorded than ictal activity in routine EEGs; ictal activity is usually associated with clinical manifestations at the time of the recording.

*Epileptiform activity in patients with seizure history.* In adults, the location of the epileptiform activity usually correlates with the seizure type. This correlation is fairly good for interictal discharges and very good for ictal discharges, especially those outside the temporal and frontotemporal areas. Focal discharges in the motor area are associated with partial seizures with motor symptoms, while focal discharges in sensory and other areas outside the temporal and frontotemporal regions are associated with partial seizures with the corresponding simple symptoms (16.2) as indicated in Table 17.1. Focal discharges in the temporal and frontotemporal areas are often associated with one or another of the partial complex seizure types. Some patients with focal epileptiform activity have generalized seizures. Although these seizures are usually due to the secondary generalization of a focal discharge, only a few of these patients show transitions between focal and generalized discharges (17.3.2) in their EEG between seizures (Fig. 17.3). Patients with secondary generalized seizures may present with a history of a mixture of partial seizures, secondary generalized seizures and apparently primary generalized seizures (16.2), or they may have a history of only one or two of these seizure types.

In a few patients, focal epileptiform discharges with or without seizure manifestations can be precipitated during the recording by activating procedures including special sensory stimuli (14.4).

Recurrent local ictal discharges are usually seen in status epilepticus but occasionally occur in patients not having clinical seizure manifestations; these patients are said to be in subclinical or electrographic status epilepticus. Periodic discharges of focal epileptiform activity (19.2) or of slow waves (19.3.2) are seen in patients with epilepsia partialis continua; in some cases, the periodic discharges are interrupted by episodes of focal seizure discharges.

The EEG can be of great value in the diagnosis of seizure disorders because clinical symptoms similar to those seen during some seizures can be caused by other conditions, namely syncope, hyperventilation, transient cerebral ischemia and psychiatric disorders. The EEG can make the diagnosis of a seizure disorder likely if it reveals epileptiform activity. The likelihood that a patient's symptoms are manifestations of seizures is further increased if the location of the focal epileptiform activity corresponds with the clinical manifestations of a patient's seizures. A positive identification of clinical symptoms as seizure manifestations can be made on those rare occasions when both an ictal discharge and the clinical manifestations of a seizure occur together during an EEG recording. Conversely, if the clinical symptoms occur during an EEG recording without being associated with epileptiform activity, it is very unlikely that they are due to a convulsive disorder.

*Epileptiform activity in persons without seizure history.* Focal epileptiform activity similar to that of patients with epilepsy may be found in the EEG of a few patients who have no history of seizures. It is possible that this abnormal EEG activity represents epileptogenic lesions which have remained below a threshold for the production of clinical seizures. In infants and children in particular, focal epileptiform activity is the expression of a great variety of pathological conditions which do not produce seizures. A few specific epileptiform patterns, for instance 14 and 6 Hz positive bursts and small sharp spikes, are commonly seen in patients without seizure disorders (19.4).

*Patients with a history of seizures but without epileptiform EEG activity.* Recordings between seizures may contain no epileptiform activity in about half of all patients with a history of seizures even if the recordings include the activation procedures of hyperventilation, photic stimulation and sleep. Both longer recording periods and repeated sampling increase the likelihood of recording epileptiform activity. The incidence of interictal activity is higher in patients with frequent seizures, in recordings made within a few days after a seizure, and in cases of partial complex seizures. The likelihood of recording epileptiform activity does not directly depend on anticonvulsant medication although it may decrease as anticonvulsants reduce the frequency of seizures. The incidence of interictal epileptiform activity varies little with the type of underlying lesion except that metastatic brain tumors are less likely to produce epileptiform activity between seizures than are other lesions producing seizures of similar frequency. Interictal focal epileptiform activity may fail to appear in the scalp EEG if the focus is small, is located deeply in the brain, or has an unusual spatial orientation with respect to the recording electrodes. These reasons may also explain the very rare instances in which recordings made during partial seizures fail to show ictal EEG activity.

**17.2.2** *Underlying cerebral abnormalities.* *Adults and adolescents* develop focal epileptiform activity often as the result of acute or chronic damage to a circumscribed area of the cerebral cortex. *Acute* damage causes epileptiform activity which usually lasts only for a few days. In general, contusions, lacerations or hemorrhages are more likely than other acute brain lesions to produce epileptiform activity, but ischemic infarcts may also be effective. *Chronic* epileptogenic lesions either are stationary, for instance scars resulting from head injuries or strokes, or are gradually progressive, as in cases of slowly growing tumors. In stationary lesions, epileptiform activity does not develop until after a period of several months or years, even in patients who have shown epileptiform activity during the few days after an acute cerebral injury. Lesions in the temporal and frontal lobes seem more likely than lesions in the parietal and occipital cortical areas to produce epileptogenic foci. In some patients with acute or chronically recurrent epileptiform activity, no historical, clinical or laboratory evidence for a lesion can be found, but it is customary to assume that such lesions are present in all adults with persistent focal epileptiform abnormalities.

*Infants and children* react with focal discharges to acute damage which is often more widespread than that which produces focal epileptiform discharges in adults. The widespread involvement of the brain is probably one reason why focal discharges in children may shift from moment to moment and do not reliably indicate a focus of circumscribed damage. Although foci do not shift so rapidly after infancy, the fact that they change location gradually and that many of them disappear before puberty would indicate that focal epileptiform activity at an early age often does not have the same significance in indicating an underlying lesion as it does in adults.

## 17.3 OTHER EEG ABNORMALITIES ASSOCIATED WITH FOCAL EPILEPTIFORM ACTIVITY

**17.3.1** *Focal sharp transients,* which have less distinct and more variable shapes than do spikes and sharp waves (9.1), may be seen in recordings which also contain focal spikes and sharp waves in the same distribution. However, sharp transients unassociated with spikes and sharp waves, although suggesting some local hyperexcitability, are not a definite indicator of an established epileptogenic focus.

**17.3.2** *Generalized epileptiform activity,* i.e. epileptiform activity which appears simultaneously on both sides, is sometimes immediately preceded by interictal or ictal focal discharges in a manner suggesting that a primary focal discharge secondarily triggers the generalized discharge. In ictal discharges, this secondary generalization is the electrographic correlate of the secondary generalization of partial seizures. Electrographic generalization has various patterns: (a) an interictal

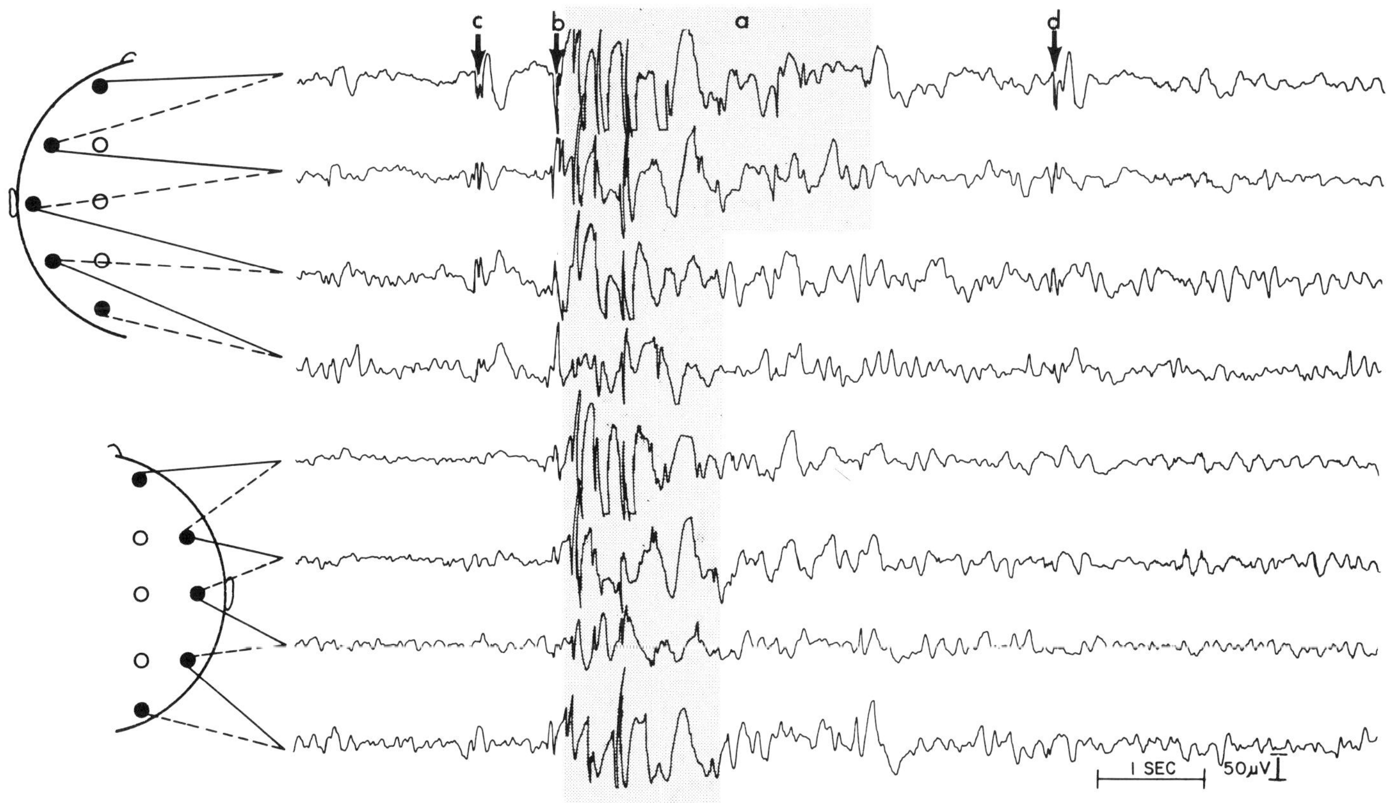


Fig. 17.3. Generalized spike-and-wave discharges (a) preceded by focal left temporal spike discharge (b). Focal left temporal spikes also appear before (c) and after (d) the generalized discharge. This 22-year-old man was hit on the head with a garbage can and passed out briefly five months before the recording; he began to have attacks of being dazed for 10–15 seconds 6 weeks before the recording and had a generalized seizure on the day of the recording.

discharge may be followed by a sudden generalized interictal or ictal discharge (Fig. 17.3); (b) an ictal focal discharge may suddenly change into a bilaterally synchronous ictal discharge; (c) an ictal focal discharge may continue to spread in the same hemisphere, then appear in some corresponding parts of the opposite hemisphere and eventually occupy most or all of both hemispheres. EEGs showing these patterns of secondary generalization must be distinguished from other EEGs showing episodes of generalized epileptiform activity which have an occasional focal onset or which occasionally remain restricted to one area. Longer recording in these instances usually shows that the location of the onset is not constant and that discharges of limited distribution also appear in other areas.

**17.3.3** *Unilateral epileptiform activity* may develop gradually or suddenly from focal interictal and ictal epileptiform activity. This unilateral form of generalization occurs practically only in infants and young children and is one of the EEG correlates of unilateral seizures (16.2).

**17.3.4** *Local slow waves* may be the result of epileptogenic cerebral damage (Fig. 20.4) or of focal epileptiform activity itself (20.6.6).

**17.3.5** *Local reduction of amplitude* of the background in the area of the focal discharge has similar connotations as do focal slow waves except that postictal depression of amplitude usually persists for only a few seconds or minutes after the end of the ictal discharge.

**17.3.6** *Generalized asynchronous and bisynchronous slow waves* may be due either to a recent secondary generalized seizure, to a condition giving rise to both epileptiform and slow wave activity, or to unrelated causes.

## 17.4 GRADING OF FOCAL EPILEPTIFORM ACTIVITY

Grading of epileptiform activity depends on the incidence of interictal and ictal discharges. The epileptiform abnormality is rated *mild* or *mildly active* if only a few interictal discharges occur in an entire recording, *moderate* or *moderately active* if discharges are more frequent and *marked* or *very active* if interictal discharges appear on most pages or if ictal discharges appear more than once or twice. The grading of focal epileptiform activity is less important than the grading of other EEG abnormalities because the incidence of epileptiform activity often does not correlate well with the severity of the underlying abnormality or with the frequency of seizures.

## 17.5 MECHANISMS UNDERLYING FOCAL EPILEPTIFORM ACTIVITY

**17.5.1** *Interictal focal epileptiform discharges* are probably the reflection of abnormally synchronized and abnormally intense fluctuations of membrane potential of neurons in the epileptogenic focus. Microelectrode recordings from neurons within a focus suggest (a) that the abnormal synchronization is accomplished by a small group of neurons ('epileptic neurons' or 'epileptic neuronal aggregate') which send intermittent bursts of action potentials to many neurons in the focus and (b) that the abnormally intense membrane fluctuation consists of a powerful paroxysmal depolarizing shift (PDS) which probably represents the response to excitatory input and is followed by a transient hyperpolarization.

The spread of interictal epileptiform activity in the focus is limited in time and space. Temporal continuation of this activity is restricted by the hyperpolarization which follows the paroxysmal depolarizing shift; spatial extension of interictal activity is limited by neurons at the periphery of the focus which show only inhibition during the interictal discharge ('surround inhibition').

**17.5.2** *Ictal focal epileptiform discharges* occur when, for reasons not yet understood, the hyperpolarization following each paroxysmal depolarizing shift weakens and is overwhelmed by depolarization. This leads to repetitive depolarizations manifested by rhythmical membrane fluctuations of neurons in the focus and by rhythmical ictal patterns in the EEG. Subcortical structures connected to the cortical focus may become involved in the seizure activity and probably serve to sustain it. Failure of surrounding inhibition can lead to the spread of focal ictal discharges to adjacent parts of the cortex.

**17.5.3** *Acute focal epileptiform activity* is produced by various kinds of cerebral lesions. It can be explained by several mechanisms all of which reduce the level of the neuronal membrane potential and thereby increase the tendency of the neuron to depolarize and to fire repetitively. Some of these mechanisms are: Mechanical deformation of neuronal membrane, changes of membrane permeability resulting in abnormal ion exchanges; changes of ion concentrations, especially increase of potassium and decrease of calcium in the extracellular space; ischemia, hypoxia and toxic products paralyzing the cellular metabolism needed to maintain the neuronal membrane potential.

**17.5.4** *Chronic focal epileptiform activity* in adults is usually due to lasting structural change. Because spikes and ictal discharges in a chronic focus usually do not vary much in shape, it can be assumed that the sequence of the underlying neuronal events in the established focus is very stereotyped, i.e. that the epileptiform neuronal aggregate is rigidly organized. The long delay of several months or years between cerebral damage and the establishment of a discharging focus suggests that extensive reorganization of local circuitry takes place during this period. Pathological studies of foci usually show scars of astrocytic gliosis at the site of the chronic epileptogenic focus. However, anatomical, histological, biochemical and other techniques have not so far been able to distinguish between lesions which produce epileptiform activity and those which do not.

The mechanisms immediately responsible for the production of epileptiform activity in the chronic focus include those listed for the acute focus. In addition, several other mechanisms have been considered important in the case of chronic focal activity. Partial deafferentation of cortical neurons may lead to altered sensitivity to synaptic transmitters. Reorganiztion of synaptic connections and collateral sprouting of axon terminals after injury may lead to increased excitation or decreased inhibition of neurons in the focus. Chronic foci without gross structural substrate may result from excessive afferent stimulation, for instance by bombardment with discharges from another epileptiform focus causing a secondary or mirror focus (17.1.2). That an abnormal input alone can generate independent, chronically recurring epileptiform activity is supported by the experimental phenomenon of kindling: Periodic electrical stimulation of the amygdaloid nucleus or other parts of the brain with stimulus intensities insufficient to induce seizures gradually leads to widespread epileptiform activity which becomes associated with clinical seizure manifestations and eventually recurs in the absence of electrical stimulation, i.e. apparently spontaneously as in human epilepsy.

## 17.6 SPECIFIC DISORDERS CAUSING FOCAL EPILEPTIFORM ACTIVITY

**17.6.1** *Degenerative, developmental and demyelinating diseases:*

(1) *Senile and presenile dementia (Alzheimer's disease)* in some patients leads to sharp transients in the same distribution as the intermittent left temporal slow waves characteristically seen in normal older persons. The sharp transients often form complexes with the slow waves. These patients generally do not have seizures.

(2) *Jakob-Creutzfeldt disease* is associated with periodic sharp wave complexes in

many cases (Fig. 19.7). The sharp waves may be localized to one part of the brain for several days before they become generalized. They are usually associated with myoclonic twitching (19.2.2).

(3) *Tuberous sclerosis* often presents with single or multiple spike foci in addition to single or multiple slow wave foci and generalized asynchronous slow waves, especially in children and adults with mental deficiency and epilepsy. Infants with tuberous sclerosis often show hypsarrhythmia (19.1.1) or multifocal independent spikes (19.1.3).

(4) *Sturge-Weber syndrome* is associated with epileptiform activity in about one-half of all cases. Local reductions of amplitude are very common (23.6.1). The epileptiform discharges may arise from one focus, from several foci near the involved area, or from the entire area. They may secondarily generalize or be generalized from the start.

(5) *Porencephaly, microgyria, pachygyria, agyria, holoprosencephaly and hydrocephaly of various causes* all can cause focal spikes although they more characteristically cause focal (20.6.1) slow waves.

(6) *Bilateral optic neuritis* in children, if causing significant visual loss, may lead to occipital spikes unassociated with seizures (19.4.6).

**17.6.2** *Metabolic and toxic encephalopathies:*

(1) *Acute metabolic encephalopathies* such as those produced by hypoglycemia, hypoxia, hyperosmolar nonketotic hyperglycemia, hypoparathyroidism and acute porphyria are most commonly characterized by generalized bisynchronous (22.6.2) and asychronous (21.6.2) slow waves. Generalized epileptiform activity is common while focal spikes or sharp waves are less common and may be due to activation of a chronic abnormality caused by earlier damage.

(2) *Cerebral lipidoses* may produce focal spikes, usually of the multifocal type (19.1).

**17.6.3** *Cerebrovascular diseases:*

(1) *Acute strokes* due to arterial thrombosis, embolism, intracerebral hemorrhage and subarachnoid hemorrhage extending into the brain may cause focal epileptiform discharges, usually associated with focal slow waves (20.6.3), generalized slow waves and amplitude asymmetries indicating recent structural damage. The focal epileptiform discharges are of the interictal and ictal types. Periodic lateralizing epileptiform discharges (19.2.1) are fairly common. Single or repetitive partial seizures, status epilepticus and epilepsia partialis continua may occur at the time of the acute damage.

(2) *Transient global amnesia* may be associated with sharp waves or slow waves (20.6.3) in the temporal areas, presumably as a result of hippocampal ischemia.

(3) *Basilar artery migraine* may be associated with posterior epileptiform activity or slow waves (20.6.3) during or even between attacks.

(4) *Old strokes* can lead to the production of chronic epileptogenic foci several months or years after the acute event. This development is slightly more likely in patients who showed focal epileptiform activity at the time of the acute event. The background of the EEG and the clinical condition of the patient may show little or no residual evidence of the stroke when the chronic focus appears.

(5) *Chronic subdural hematoma* rarely causes focal epileptiform activity in the area of focal slow waves (20.6.3) or amplitude reduction (23.6.3); such activity and partial seizures may, however, develop after surgical evacuation of the hematoma.

**17.6.4** *Cerebral trauma:*

(1) *'Traumatic seizures' or 'early posttraumatic seizures'* may occur during the first 1 or 2 weeks after head injuries of sufficient strength to produce cortical damage. The EEG may show focal spikes and sharp waves which are practically always associated with other EEG abnormalities (20.6.4, 23.6.4). Similar abnormalities may occur after brain surgery. In children, early posttraumatic epilepti-

form activity is more common, more dramatic and more persistent than in adults; multiple shifting or stationary foci (19.1) are a common indicator of cerebral damage in infants and young children.

(2) *'Posttraumatic epilepsy' or 'late traumatic epilepsy'* may develop several months or years after severe head injuries, especially after injuries which penetrate into the brain. Spike foci develop not only in patients with this form of epilepsy but also in some patients with similar head injuries which do not lead to posttraumatic epilepsy. Focal epileptiform EEG discharges and epilepsy may also develop after brain surgery, especially after operations associated with major cortical damage; however, both abnormalities may occur after operations producing only minor cortical damage, for instance the insertion of a ventricular shunt or of stereotaxic probes, although they occur more often after major cortical damage. Skull defects may enhance the local sharp activity (23.6.4).

Posttraumatic, postoperative and other spike foci may require surgical excision if they generate a disabling seizure disorder which cannot be controlled medically. Before surgery, activation with convulsant drugs (14.5) and special recording methods are often used to evaluate the role of a focus in the production of seizures. During surgery, recordings from electrodes on the cortical surface can guide the excision of spike foci.

**17.6.5** *Brain tumors.* *Supratentorial tumors* are most likely to produce a focus of epileptiform activity if they grow slowly and near the cortex. Spike foci are therefore most common in oligodendrogliomas and angiomas, fairly common in astrocytomas and meningiomas, and least common in the faster growing glioblastomas and metastases. Spike foci due to tumors are not always associated with clinical seizures; the association depends on the type of tumor. While seizures are most common in oligodendrogliomas and angiomas, they are also fairly common in meningiomas and metastases and least common in astrocytomas and glioblastomas.

**17.6.6** *Focal epileptiform activity in seizure disorders without known underlying diseases and in normal persons:*

(1) *Benign epilepsy of childhood with rolandic spikes,* also called 'Rolandic epilepsy' or 'Sylvian seizures', is a fairly distinct and common convulsive disorder of childhood which begins between 2 and 12 years of age. It is benign in that it usually disappears before or at puberty. History, clinical findings and laboratory tests give no evidence of a local brain lesion in spite of the clearly focal origin of epileptiform activity and seizures. The EEG shows spikes which are often followed by slow waves and tend to recur at rates up to 2 Hz (Fig. 17.4). They are located in the central or temporal areas and may shift slightly in distribution. They may be present on both sides, usually firing independently. They are facilitated by drowsiness and light sleep. Children with these rolandic spikes often have partial seizures with simple motor symptoms. The seizures are usually tonic or clonic, often involve half of the face or other parts of the body and may consist of speech arrest or pharyngeal manifestations. The seizures tend to secondarily generalize. Seizures often occur at night and may go unnoticed unless they become generalized.

(2) *Normal subjects* may show certain epileptiform patterns which have no clearly proven pathological significance and therefore must be distinguished from other epileptiform activity (19.4).

**17.6.7** *Infectious diseases:*

(1) *Meningitis and encephalitis* produce focal spikes only rarely in adults. Because infants are likely to react to widespread cerebral damage with focal spikes, such spikes may be seen in neonatal meningitis, syphilis and cytomegalic inclusion body disease; they may be associated with partial, unilateral or generalized seizures.

(2) *Cerebral abscesses* rarely produce interictal or ictal focal epileptiform abnormalities in adults.

(3) *Thrombophlebitis* of the cerebral venous sinus systems can produce focal or

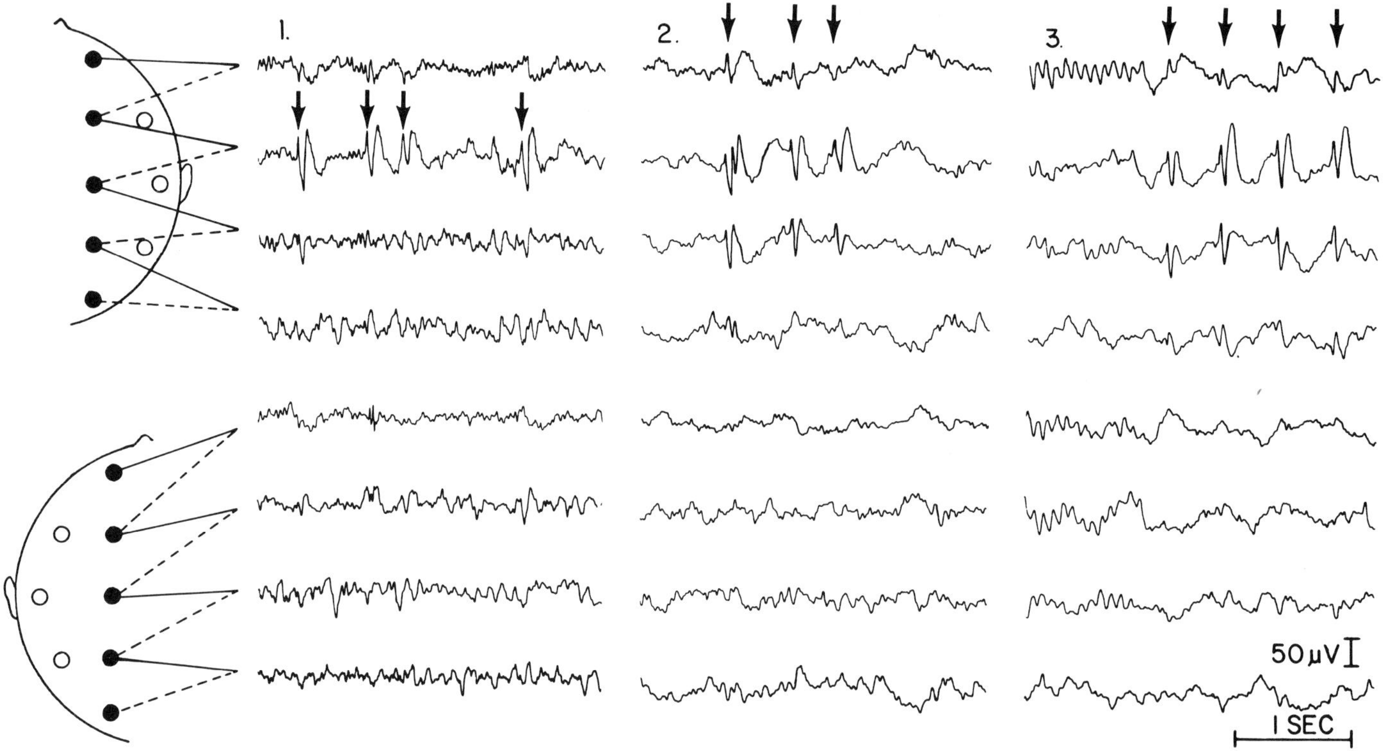


Fig. 17.4. Spikes (arrows), usually followed by slow waves and repeating in brief bursts at 1–2 Hz in the right fronto-central regions ('Rolandic spikes'). 1. Awake: Spikes limited to the area between frontal and central electrode; 2. Light sleep: Slightly wider distribution and occasional polyphasic spikes; 3. Deeper sleep: Widest distribution. This 6-year-old girl had her first seizure a few hours before the EEG recording. The seizure began in the left side of the face and then generalized. History, clinical examination and other test results were normal.

unilateral spikes in addition to decreased amplitude and slow waves. Septic phlebitis of the lateral or cavernous sinus may lead to the syndrome of hemiconvulsions, hemiplegia and epilepsy (HHE syndrome) in children. The acute phase of this syndrome is characterized by long-lasting and repetitive seizures of unilateral onset; this phase may be followed by epilepsy with partial complex seizures at a later age.

(4) *Herpes simplex encephalitis* often leads to periodic sharp waves in the temporal regions (19.2.5).

(5) *Subacute sclerosing panencephalitis* is usually associated with periodic sharp wave complexes which may begin locally (19.2.3).

(6) *Sydenham's chorea* may be associated with local spikes in some cases, although generalized asynchronous slow waves are more common (21.6.7).

**17.6.8** *Psychiatric diseases. Behavior disorders and episodic psychotic or psychopathic behavior in children* have been found in association with focal spikes, especially in the temporal lobes, in many patients with these disorders. However, because the relationship between spike foci and the psychiatric abnormalities is unclear, focal cerebral lesions must be searched for in these patients.

## REFERENCES


Ajmone Marsan, C. and Zivin, L.S. (1970) Factors related to the occurrence of typical paroxysmal abnormalities in the EEG records of epileptic patients. Epilepsia 11: 361–381.

Beaussart, M. (1972) Benign epilepsy of children with Rolandic (centro-temporal) paroxysmal foci. A clinical entity. Study of 221 cases. Epilepsia 13: 795–811.

Binnie, C.D., Batchelor, B.G., Gainsborough, A.J., Lloyd, D.S.L., Smith, D.M. and Smith, G.F. (1979) Visual and computer-assisted assessment of the EEG in epilepsy of late onset. Electroenceph. clin. Neurophysiol. 47: 102–107.

Camfield, P.R., Metrakos, K. and Andermann, F. (1978) Basilar artery migraine, seizures, and severe epileptiform EEG abnormalities. Neurology 28: 584–588.

Falconer, M.A. (1974) Mesial temporal (Ammon's horn) sclerosis as a common cause of epilepsy. Aetiology, treatment, and prevention. Lancet 2: 767–770.
Gastaut, H., Poirier, F., Payan, H., Salamon, G., Toga, M. and Vigouroux, M. (1960) H.H.E. syndrome: Hemiconvulsions, hemiplegia, epilepsy. Epilepsia 1: 418–447.
Geier, S., Bancaud, J., Talairach, J., Bonis, A., Szikla, G. and Enjelvin, M. (1977) The seizures of frontal lobe epilepsy. A study of clinical manifestations. Neurology 27: 951–958.
Geiger, L.R. and Harner, R.N. (1978) EEG patterns at the time of focal seizure onset. Arch. Neurol. 35: 276–286.
Jennett, B. (1975) Epilepsy After Non-Missile Head Injuries. 2nd Ed., William Heinemann Medical Books, Chicago.
Jensen, I. and Klinken, L. (1976) Temporal lobe epilepsy and neuropathology. Acta Neurol. Scand. 54: 391–414.
King, D.W. and Ajmone Marsan, C. (1977) Clinical features and ictal patterns in epileptic patients with EEG temporal lobe foci. Ann. Neurol. 2: 138–147.
Klass, D.W. (1975) Electroencephalographic manifestations of complex partial seizures. In: Penry, J.K. and Daly, D.D. (Eds.), Advances in Neurology, Vol. 11, Raven Press, New York, pp. 113–140.
Lerman, P. and Kivity, S. (1975) Benign focal epilepsy of childhood. Arch. Neurol. 32: 261–264.
Ludwig, B.I. and Ajmone Marsan, C. (1975) Clinical ictal patterns in epileptic patients with occipital electroencephalographic foci. Neurology 25: 463–471.
Markand, O.N., Wheeler, G.L. and Pollack, S.L. (1978) Complex partial status epilepticus (psychomotor status). Neurology 28: 189–196.
Michel, B., Gastaut, J.L. and Bianchi, L. (1979) Electroencephalographic cranial computerized tomographic correlates in brain abscess. Electroenceph. clin. Neurophysiol. 46: 256–273.
Prince, D.A. (1978) Neurophysiology of epilepsy. Ann. Rev. Neurosci. 1: 395–415.
Purpura, D.P., Penry, J.K. and Walter, R.D., eds. (1975) Neurosurgical Management of the Epilepsies. Advances in Neurology, Vol. 8, Raven Press, New York.
Scheibel, M.E., Crandall, P.H. and Scheibel, A.B. (1974) The hippocampal-dentate complex in temporal lobe epilepsy. Epilepsia 15: 55–80.
Schwartzkroin, P.A. and Wyler, A.R. (1980) Mechanisms underlying epileptiform burst discharge. Ann. Neurol. 7: 95–107.
Swanson, J.W. and Vick, N.A. (1978) Basilar artery migraine. Neurology 28: 782–786.
Trojaborg, W. (1968) Changes of spike foci in children. In: Kellaway, P. and Petersén, I. (Eds.), Clinical Electroencephalography of Children. Stockholm, Almqvist and Wiksell, pp. 213–225.
van der Drift, J.H.A. (1957) The Significance of Electroencephalography for the Diagnosis and Localization of Cerebral Tumours. Stenfert Kroese, Leiden.
Walker, E.A., Caveness, W.F. and Critchley, M. (1969) The Late Effects of Head Injury. Thomas, Springfield.
Zivin, L. and Ajmone-Marsan, C. (1968) Incidence and prognostic significance of 'epileptiform' activity in the EEG of non-epileptic subjects. Brain 91: 751–778.

# Generalized epileptiform patterns

SUMMARY

(18.1) *The patterns* of generalized epileptiform activity (Table 18.1) differ from those of focal epileptiform activity in that they appear over most or all parts of both hemispheres and usually have similar shape, amplitude and timing in corresponding areas. Generalized discharges resemble focal ones in that they consist of sharp waves, spikes, polyspikes and their combinations with slow waves. Generalized interictal discharges, more commonly than local interictal discharges, consist of brief repetitive discharges, often of spike-and-wave complexes, at regular intervals. Generalized ictal patterns consist either of longer repetitions of interictal patterns, or of patterns containing different, progressively changing elements.

(18.2.1) *Clinical correlates* of generalized epileptiform activity (Table 18.1) are generalized seizures. There is some correspondence between the type of seizure and the type of ictal discharge. Like patients with partial seizures and focal epileptiform discharges, many patients with a history of generalized seizures have normal EEGs whereas others have generalized epileptiform activity in their EEG without having had any seizures.

(18.2.2) *Causes* of generalized epileptiform activity cannot be found in a large portion of patients, especially those who have symmetrical and synchronous epileptiform activity and no other EEG and clinical abnormalities; such patients are said to have idiopathic epilepsy. Other patients have epilepsy as a manifestation of widespread, lasting cerebral diseases which cause other clinical and EEG abnormalities as well. Another group of patients, not usually said to have epilepsy, have generalized epileptiform discharges, with or without generalized seizures, as a result of transient cerebral diseases or as the result of toxic, metabolic or other primary extracerebral disorders.

(18.3) *Other EEG abnormalities* do not usually occur in patients with idiopathic epilepsy. The appearance of other EEG abnormalities may therefore indicate underlying cerebral or extracerebral pathology.

(18.4) *Grading* of generalized epileptiform activity is similar to that of focal epileptiform activity (17.4).

(18.5) *Mechanisms* underlying generalized epileptiform discharges are poorly understood. An increased familial incidence of epilepsy in patients with primary generalized seizures suggests a hereditary predisposition. The widespread and bilaterally synchronous appearance of epileptiform activity may be secondary to the action of a central, subcortical, pacemaker ('centrencephalic' or 'primary subcortical' seizures) which may be activated by a focal abnormality in at least some cases. In other cases, generalized epileptiform activity is due to a diffuse cortical abnormality.

(18.6) *Specific disorders* causing generalized epileptiform activity include degenerative, metabolic and toxic, vascular and inflammatory disorders which involve large parts of the brain.

## **18.1** DESCRIPTION OF PATTERNS

**18.1.1** *Generalized epileptiform activity* differs from focal epileptiform activity mainly in distribution and slightly in configuration. It appears over corresponding parts of both hemispheres or the entire head. The waveforms usually have similar configuration, symmetrical amplitude, simultaneous onset and synchronous timing in corresponding parts of the two hemispheres, but may differ slightly in different parts of the same hemisphere. In many patients, the epileptiform discharges at some times have a higher amplitude or are apparent only in one area of the brain, but discharges with local predominance are usually transient and may be followed by discharges having greater prominence in other areas. In other patients, generalized discharges begin consistently in the same area and often have higher amplitude and greater persistence in that area. These generalized discharges with focal emphasis suggest a focal origin of the generalized discharges, but this remains unproven unless focal discharges either consistently precede the generalized discharges or appear independent of the generalized discharges.

Like localized epileptiform activity, generalized discharges usually contain spikes and sharp waves, often in combination with slow waves, and can be divided into interictal activity lasting less than a few seconds and ictal activity which lasts longer (Table 18.1). Generalized interictal discharges, in contrast to localized interictal discharges, often consist of spike-and-wave and other complexes which repeat at regular rates. Generalized ictal discharges, more often than focal ictal discharges, consist of long repetitions of interictal patterns. The shape of generalized ictal

TABLE 18.1
Generalized epileptiform activity

| Interictal epileptiform pattern | Ictal epileptiform pattern | Clinical seizure type | Underlying brain lesion |
|---|---|---|---|
| Usually complexes of spike-and-waves or polyspike-and-waves, often repetitive; rarely single spikes and sharp waves | Episodes of prolonged activity of interictal type or of progressively changing activity | Generalized seizures | Unknown ('idiopathic') or widespread structural or metabolic diseases |
| 1. Three hertz spike-and-waves or polyspike-and-waves, symmetrical and synchronous | Same as interictal pattern, but longer | *Absences* ('petit mal seizures')[a] | Unknown |
| 2. Polyspike-and-waves, spike-and-waves, mono- and polyphasic sharp waves | Same as interictal, but repetitive | Bilateral massive epileptic myoclonus[a,c] | Unknown or widespread structural or metabolic diseases |
| 3. Hypsarrhythmia and other patterns (Table 19.1) | (Table 19.1) | Infantile spasms[b] | As above |
| 4. Spike-and-waves or polyspike-and-waves | Mixture of fast waves of over 10 Hz and slow waves with occasional spike-and-wave patterns | Clonic seizures[a] | As above |
| 5. Slow spike-and-waves and other patterns (Table 19.1) | Rhythm of 10 Hz or more with increasing amplitude and decreasing frequency | Tonic seizures[b] | As above |
| 6. Spike-and-waves or polyspike-and-waves | Rhythm of 10 Hz or more with increasing amplitude and decreasing frequency, later interrupted by slow waves | *Tonic clonic seizures*[a] ('grand mal seizures') | As above |
| 7a. Polyspike-and-waves or spike-and-waves | Polyspike-and-waves | Brief atonic seizures (epileptic drop attacks) | As above |
| 7b. Polyspike-and-waves, spike-and-waves | Mixed fast and slow waves with occasional spike-and-wave patterns | Long atonic seizures[a] (incl. atonic absences) | As above |
| 8. Polyspike-and-waves | Mixed fast and slow waves with occasional spike-and-wave patterns | Akinetic seizures[a] | As above |

[a] Also occur with special infantile patterns (Table 19.1).
[b] Usually occur with special infantile patterns (Table 19.1).
[c] Also occur with periodic complexes (Table 19.2).

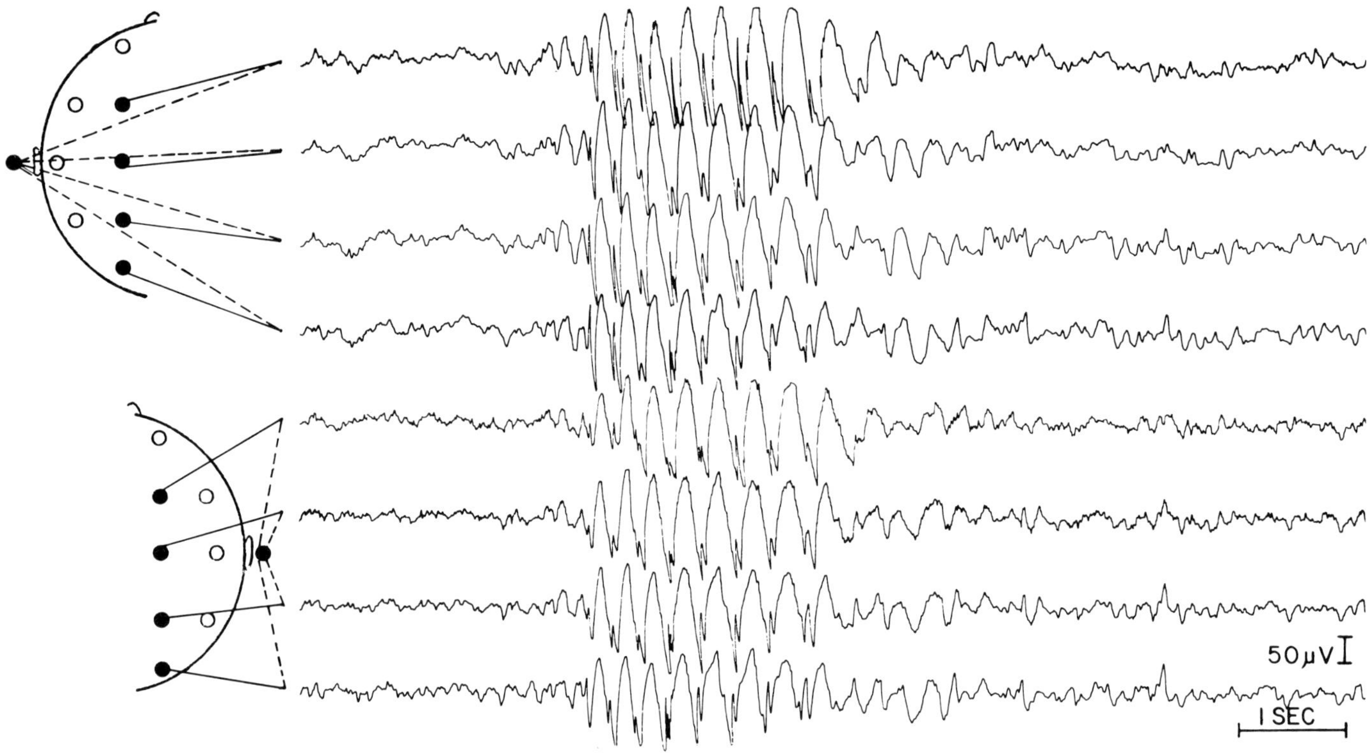


Fig. 18.1. Interictal generalized 3 Hz spike-and-wave discharge, unassociated with clinical manifestations; the patient remembered a test word given during the discharge. This 22-year-old woman has a history of absence attacks since age 12 and of generalized tonic-clonic seizures since age 18.

patterns is of greater clinical importance than that of localized ictal patterns because it correlates fairly well with clinical seizure type whereas the correlation between generalized interictal discharges and seizure types is poor.

**18.1.2** *Interictal patterns:*

(1) *3 Hz spike-and-wave discharges,* formerly called 'petit mal pattern', consist of complexes containing a spike of high amplitude followed by a slow wave. The spike-and-wave complexes repeat at a frequency of about 3 Hz (Fig. 18.1). The slow wave usually immediately follows the spike, but the spike may be superimposed on various parts of the slow wave and the time relation between spike and wave may differ in different derivations and may shift during the same discharge. Although the frequency is constant in most cases, some bursts begin at rates of 3–4 Hz and end at 2–3 Hz.

The discharges may have a frontal maximum, showing phase reversal in bipolar recordings from anterior-posterior electrode chains. The background may contain bisynchronous slow wave bursts at 3 Hz resembling 3 Hz spike-and-wave complexes without spikes. Other abnormalities of the background are very uncommon. Three hertz spike-and-wave discharges are usually facilitated by hyperventilation and often precipitated by photic stimulation. The sleep record often shows complexes of polyspikes which are separated from each other by smaller slow waves than those in paroxysms of the waking record (Fig. 18.2); these complexes may or may not repeat at 3 Hz. During wakefulness, polyspikes may also replace single spikes intermittently in 3 Hz spike-and-wave complexes. However, if all interictal complexes show polyspikes, the pattern is more appropriately classified as polyspike-and-wave complexes (see below).

(2) *Spike-and-wave and polyspike-and-wave discharges* often differ from the classical 3 Hz spike-and-wave pattern by being less regular or having different frequency. The frequency of spikes may vary in a burst or between bursts (Fig.

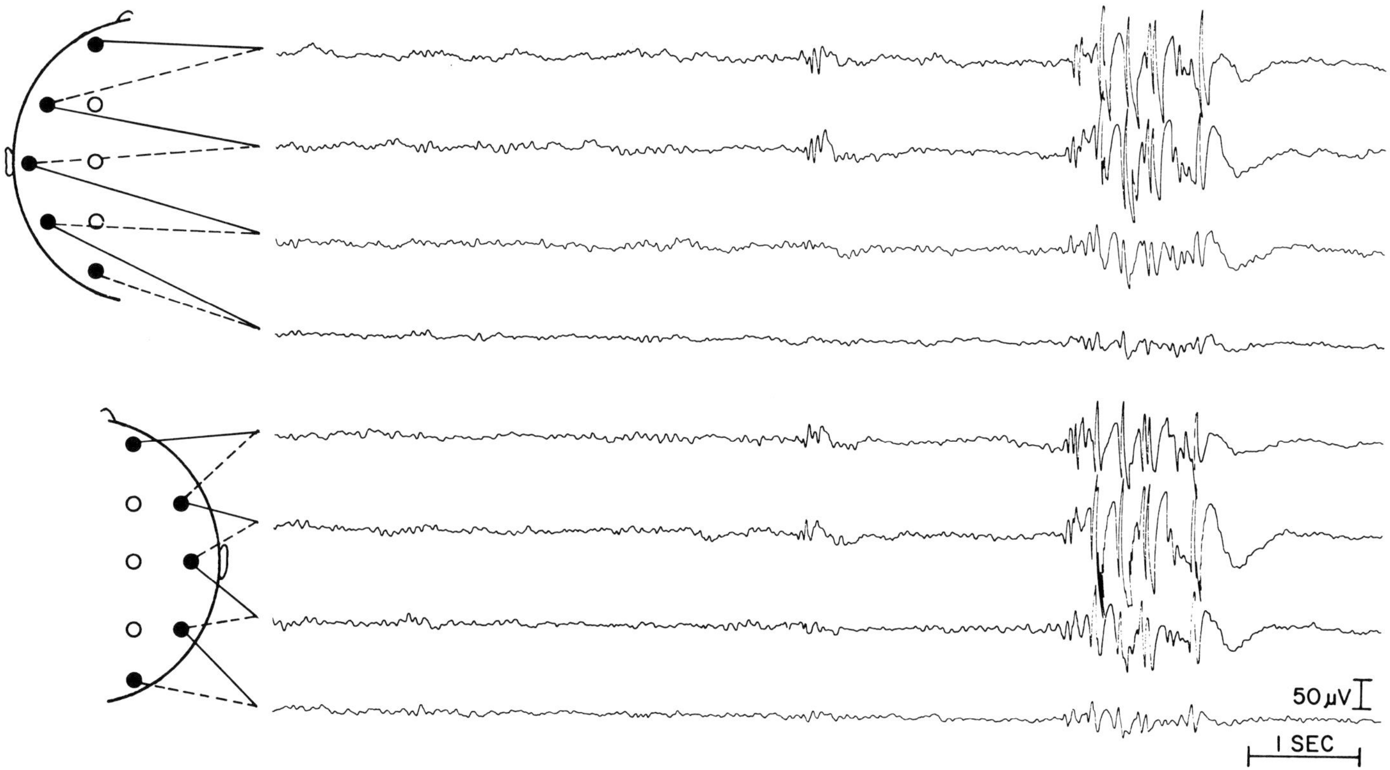


Fig. 18.2. Paroxysm of generalized 3–4 Hz spike-and-wave and polyspike-and-wave complexes during light sleep. Same patient as in Fig. 18.1.

18.3). If the frequency reaches 6 Hz (Fig. 18.3, Part 2), these complexes must be distinguished from 6 Hz spike-and-slow-wave discharges (19.4.1) which are smaller, shorter lasting and usually not widely distibuted (Fig. 19.10).

(3) *Slow spike-and-wave discharges* (Fig. 19.3) are similar to the 3 Hz spike-and-wave complexes except that (a) they repeat at rates of less than 3 Hz, usually at 1.5–2.5 Hz; (b) the first component may be a sharp wave rather than a spike in which case the discharges are called 'sharp-and-slow-wave complexes'; (c) the discharges may have focal preponderance or consistently focal onset in one area; (d) they are usually not facilitated by hyperventilation. The pattern of slow spike-and-wave discharges is discussed in the next chapter (19.1.2).

(4) *Hypsarrhythmia* is described in the next chapter (19.1.1).

(5) *Intermittent spikes, polyspikes and sharp waves* occur either sporadically as rudiments of other interictal patterns or periodically as elements of periodic complexes (19.2). These elements are seen much less often as interictal generalized epileptiform activity than as interictal focal epileptiform activity.

**18.1.3** *Ictal patterns* are of many different types (Table 18.1). Some of the more common patterns have fairly reliable associations with clinical seizure types. The most common ictal patterns are described below.

(1) *3 Hz spike-and-wave discharges* are repetitions of the interictal 3 Hz spike-and-wave pattern and last more than a few seconds. Most patients with this ictal pattern have the same interictal pattern, but not all patients with interictal 3 Hz spike-and-wave discharges show this ictal pattern. Patients having ictal 3 Hz discharges almost always suffer from absence attacks. Patients in absence status show less regular spike-and-wave complexes, sometimes polyspike-and-wave complexes; this is true both of children and of elderly persons who may suddenly develop absence status (16.2 and Fig. 18.4).

(2) *Slow spike-and-wave discharges and sharp-and-slow-wave discharges* are

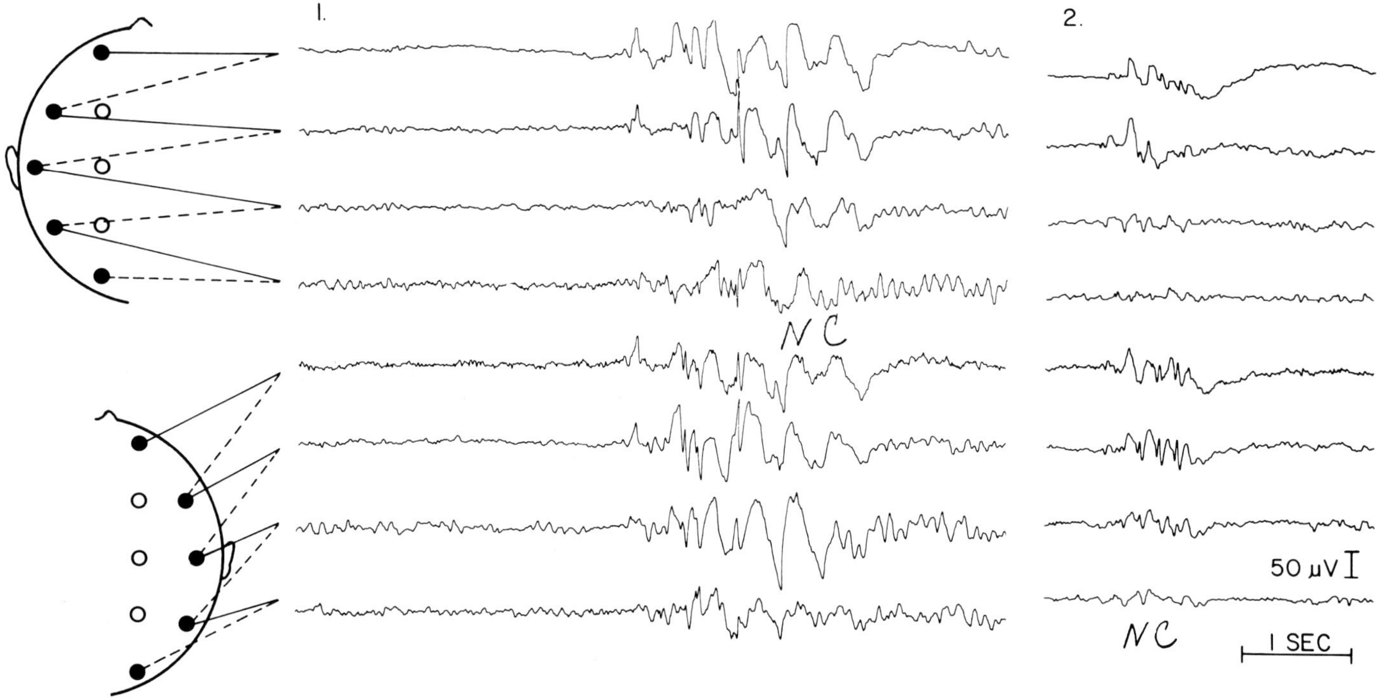


Fig. 18.3. Interictal generalized spike-and-wave discharges. 1. Irregular discharges during drowsiness; 2. Regular discharges at 6 Hz during light sleep. This 24-year-old woman has a history of generalized tonic-clonic seizures since the age of 4.

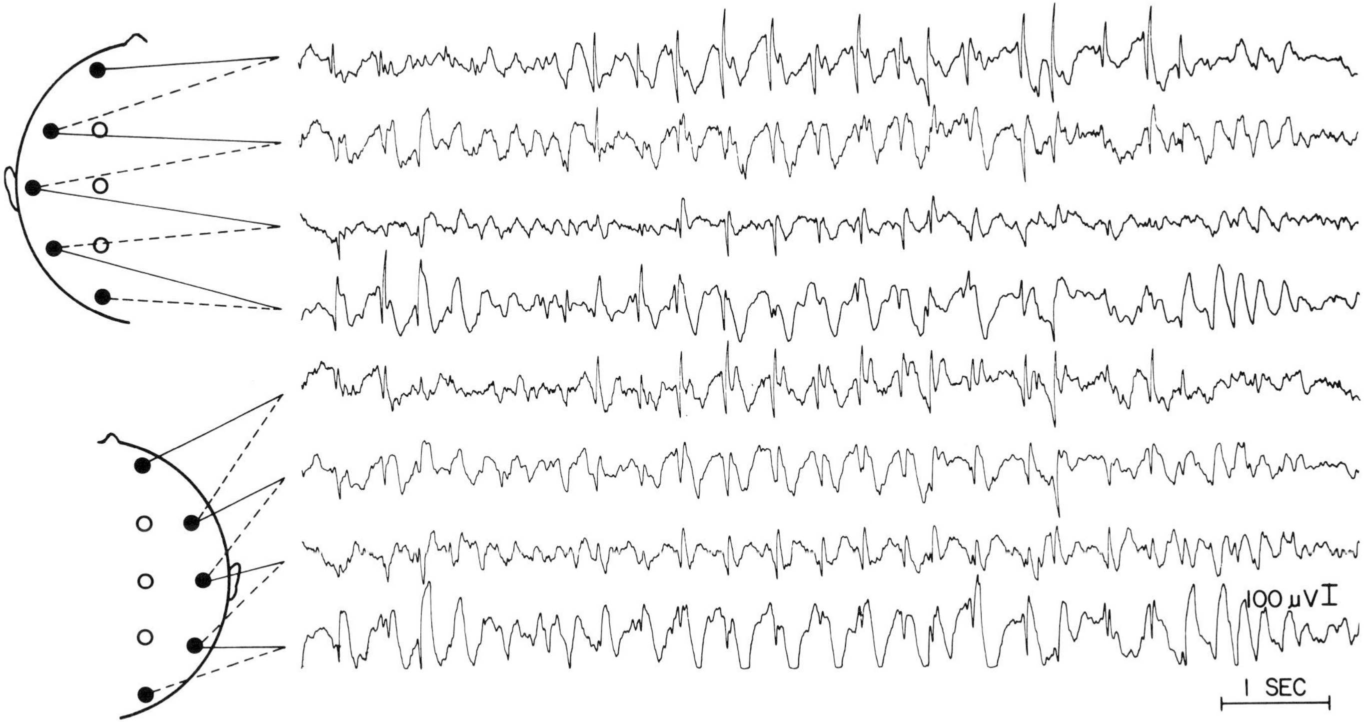


Fig. 18.4. Ictal generalized spike-and-wave discharges at 2–3 Hz. This 60-year-old woman has a history of generalized tonic-clonic seizures since childhood with sudden onset of absence status two days before this recording.

repetitions of the corresponding interictal patterns. They are often associated with atypical absence attacks. They are related to infantile patterns and are further described in the next chapter (19.1.2).

(3) *A rhythm of 10 Hz or more* increases in amplitude and decreases in frequency to form repetitive spikes which are occasionally interrupted by slow waves before the discharge ends. A discharge of this kind forms the first of the two phases associated with generalized tonic-clonic seizures (Fig. 18.5). A similar discharge is often associated with tonic seizures (Fig. 19.4) and appears mainly in patients with interictal patterns described in the next chapter (19.1.2).

(4) *Polyspike-and-wave discharges and spike-and-wave discharges* which are usually less regular than the 3 Hz spike-and-wave discharges appear in patients who often have interictal discharges of similar shape and suffer from a variety of different seizures. Similar discharges form the second phase of the diphasic discharge associated with generalized tonic-clonic seizures (Figs. 18.5–18.7).

(5) *A biphasic discharge,* often associated with tonic-clonic seizures, consists of a sequence of the two last-described patterns (Figs. 18.5–18.7). A rhythm of 10 Hz or more which increases in amplitude and decreases in frequency corresponds with the tonic phase of the seizure; it lasts about 10–20 seconds. At the end, it may be interrupted by slow waves which appear at regular intervals and lead to a gradual development of the second phase. This clonic phase is characterized by high amplitude spike-and-wave or polyspike-and-wave complexes which repeat at 1–4 Hz for about 30 seconds, having a faster rate initially and then becoming slower. When they stop, the record usually shows no distinguishable activity for many seconds or a few minutes before slow waves of low amplitude begin to appear. The waves gradually increase amplitude and frequency until pre-ictal patterns eventually reappear. Postictal slow waves may remain as a residual EEG abnormality for up to several days after a seizure.

Most patients with this ictal pattern have interictal patterns of spike-and-wave

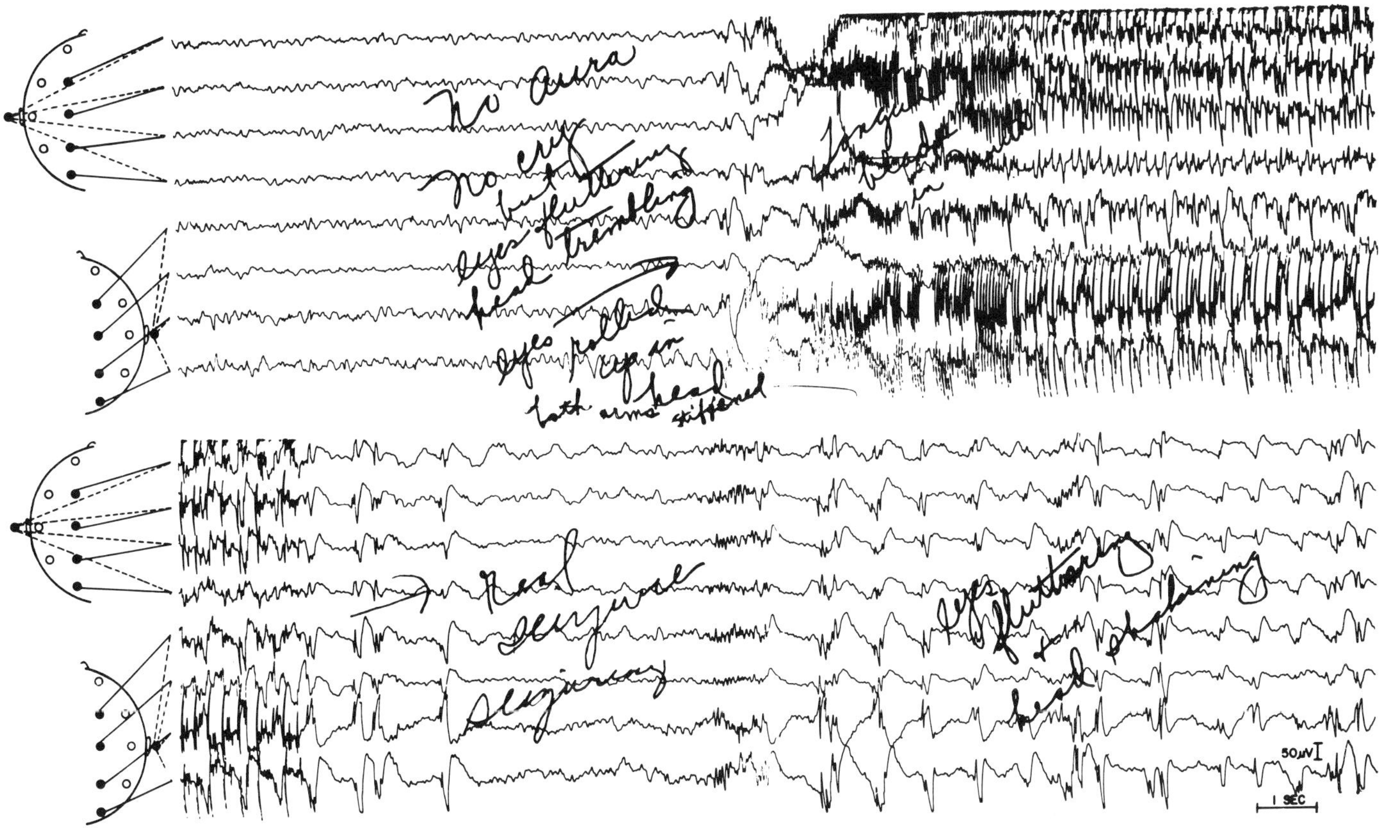


Fig. 18.5. Generalized tonic-clonic seizure in an 18-year-old girl with a life-long history of major and minor generalized seizures. *Top*: Pattern of slight drowsiness, suddenly interrupted by intermittent spikes and movement artifacts at the onset of a rhythm of generalized repetitive spikes of increasing amplitude and decreasing frequency which lasts about 10 seconds. Technician's comments read: 'No aura, no cry, but eyes fluttering, head trembling, eyes rolled up in head, both arms stiffened. Tongue blade in mouth'. This represents the tonic phase of the tonic-clonic seizure. *Bottom*: Spikes begin to be interrupted by slow waves. This signals the beginning of the clonic phase which starts with rhythmical high amplitude polyspike-and-wave and spike-and-wave complexes at about 1 Hz. Technician's notes read: 'Real seizure, seizuring. Eyes fluttering + head shaking'.

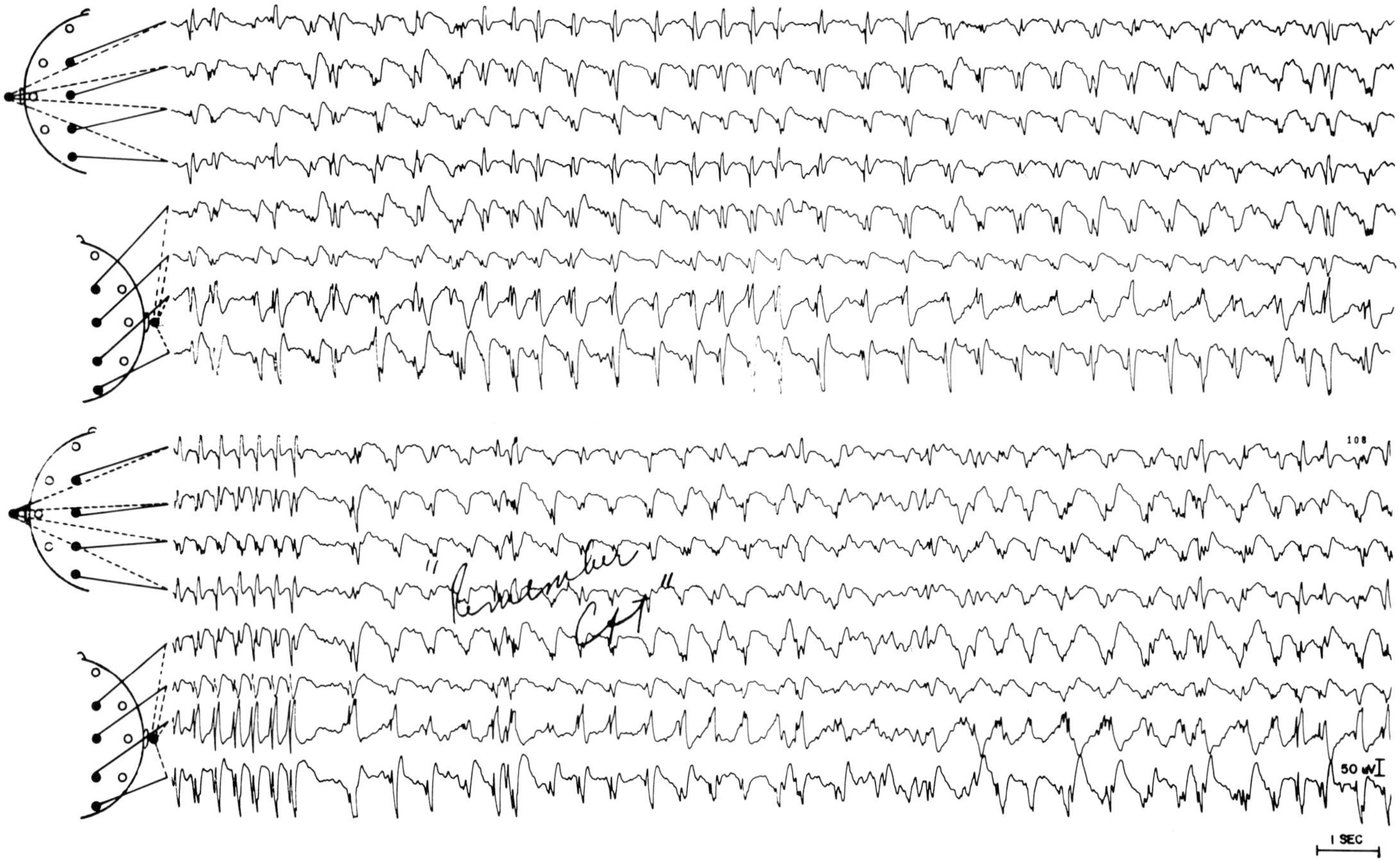


Fig. 18.6. Continuation of the generalized seizure shown in Fig. 18.5. High amplitude spike-and-wave discharges continue during the clonic phase. Top part is continuous with the bottom part of Fig. 18.5. Technician's note reads: 'Remember Cat', indicating that the technician was testing the patient's ability to remember a test word; the patient later did not recall anything.

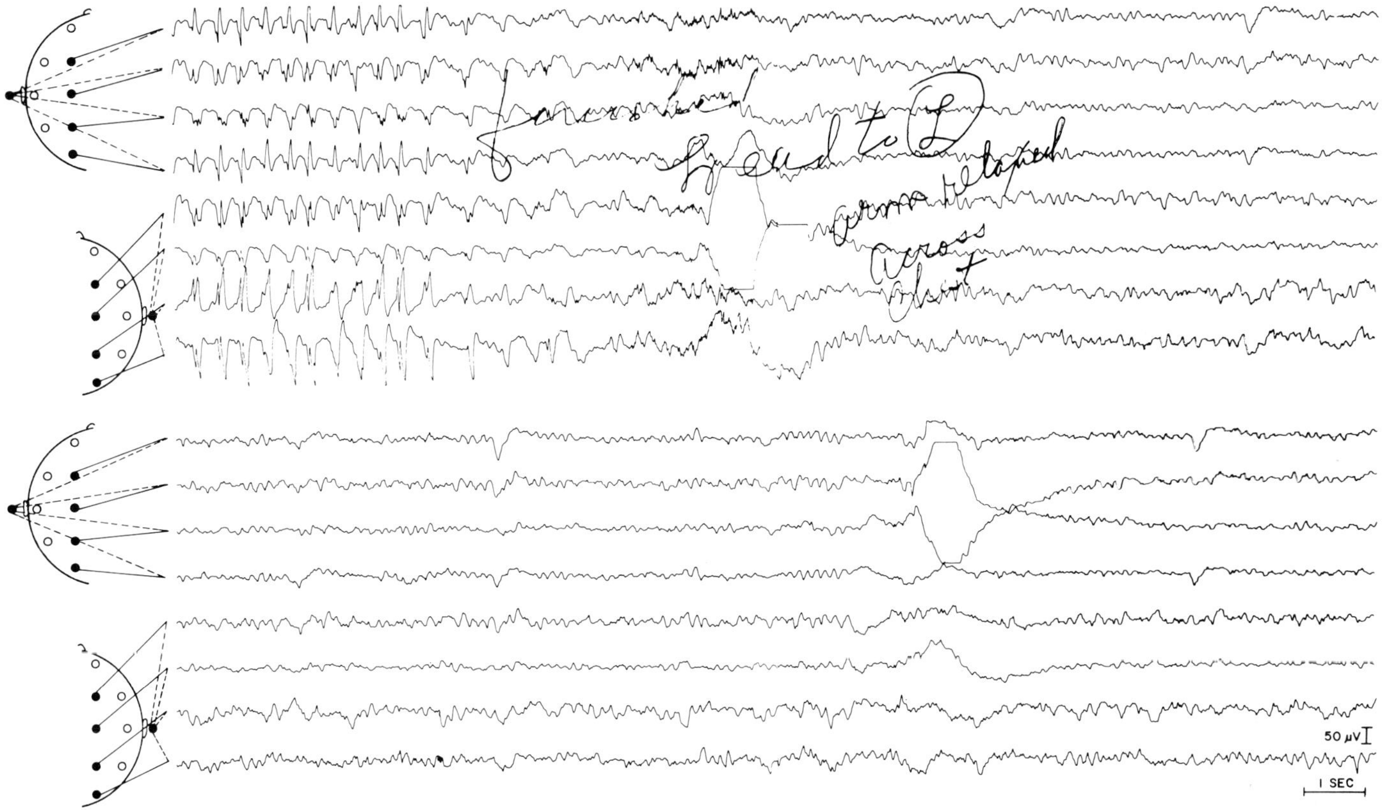


Fig. 18.7. End of the generalized seizure shown in Figs. 18.5. and 18.6. Top part is continuous with bottom part of Fig. 18.6. The end of the high amplitude generalized bisynchronous spike-and-wave complexes represents the end of the clonic phase of the seizure. This is followed by slow waves, movement artifacts and gradual return of normal background activity. Technician's notes read: 'Head to left, arms relaxed across chest'. This was a mild generalized seizure. More violent seizures are usually followed by postictal depression of amplitude and longer lasting slow waves of lower frequency. Violent seizures can usually not be recorded completely because the recording electrodes become dislodged.

complexes of any frequency although some patients show no interictal abnormalities at all.

(6) *A sudden transient decrease of amplitude* of all activity or a paroxysmal appearance of *generalized fast waves* are ictal patterns mainly seen in infants and very young children (19.1).

## 18.2 CLINICAL SIGNIFICANCE OF GENERALIZED EPILEPTIFORM ACTIVITY

### 18.2.1 *Association with seizures and epilepsy*

*Epileptiform activity associated with seizures.* Most patients with generalized epileptiform EEG activity, similar to patients with focal epileptiform activity (17.2.1) in this regard, have a history of seizures, and many patients with a seizure history show generalized epileptiform activity in the EEG. Most ictal discharges and some interictal discharges in the EEG are accompanied by clinical seizure manifestations. In some patients, generalized epileptiform discharges and seizure manifestations are precipitated by particular sensory and other stimuli (14.4). In contrast to patients with precipitated focal discharges and partial seizures, patients with precipitated generalized discharges and seizures are more susceptible to simple stimuli. Their response depends on stimulus intensity, and has a sharp latency from the time of the stimulus presentation.

*Epileptiform activity without seizures.* Like patients with local epileptiform activity, some patients with generalized epileptiform activity have no clinical evidence of seizures. This is true especially of some patients with toxic and metabolic encephalopathies, including that due to alcohol withdrawal. A few patients with structural brain diseases may develop generalized epileptiform activity in the EEG before or without developing seizures. The epileptiform patterns of 6 Hz spike-and-slow-wave and of 14 and 6 Hz positive bursts (19.4) have no associated ictal patterns and no proven relation to seizures.

*Epilepsy and seizures without epileptiform activity* may occur for several reasons. EEG recordings made between seizures may fail to show epileptiform activity for reasons discussed in connection with local epileptiform activity (17.2.1). Patients with generalized seizures due to drug withdrawal or other toxic and metabolic encephalopathies are unlikely to show epileptiform activity between these disorders but may show it during the periods of heightened susceptibility to seizures. EEG recordings made during generalized seizures nearly always show epileptiform activity (19.3).

**18.2.2** *Underlying cerebral abnormality in adults and adolescents. No demonstrable lesion* is found in the majority of adults and adolescents with primary generalized epileptiform activity, especially in those who have bilaterally synchronous and symmetrical epileptiform patterns and no other EEG abnormalities. There is no history, clinical or laboratory evidence of cerebral damage. These patients have idiopathic epilepsy (18.6.6).

*Widespread lasting structural damage* is present in some patients with primary generalized epileptiform activity. Most patients in this group have a history, clinical signs or laboratory findings pointing to the cause of the lesions; they may have suffered widespread cerebral injury, anoxia or encephalitis. The EEG may show other abnormalities in addition to generalized epileptiform discharges. These discharges are generally less symmetrical and synchronous than those of patients without obvious cerebral lesions.

*Transient conditions causing seizures,* for instance acute anoxia, recent severe head injury, hypoglycemia, withdrawal from chronic use of alcohol, barbiturates and CNS depressant drugs, renal, hepatic and other metabolic encephalopathies, are seen in a third group of patients with primary generalized epileptiform activity. Their EEG at the time of the acute derangement usually shows other abnormalities

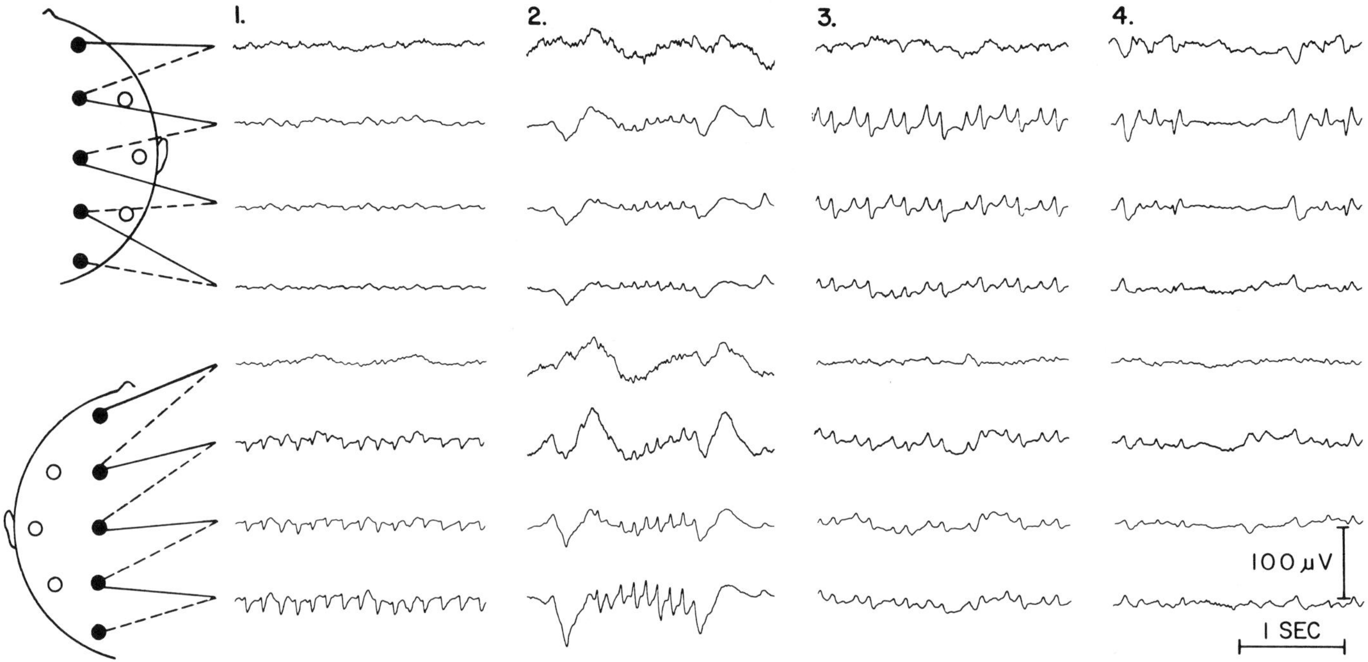


Fig. 18.8. Neonatal status epilepticus with seizure discharges on alternating sides in a 1-day-old full-term infant following an anoxic episode at birth. 1. Seizure discharge of rhythmical waves of 6–7 Hz, mainly on the left side; 2. One minute later, the left-sided seizure discharge consists of polyspikes, separated by high amplitude slow waves; similar discharges of lower amplitude appear on the right side; 3. Two minutes later, the seizure discharge on the left side abates and seizure discharges on the right side are at their height; 4. One minute later, the seizure discharge on the right side diminishes.

in addition to the generalized epileptiform activity, especially disappearance of alpha rhythm and appearance of generalized slow waves. The epileptiform activity in some of these patients consists of periodic complexes (19.2). When the underlying transient abnormality disappears, both the epileptiform and other EEG abnormalities may also disappear without residuals.

**18.2.3** *Infants and young children* rarely show bilaterally synchronous and symmetrical generalized epileptiform activity. More often they show multifocal, unilateral, or alternating epileptiform activity. In newborns, this activity may migrate from one part of the cortex to another in correspondence with the shifting, disorderly migration of clinical seizure manifestations (Fig. 18.8). This activity is often due to acute or recent widespread structural damage or toxic, metabolic, endocrine or electrolytic disturbances. Some specific infantile patterns are described in the next chapter (19.1).

## 18.3 OTHER EEG ABNORMALITIES ASSOCIATED WITH GENERALIZED EPILEPTIFORM ACTIVITY

**18.3.1** *Focal epileptiform discharges* in a record also showing generalized epileptiform discharges strongly suggest that the generalized epileptiform activity is triggered by a focal discharge. This is supported if generalized discharges consistently follow the focal discharges (17.3.2).

**18.3.2** *Focal slow waves* or a *local decrease of background amplitude* may suggest a focal brain lesion related to the generalized epileptiform discharges.

**18.3.3** *Generalized asynchronous and bisynchronous slow waves and generalized decrease of amplitude* may indicate a generalized cerebral abnormality giving rise to generalized epileptiform discharges (e.g. metabolic encephalopathy, postanoxic myoclonus, Jakob-Creutzfeldt disease). However, similar abnormalities may be the result of a generalized seizure discharge; mild postictal slow waves may persist for several days after a seizure.

### 18.4 GRADING OF GENERALIZED EPILEPTIFORM ACTIVITY

*Grading of generalized epileptiform activity* may use the same criteria and has the same implications as the grading of focal epileptiform activity (17.4).

### 18.5 MECHANISMS UNDERLYING GENERALIZED EPILEPTIFORM ACTIVITY

**18.5.1** *The involvement of intact cortex by epileptiform activity* distinguishes generalized from focal abnormalities. While most focal discharges are the result of circumscribed lesions causing local disturbances of neuronal function, generalized epileptiform discharges involve the entire brain, including areas which are not primarily diseased. Although the excessive depolarization and insufficient hyperpolarization, described for focal discharges (17.5.1), may also be the immediate cause of generalized discharges, it is not understood what brings these mechanisms into play. It is known that generalized discharges can be induced in healthy cortex by a variety of manipulations, for instance electrical stimulation, convulsant drugs and electrolyte changes. The ability to develop and sustain epileptiform activity therefore seems a basic property of the neuronal organization of normal cerebral cortex. Primary generalized seizures can therefore be considered a nonspecific reaction of the brain to a wide variety of pathological conditions.

**18.5.2** *The simultaneous appearance of epileptiform activity* in both hemispheres has prompted several explanations, each of which probably applies in different groups of patients.

*A central pacemaker* has been postulated to explain the sudden, bilaterally synchronous and symmetrical appearance of epileptiform discharges in generalized seizures, especially those of idiopathic epilepsy. Generalized seizures of this type have therefore been called 'centrencephalic seizures' or 'primary subcortical seizures'. These concepts imply that the primary fault lies in the pacemaking system itself and that the cortex of the cerebral hemispheres is involved only secondarily, generating widespread epileptiform activity in response to the faulty impulses from the pacemaker. Because the midbrain reticular formation has diffuse projections to the cerebral cortex, this structure is often thought to be an essential part of the pacemaker system.

*Secondary bilateral synchrony* is an EEG concept which hypothesizes that an epileptogenic focus bombards the presumed centrencephalic pacemaker system so that this system distributes the abnormal impulses to the cerebral cortex and thus produces generalized epileptiform discharges. This concept could explain many cases of partial seizures with secondary generalization (16.2; 17.3.2) and it may also be the basis for primary generalized seizures with bisynchronous and symmetrical epileptiform activity which could be triggered by a small or otherwise undetectable focus.

*Diffuse cortical epilepsy* is a concept introduced to explain the mechanism of seizure production in cases of obvious widespread cortical disease with epileptiform activity which is less symmetrical, synchronous and regular than that seen in patients with idiopathic epilepsy. In these cases, the diseased cortex with its inter-cortical and interhemispheric connections may play the leading role in seizure production; the centrencephalic distributor system is involved probably only to the extent that the epileptiform activity is symmetrical and synchronous. The name 'cortico-reticular seizures' expresses the possibility that a primary cortical abnormality contributes to, or initiates, the production of these seizures.

*Hereditary predisposition* probably plays an important role in the genesis of epilepsy with primary generalized seizures; the incidence of epilepsy in family members is higher than in the general population. The hereditary factor seems most important in cases with least evidence of cerebral disease. More than one epileptogenic factor is probably required to cause epilepsy in a patient; the constellation of factors probably varies widely between patients with this 'multifactorial' disorder.

## 18.6 SPECIFIC DISORDERS CAUSING GENERALIZED EPILEPTIFORM ACTIVITY

**18.6.1** *Degenerative, developmental and demyelinating diseases:*

(1) *Unverricht-Lundborg's myoclonus epilepsy* is associated with interictal multiple spikes or bursts of spike-and-waves at 3–6 Hz which last for 1–2 seconds. The background contains theta and delta activity with superimposed beta waves. Photic stimulation may elicit multiple generalized spikes and waves with or without myoclonic jerks.

(2) *Lafora's inclusion body epilepsy* may show spikes, polyspikes and spike-and-wave complexes with focal or bilaterally synchronous distribution and with limited correlation to myoclonic jerks. The background may show diffuse asynchronous and bisynchronous delta waves of high amplitude.

(3) *Jakob-Creutzfeldt disease* often shows generalized periodic sharp waves (19.2.2).

(4) *Ramsey Hunt's syndrome of dyssynergia cerebellaris myoclonica* may be associated with spikes, spike-and-waves, polyspike-and-waves at 4–6 Hz, with an anterior maximum. Photic stimulation often elicits a paroxysmal response with jerks. Focal spikes may appear in sleep. Seizures are tonic-clonic or only clonic.

(5) *Sturge-Weber syndrome* may show bilateral spikes although it is often associated with local reduction of amplitude (23.6.1) and local spikes (17.6.1).

(6) *Riley-Day's familial dysautonomia* may be associated with generalized epileptiform activity.

(7) *Microgyria, agyria and holoprosencephaly* may show generalized spikes, spike-and-waves as well as focal slow waves (20.6.1), focal spikes, hypsarrhythmia and multifocal spikes (19.1).

**18.6.2** *Metabolic and toxic encephalopathies.* Generalized spikes or sharp waves occur in many of these encephalopathies, usually on a background of widespread bisynchronous and asychronous slow waves (22.6.2) and other abnormalities. Generalized epileptiform discharges occasionally repeat at regular intervals, and may form complexes resembling spike-and-wave discharges. Regular, organized and sustained spike-and-wave patterns are rarely seen in adults except in some cases of dialysis encephalopathy. Periodic epileptiform discharges in the form of triphasic waves may occur especially in hepatic and uremic encephalopathy (19.2.6). In infants and children, metabolic encephalopathies may be associated with multifocal or generalized epileptiform discharges of special types (19.1).

The following metabolic and endocrine encephalopathies may be associated with generalized epileptiform activity: Addison's disease, dialysis encephalopathy, hyperglycemia without ketoacidosis, hypoglycemia, hypocalcemia due to hypoparathyroidism of pseudohypoparathyroidism, hyponatremia, acute intermittent porphyria, pyridoxine deficiency and uremia (Table 22.1).

A very great number of toxic agents are capable of producing generalized epileptiform activity. Among the more common agents are high doses of therapeutic agents, such as phenothiazines, haloperidol, rauwolfia derivatives, INH, tricyclic antidepressants, environmental agents and organic solvents such as methyl bromide and chloride, pesticides, DDT, lead and mercury.

Withdrawal from chronic use of drugs depressing central nervous function can induce generalized epileptiform activity for a few days after withdrawal; photoconvulsive responses are often seen in this condition. The most common agents are barbiturates and alcohol.

Hyperthermia can induce or precipitate generalized epileptiform activity, especially in young children who tend to have seizures during febrile illnesses. These *febrile seizures* are usually tonic or clonic. Most of these children show no epileptiform EEG activity between seizures, but some of them develop such activity, and recurring generalized seizures, independent of fever.

**18.6.3** *Cerebrovascular diseases:*

(1) *Postanoxic encephalopathy* may produce generalized epileptiform activity among many other EEG abnormalities (21.6.3). A special form of this activity consists of periodic sharp waves which are seen in cases of postanoxic myoclonus (19.2.2).

(2) *Cerebral infarcts* rarely cause generalized epileptiform activity, but bilateral periodic lateralizing epileptiform discharges may be seen in some acute strokes (19.2.1).

(3) *Vertebro-basilar migraine* may be associated with epileptiform activity during and between attacks. This activity usually appears over the posterior head regions and is often bilaterally synchronous; focal epileptiform activity and slow waves (20.6.3) may also be seen.

**18.6.4** *Cerebral trauma.* Severe head injuries can lead to generalized epileptiform activity and seizures. Like focal epileptiform abnormalities (17.6.4), the generalized abnormalities may appear soon after the injury or with a delay. The effects of cerebral injury on the EEG are especially pronounced in infants and young children who may react with special epileptiform patterns (19.1).

**18.6.5** *Brain tumors.* The incidence of generalized epileptiform activity may be increased very slightly compared with that encountered in the general population.

**18.6.6** *Generalized epileptiform activity in seizure disorders without known underlying diseases and in normal persons.* *Idiopathic epilepsy* is the diagnosis of many cases of generalized epileptiform seizures without known cause, especially in cases of typical absence attacks associated with interictal and ictal 3 Hz spike-and-wave patterns, and in cases of generalized tonic-clonic seizures.

In practice, this diagnosis requires exclusion of organic disorders known to cause generalized seizures. Organic lesions must be suspected in patients who have (a) EEG findings of asynchronous and asymmetrical generalized epileptiform activity and of abnormal background activity; (b) a history of cerebral injuries or diseases at any time from before birth to before the onset of seizures; (c) abnormal findings on neurological examination; (d) a general medical condition capable of causing generalized seizures. *Normal subjects* may show specific patterns of generalized epileptiform activity (19.4).

**18.6.7** *Infectious diseases* produce generalized epileptiform activity only rarely and then mainly in the form of periodic complexes seen in subacute sclerosing panencephalitis, Jakob-Creutzfeldt disease and herpes simplex (19.2) or of infantile patterns (19.1).

**18.6.8** *Psychiatric diseases* are not characterized by generalized epileptiform activity although widespread interictal discharges have been reported in small fractions of large groups of patients with various diseases. The possibility of causes other than non-organic psychiatric disorders must be evaluated in every case.

## REFERENCES

Bancaud, J., Talairach, J., Morel, P., Bresson, M., Bonis, A., Geier, S., Hemon, E. and Buser, P. (1974) "Generalized" epileptic seizures elicited by electrical stimulation of the frontal lobe in man. Electroenceph. clin. Neurophysiol. 37: 275–282.

Belafsky, M.A., Carwille, S., Miller, P., Waddell, G., Boxley-Johnson, J. and Delgado-Escueta, A.V. (1978) Prolonged epileptic twilight states: Continuous recordings with nasopharyngeal electrodes and videotape analysis. Neurology 28: 239–245.

Dalby, M.A. (1969) Epilepsy and 3 per second spike and wave rhythms. Acta Neurol. Scand., Suppl. 40: 1–183.

Ellis, J.M. and Lee, S.I. (1978) Acute prolonged confusion in later life as an ictal state. Epilepsia 19: 119–128.

Forster, F.M. (1977) Reflex Epilepsy, Behavioral Therapy and Conditional Reflexes. Thomas, Springfield.

Gloor, P. (1979) Generalized epilepsy with spike-and-wave discharge: A reinterpretation of its electrographic and clinical manifestations. Epilepsia 20: 571–588.

Janeway, R., Ravens, J.R., Pearce, L.A., Odor, D.L. and Suzuki, K. (1967) Progressive myoclonus epilepsy with Lafora inclusion bodies. Arch. Neurol. 16: 565–582.

Lederman, R.J. and Henry, C.E. (1978) Progressive dialysis encephalopathy. Ann. Neurol. 4: 199–204.

Lombroso, C.T. and Erba, G. (1970) Primary and secondary bilateral synchrony in epilepsy. Arch. Neurol. 22: 321–334.

Mancardi, G.L., Primavera, A., Leonardi, A., De Martini, I., Salvarani, S. and Bugiani, O. (1979) Tendency to periodic recurrence of EEG changes in Lafora's disease. Eur. Neurol. 18: 129–135.

Niedermeyer, E., Fineyre, F., Riley, T. and Uematsu, S. (1979) Absence status (petit mal status) with focal characteristics. Arch. Neurol. 36: 417–421.

Noriega-Sanchez, A., Martinez-Maldonado, M. and Haiffe, R.M. (1978) Clinical and electroencephalographic changes in progressive uremic encephalopathy. Neurology 28: 667–669.

Penry, J.K., Porter, R.J. and Dreifuss, F.E. (1975) Simultaneous recording of absence seizures with video tape and electroencephalography. A study of 374 seizures in 48 patients. Brain 98: 427–440.

Rodin, E., Smid, N. and Mason, K. (1976) The grand mal pattern of Gibbs, Gibbs and Lennox. Electroenceph. clin. Neurophysiol. 40: 401–406.

Rose, A.L. and Lombroso, C.T. (1970) Neonatal seizure states. A study of clinical, pathological, and electroencephalographic features in 137 full-term babies with long-term follow-up. Pediatrics 45: 404–425.

Tükel, K. and Jasper, H. (1952) The electroencephalogram in parasagittal lesions. Electroenceph. clin. Neurophysiol. 4: 481–494.

Wilkins, A.J., Darby, C.E. and Binnie, C.D. (1979) Neurophysiological aspects of pattern-sensitive epilepsy. Brain 102: 1–25.

# Special epileptiform patterns

# 19

SUMMARY

This chapter joins several groups of interictal and ictal patterns which are clearly distinguished from the epileptiform patterns described in the preceding chapters.

(19.1) *Hypsarrhythmia, slow spike-and-wave complexes and multifocal independent spikes* have features of both focal and generalized epileptiform activity and appear at slightly different ages in infants and young children as the result of a great variety of organic brain disorders.

(19.2) *Periodic complexes* are characterized by the fairly regular recurrence of paroxysmal activity of various forms.

(19.3) *Ictal patterns without spikes and sharp waves* occur in patients with various focal and generalized interictal patterns which have been described in other sections.

(19.4) *Pseudo-epileptogenic patterns* contain epileptiform activity but have no proven relation to epilepsy and seizures.

## 19.1 THE INFANTILE AND JUVENILE PATTERNS OF HYPSARRHYTHMIA, SLOW SPIKE-AND-WAVE DISCHARGES AND MULTIFOCAL INDEPENDENT SPIKES

These patterns (Table 19.1) are similar to each other in that (1) they usually have some focal or multifocal interictal features even though many of their ictal patterns are generalized from the start; (2) they are often associated with neurological abnormalities in the form of mental retardation and seizures; (3) they are the result of a great variety of prenatal, perinatal and postnatal pathological conditions most of which produce widespread or multifocal cerebral damage; (4) they depend more on the age of the patient and the severity of the underlying condition than on the particular type of the lesion. Hypsarrhythmia begins between the ages of 6 months to 2 years and may be replaced by one of the other patterns. The slow spike-and-

Table 19.1
Special infantile and juvenile epileptiform patterns

| Interictal epileptiform pattern | Ictal epileptiform pattern | Clinical seizure type | Underlying brain lesion |
|---|---|---|---|
| A. *Hypsarrhythmia:* Multiple spikes with shifting foci, on high amplitude, generalized asynchronous and bisynchronous slow waves | 1. Sudden attenuation of amplitude, often preceded by a large slow wave or a sharp-and-slow-wave complex<br>2. A sharp-and-slow-wave complex or large slow wave only<br>3. Fast activity during amplitude attenuation | Infantile spasms<br>Tonic seizures | *Prenatal*<br>Prematurity<br>Complicated pregnancy<br>Meningocele<br>Encephalocele<br>Hydrocephalus<br>Microcephaly<br>Tuberous sclerosis<br>Toxoplasmosis |
| B. *Slow spike-and-wave* ('Petit mal variant'): Spike-and-wave or sharp-and-slow-wave at 1.5–2.5 Hz; synchronous and symmetrical or not | 1. Long slow-spike-and-wave discharge<br>2. Low voltage fast<br>3. Rhythmic 10 Hz discharge with increasing amplitude and decreasing frequency<br>4. Mixed fast and slow<br>5. Flattening<br>6. Slow waves<br>7. Pattern as in tonic-clonic seizures (Table 18.1) | Absences<br>Bilateral massive epileptic myoclonus<br>Tonic seizures<br>Long atonic seizures<br>Akinetic seizures<br>Tonic-clonic seizures | Cerebromacular degeneration<br>Phenylketonuria<br>Sturge-Weber<br><br>*Perinatal*<br>Birth injury<br>Anoxia<br>Ischemia<br>Hypoglycemia |
| C. *Independent multifocal spikes:* Spikes from more than two foci of constant location | Focal or generalized seizure discharges similar to those of adults (Tables 17.1, 18.1) | Partial simple seizures<br>Partial complex seizures<br>Generalized tonic, clonic, tonic-clonic seizures | *Postnatal*<br>Infections<br>Head injuries<br>Cerebrovascular disease<br>Metachromatic leukodystrophy<br>Pyridoxine deficiency |

wave pattern begins at the age of 2 to 4 years and may continue through early childhood. The pattern of multifocal independent spikes may develop from either one of the other patterns, or appear at the same ages as the other patterns in which case it usually represents less severe damage.

**19.1.1** *Hypsarrhythmia.* *The interictal pattern* differs from most other interictal patterns in that it is continuously abnormal (Fig. 19.1). It shows asynchronous and bisynchronous slow waves of high amplitude with superimposed focal spikes and sharp waves in various parts of the brain. Hypsarrhythmia differs from other patterns of multifocal epileptiform discharges in that the locations of the focal spikes and sharp waves are not constant but shift from moment to moment.

*The ictal patterns* consist usually of (1) sudden attenuation of amplitude, often preceded by a paroxysmal slow wave of high amplitude and frontal dominance or by a generalized sharp-and-slow-wave complex; (2) a generalized sharp-and-slow-wave complex or a generalized paroxysmal slow wave only; or (3) fast activity appearing during the period of amplitude attenuation (Fig. 19.2).

*Clinical seizures* consist of infantile spasms and tonic seizures (16.2). Infants and children with this pattern often show arrest of development of perceptual and motor skills. The combination of infantile spasms, retardation and hypsarrhythmia is called 'West syndrome'.

*Clinical conditions causing hypsarrhythmia* comprise a great variety of disorders of prenatal, perinatal or postnatal onset (Table 19.1, Column 4). Most are due to diffuse structural damage, but a few are due to metabolic disorders and are reversible, for instance hypoglycemia, pyridoxine deficiency and phenylketonuria. Rarely, local cerebral lesions such as choroid plexus papilloma or the lesions seen in Sturge-Weber syndrome may be associated with hypsarrhythmia.

**19.1.2** *Slow spike-and-wave pattern* (formerly called 'petit mal variant'). *The*

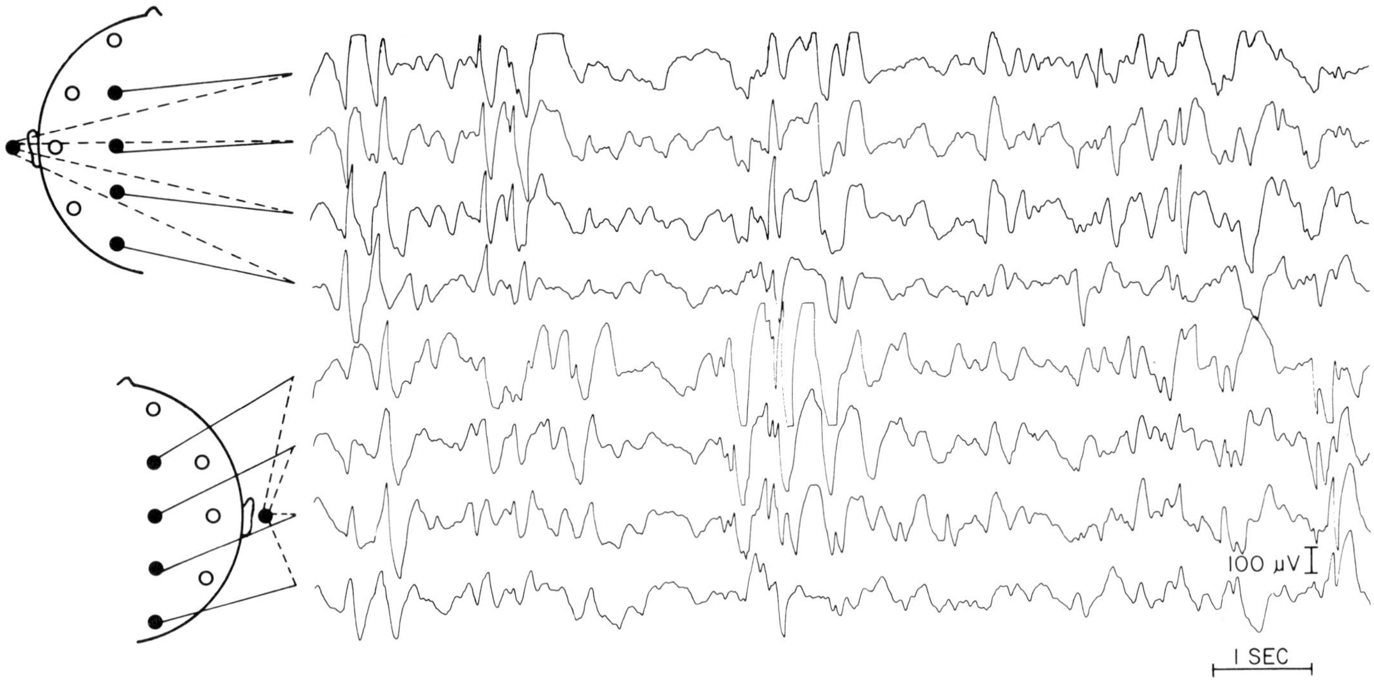


Fig. 19.1. Pattern of hypsarrhythmia. Interictal continuous spikes and slow waves of high amplitude in a shifting distribution. The patient is a 6-month-old infant with dysplasia of the left posterior fossa, hypotonia and infantile spasms.

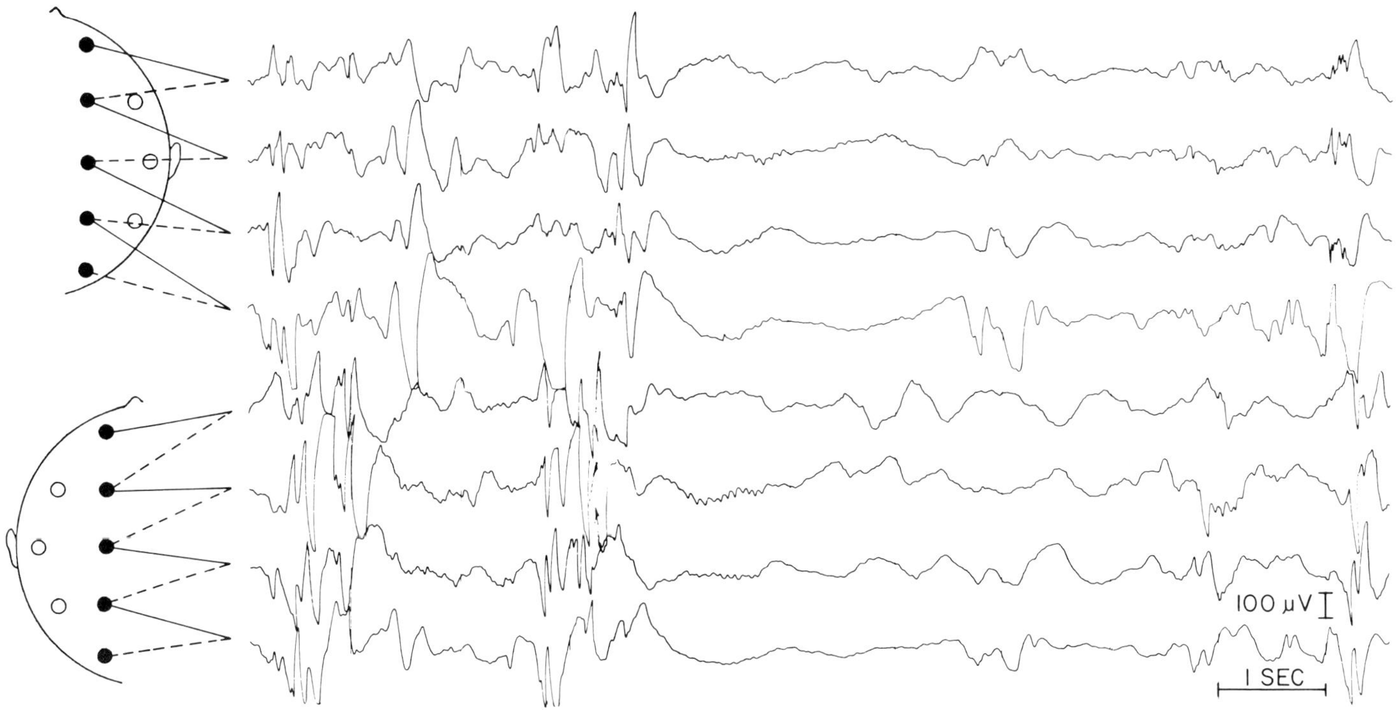


Fig. 19.2. Pattern of hypsarrhythmia interrupted by an electrodecremental seizure in the same patient as in Fig. 19.1. The hypsarrhythmic pattern at the beginning is abruptly replaced by very slow waves of much lower amplitude which were associated with mild spasmodic flexion of the arms.

*interictal pattern* consists of spike-and-wave complexes, polyspike-and-wave complexes or sharp-and-slow wave complexes which occur intermittently or repeat at about 1.5–2.5 Hz for up to a few seconds (Fig. 19.3). They may be symmetrical and bisynchronous, or asymmetrical and even asynchronous. They may have a focal onset but in most cases differ from focal discharges with secondary generalization in that there are no intermittent focal discharges which do not generalize.

*The ictal patterns* are generalized and consist of (1) repetition of the interictal discharges for more than a few seconds, often up to 1 minute; (2) low amplitude fast activity of about 20 Hz with increasing amplitude; (3) rhythmical activity of about 10 Hz with increasing amplitude and decreasing frequency, occasionally interrupted by rhythmical slow waves and forming polyspike-and-wave or spike-and-wave complexes (Fig. 19.4); (4) a mixture of rhythmical slow waves and fast waves occasionally forming spike-and-wave patterns; (5) a simple reduction of amplitude leading to apparent flattening of the EEG; (6) generalized slow waves of delta or theta frequency; (7) a biphasic discharge of the type associated with generalized tonic-clonic seizures in adults.

Clinical seizures are of various types. Absence attacks may occur with the ictal patterns (1), (2) or (3). These attacks have been called ‘atypical absences’ in contrast to ‘typical absences’ (16.2) associated with bilaterally synchronous and symmetrical 3 Hz spike-and-wave discharges (18.1.3). Tonic, clonic and other generalized motor seizures occur with patterns (2)–(6). Pattern (7) is associated with tonic-clonic seizures similar to those of adults (16.2). Many patients have more than one type of seizure.

The combination of the EEG pattern of slow spike-and-waves, intractable seizures and mental retardation has the name ‘Lennox syndrome’ or ‘Lennox-Gastaut syndrome’.

*Clinical conditions causing slow spike-and-wave discharges* are the same as those causing hypsarrhythmia in younger patients. Subacute sclerosing panencephalitis may cause slow spike-and-wave patterns in exceptional cases.

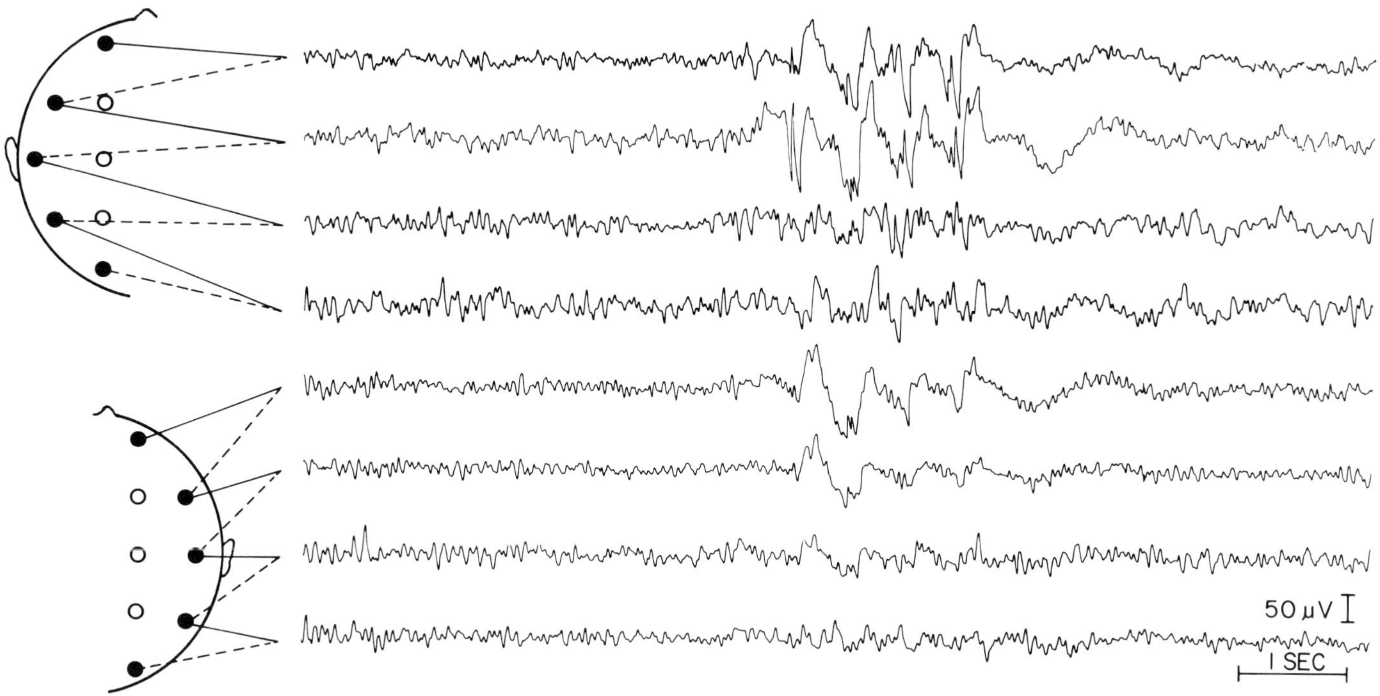


Fig. 19.3. Pattern of slow spike-and-waves at 1.5–2 Hz, maximal over the left anterior head. This 8-year-old girl has a history of generalized seizures of many types since birth; she is slightly retarded but without other neurological abnormalities.

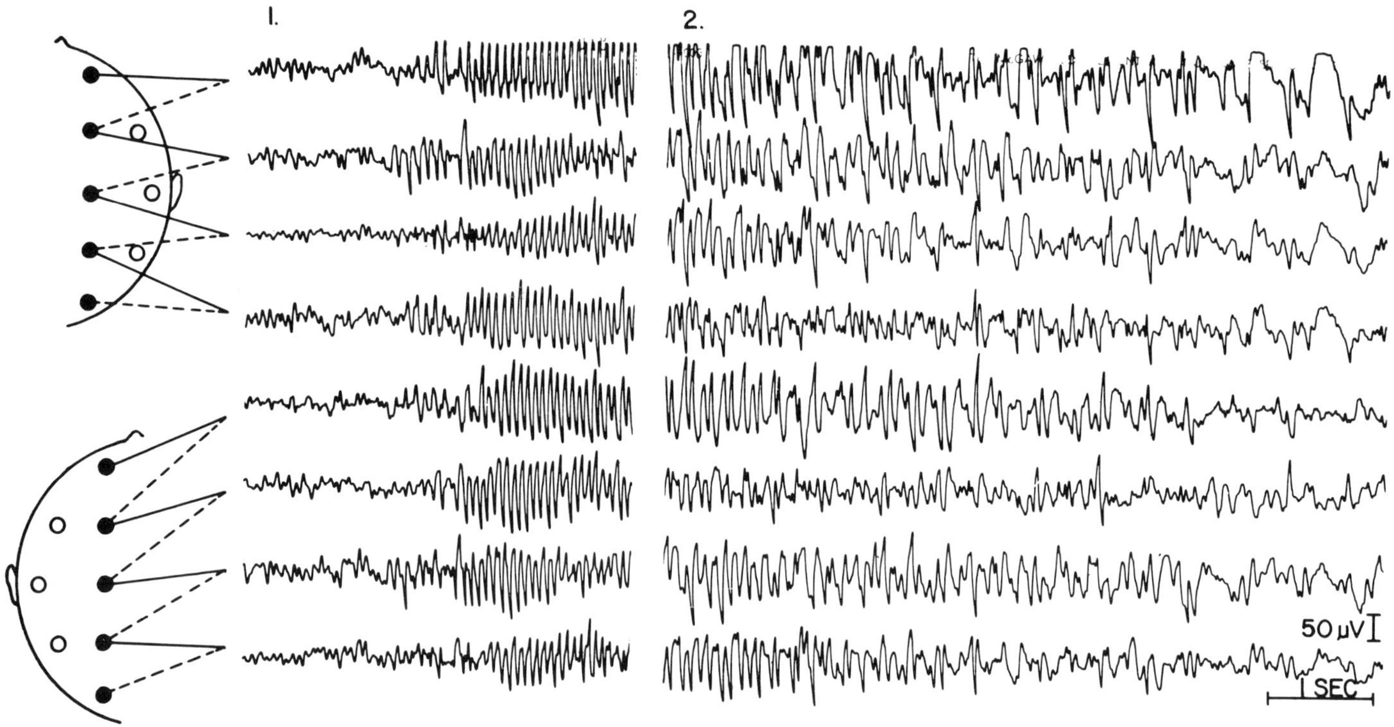


Fig. 19.4. Generalized seizure discharge in the same patient as in Fig. 19.3. 1. Generalized rhythm of high amplitude spikes at 12–14 Hz; 2. Fifteen seconds after the end of Part 1, the frequency of the spikes has slowed and slow waves begin to interrupt the spikes. This episode was associated with a mild generalized tonic seizure.

**19.1.3** *Independent multifocal spikes.* *The interictal pattern* shows spikes arising independently from more than two foci (Fig. 19.5). In contrast to hypsarrhythmia, the foci of the spike discharges are constant, i.e. they do not shift in the same recording; the background shows less abnormal slow wave activity or is normal. Some spike foci may disappear and other, new, foci may appear from one recording to the next to give the appearance of migrating foci.

*The ictal patterns* vary widely and include both focal and generalized seizure discharges of all types seen in adults (Tables 17.1 and 18.1, Column 2).

*Clinical seizures* also vary widely and include partial, secondary and primary generalized seizures of most types (Tables 17.1 and 18.1, Column 3). Most patients have generalized motor seizures, and many have more than one type of seizure. As is true for patients with hypsarrhythmia and slow spike-and-waves, the majority of patients with multifocal independent spikes suffers from combinations of seizures and mental retardation indicating severe and widespread cerebral damage.

*Clinical conditions causing multiple independent focal spikes* are the same as those causing hypsarrhythmia in younger or more severely involved patients.

## 19.2 PERIODIC COMPLEXES

The patterns described in this section (Table 19.2) are similar to each other in that (1) they consist of complexes which recur at fairly regular intervals on a background of slow waves of usually low amplitude; (2) most of them are generalized or widespread in distribution and synchronous in timing over different parts of the head; (3) the complexes are due to acute or subacute structural cerebral damage except in most cases of triphasic waves; (4) longer, ictal EEG discharges and clinical seizure episodes are rare: periodic complexes essentially are interictal activity; (5) some of the complexes caused by structural damage are associated with myoclonic jerks. The

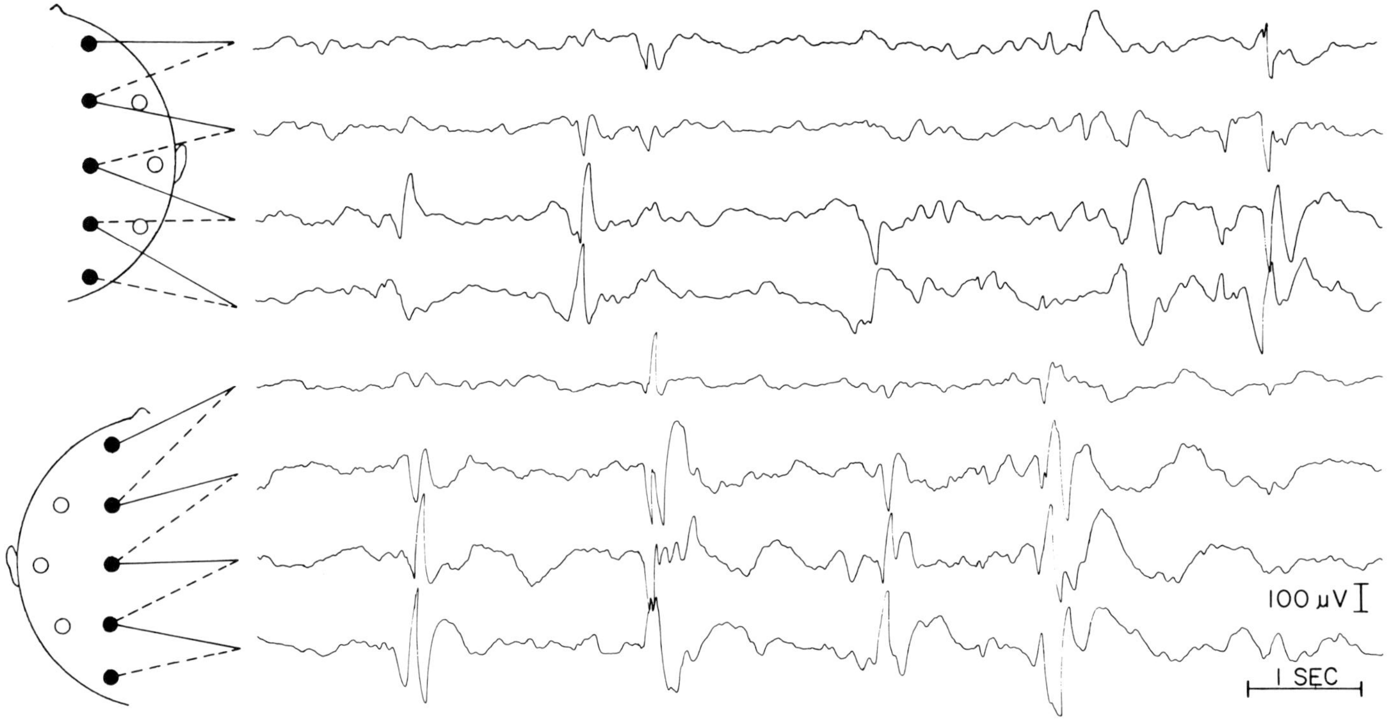


Fig. 19.5. Multifocal independent spikes. This EEG is of the same patient as in Figs. 19.1 and 19.2, now at an age of 13 months.

TABLE 19.2
Periodic complexes

| Pattern name | Wave shape | Wave duration | Interval activity | Interval duration | Distribution | Clinical seizure manifestations | Underlying lesion | Special features |
|---|---|---|---|---|---|---|---|---|
| 1. Periodic lateralizing epileptiform discharges ('PLEDs') | Di- or polyphasic sharp waves or spikes | 0.06–0.5 sec | Low amplitude delta, or no activity at regular gain | 1–2 sec | Focal, unilateral or bilateral with unilateral maximum | Epilepsia partialis continua | Fresh infarct, tumor, subdural hematoma, other superficial lesions | Not reactive to stimuli; persist in sleep |
| 2. Periodic generalized sharp waves, often associated with Jakob-Creutzfeldt disease | Mono-, di- or triphasic sharp waves | 0.15–0.6 sec | Low amplitude slow | 0.5–2 sec | Generalized, bisynchronous | Myoclonic jerks | Jakob-Creutzfeldt disease, post-anoxic encephalopathy, fat embolism | Triggered by loud noise, flashes |
| 3. Periodic generalized complexes, often associated with SSPE | One or more polyphasic sharp waves, with delta waves | 0.5–3 sec | Asynch. and bisynch. theta and delta; focal spikes and slow waves | 3–20 sec | Generalized, symmetrical, synchronous | Myoclonic jerks | SSPE, postanoxic myoclonus | Usually not triggered by stimuli; sleep may enhance or obscure the pattern |
| 4. Burst suppression | Irregular or regular slow waves, with or without sharp waves | 1–3 sec | Low amplitude delta, or no activity at regular gain | 2–10 sec (many minutes) | Bilateral, unilateral, regional | None | Anesthesia, CNS depressant drugs, hypothermia, postanoxic encephalopathy, isolated cortex | Unreactive to stimuli |
| 5. Periodic temporal sharp waves, often associated with herpes simplex encephalitis | Mono- or polyphasic sharp waves | 0.1–1.5 sec | Diffuse or focal slow waves, may have low amplitude | 1–5 sec | Unilateral or bilateral temporal, may extend to frontal | May have myoclonic jerks | After first few days and during first 2 weeks of herpes simplex encephalitis | |
| 6. Triphasic waves | Major positive sharp wave, preceded and followed by minor negative waves | 0.15–0.25 sec | Asynchronous and bisynchronous slow waves | 0.5–2 sec | Generalized, maximal frontal or occipital | None | Hepatic, uremic and other metabolic encephalopathies, post-anoxic encephalopathy | May have anterior–posterior delay |

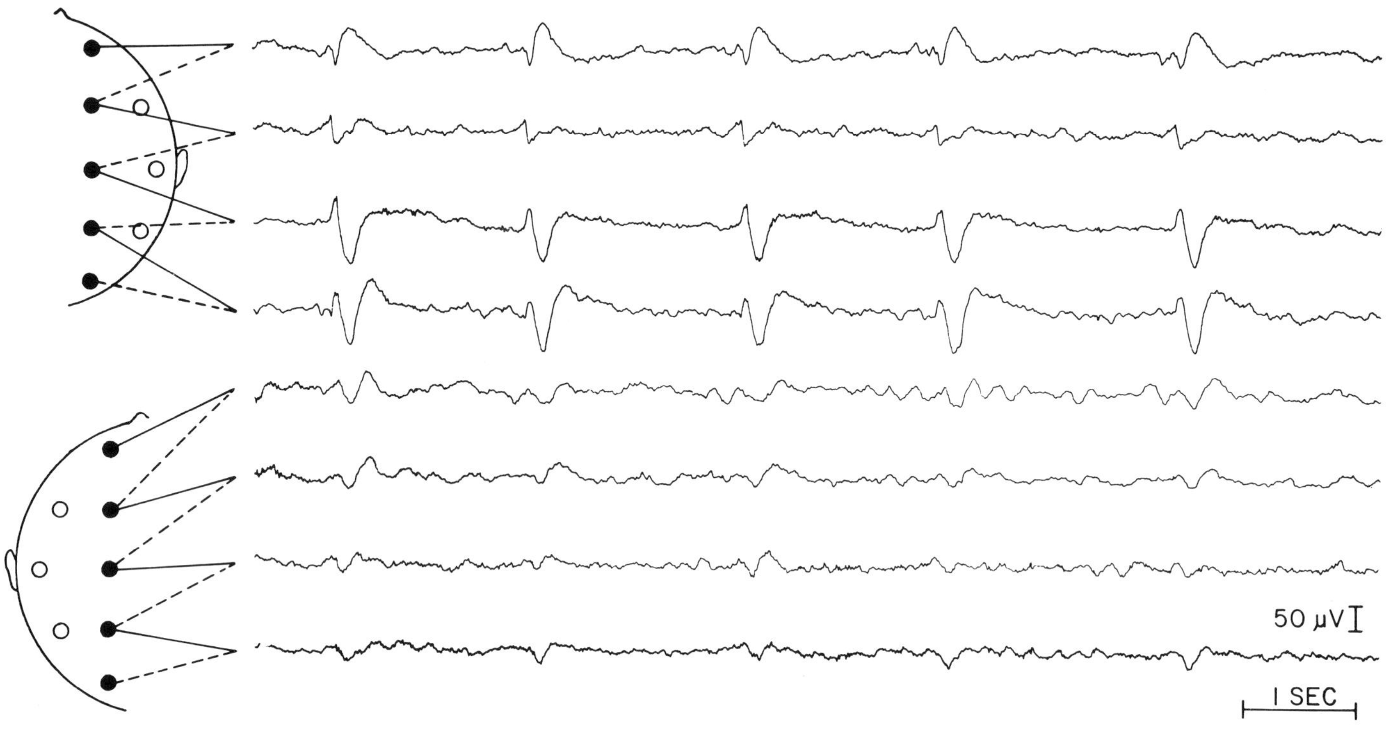


Fig. 19.6. Pattern of periodic lateralizing epileptiform discharges (PLEDs) on the right side. This 70-year-old woman suddenly developed weakness and rhythmical twitching of the left arm on the day of the recording; her condition was later diagnosed as a cerebral infarct.

jerks may occur before, during or after the complexes or have a variable time relation; jerking may disappear with or without change of the complexes, but rarely do jerks appear without complexes.

**19.2.1** *Periodic lateralizing epileptiform discharges (PLEDs).* *The EEG pattern* shows complexes which consist of a di- or polyphasic spike or sharp wave and may include a slow wave (Fig. 19.6). Complexes usually last for only a fraction of a second. They commonly appear in a wide distribution on one side of the head. In some instances, they have a focal origin and in others, they are bilateral but usually with a clear maximum on one side. They may have a different shape in different areas and they often vary in the same patient with time. The complexes recur every 1–2 seconds and are separated by low amplitude slow waves or by no detecable activity at regular gain. The background in regions not showing PLEDs is often abnormal. PLEDs may be interrupted by the appearance of a focal seizure discharge which may generalize.

*Clinical conditions causing PLEDs* are mainly fresh cerebral infarcts, but also cerebral tumors, meningitis, encephalitis, subdural hematoma, cerebral abscess, sickle cell anemia and other conditions causing fairly acute damage to an area near the cerebral cortex. PLEDs usually persist during the acute phase of these conditions but disappear after days or weeks. Patients with PLEDs often have a reduced level of alertness. Most patients with PLEDs recover from their acute disorders, but not necessarily without clinical residuals.

*Seizure manifestations* are often absent. However, epilepsia partialis continua may occur if the PLEDs involve motor areas of the brain. Then each complex in the EEG may be associated with a myoclonic jerk on the opposite side of the body. Large or small muscle groups may be involved at different times and the jerking may cease intermittently. Focal or generalized seizure discharges interrupting PLEDs may be associated with partial or generalized seizures. These episodes may recur frequently enough to form status epilepticus.

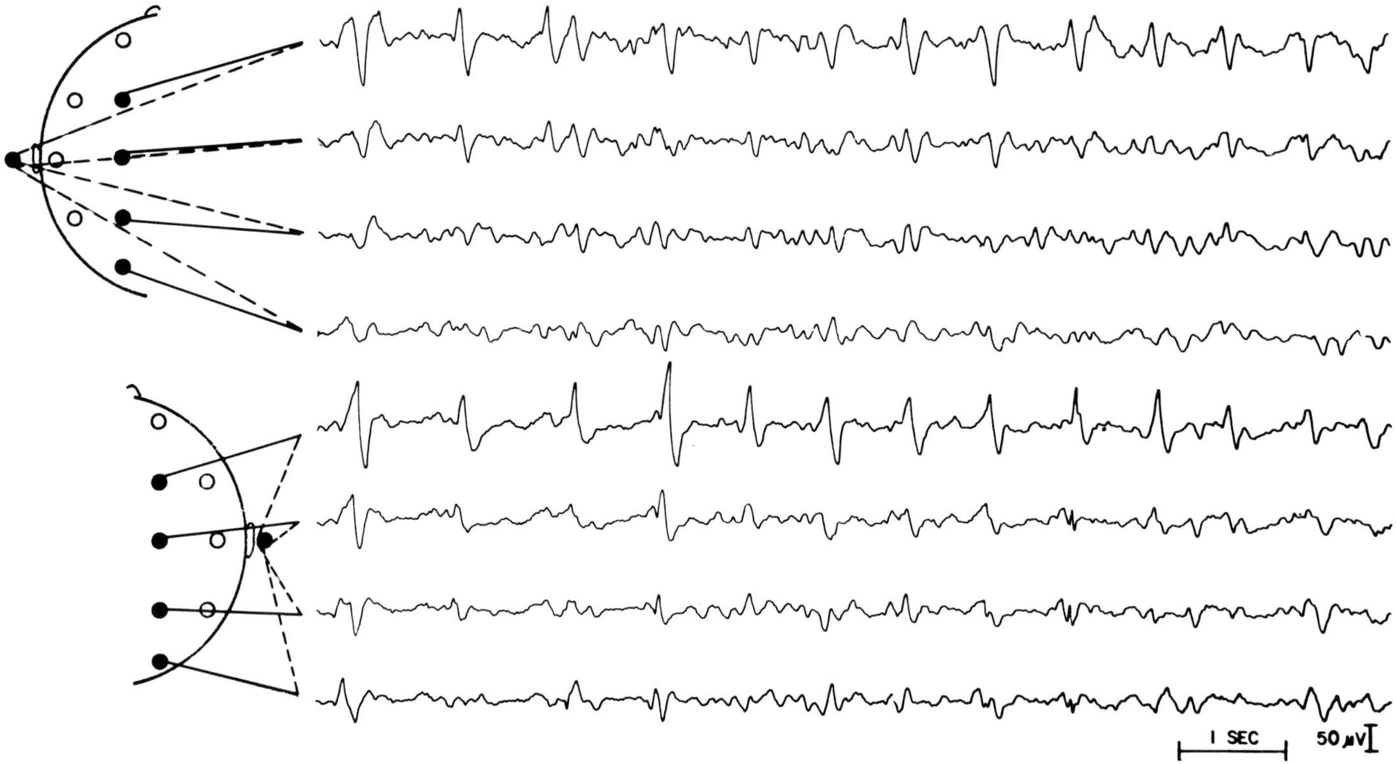


Fig. 19.7. Periodic bilateral sharp waves at about 1 Hz with a frontal maximum and variable posterior extension in a patient with Jakob-Creutzfeldt disease. This 83-year-old woman began to become confused 5 months earlier and then gradually developed dressing apraxia and illusions of a spatial distortion of objects in her left visual field. Startle myoclonus and spontaneous generalized myoclonus began soon after this EEG recording. She died 3 weeks later and her autopsy confirmed the clinical diagnosis of Jakob-Creutzfeldt disease.

**19.2.2** *Periodic generalized sharp waves, often associated with Jakob-Creutzfeldt disease.* *The EEG pattern* is dominated by sharp waves which usually have one, two or three phases and last up to 0.6 seconds (Fig. 19.7). When fully developed, the sharp waves appear synchronously in a wide distribution over both hemispheres, sometimes with a frontal maximum; while they develop, they may be focal or unilateral. The background is usually highly abnormal and consists of generalized asynchronous slow waves of low amplitude. Sharp waves may be triggered by startling stimuli and by light flashes.

*Clinical conditions causing these sharp waves* include mainly Jakob-Creutzfeldt disease. The sharp waves appear usually within 12 weeks of the onset of clinical symptoms and are present during the fully developed disease in over 90% of all patients; they persist through the course of the disease and at the end become slower and disappear in a background of low amplitude. Similar sharp waves are occasionally seen in postanoxic encephalopathy and in cerebral fat embolism.

*Seizure manifestations* consist of widespread myoclonic jerks associated with the complexes. Startling and flash stimuli which produce sharp waves often also induce myoclonic jerks.

**19.2.3** *Periodic generalized complexes, often associated with subacute sclerosing panencephalitis (SSPE).* *The EEG pattern* consists of complexes containing one or more sharp waves and delta waves. Complexes last 0.5–3 seconds and recur every 3–20 seconds. The background consists of asynchronous and bisynchronous theta and delta waves; bisynchronous slow spike-and-wave discharges, focal spikes and slow waves may also be present. Early in the course of the disease, the background may be fairly normal and the complexes may appear in a limited distribution. Later, however, the complexes usually become generalized, symmetrical and synchronous. Their shape may change with time and become disorganized before death. The complexes are usually not triggered by sensory stimuli. Sleep may enhance or obscure them.

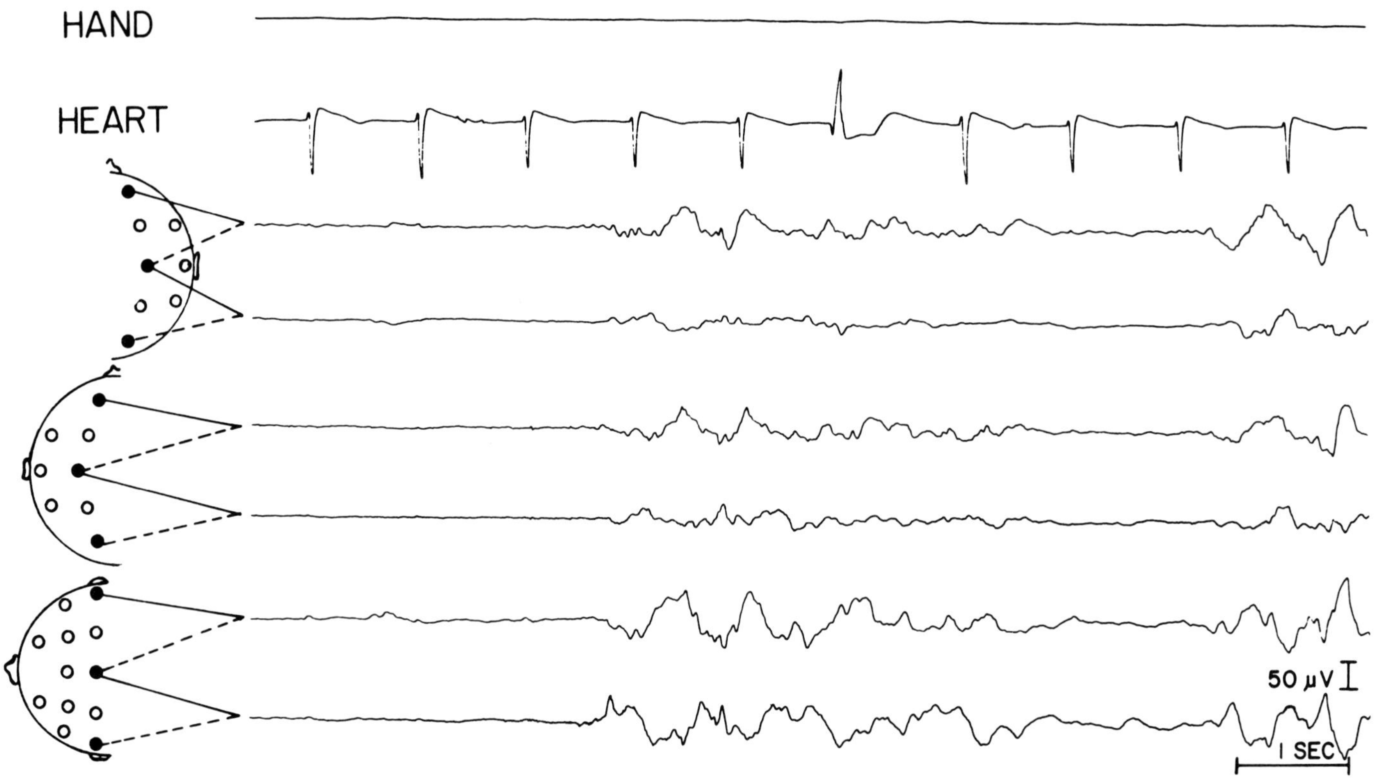


Fig. 19.8. Burst-suppression pattern recorded from a 60-year-old man in deep coma from a lethal barbiturate overdose. This recording was made in the intensive care unit with widely spaced electrodes and with monitoring of hand movement and heart beat.

*Seizure manifestations* consist of myoclonic jerks occurring with the complexes. Tonic seizures may occur with electrodecremental ictal patterns (19.3.3).

*Clinical conditions* causing these complexes include mainly subacute sclerosing panencephalitis (SSPE). The complexes may appear at any stage of the disease. Similar complexes may be seen in postanoxic encephalopathy, after head injury, in drug intoxications, lipidoses, herpes simplex encephalitis and a few other conditions.

**19.2.4** *Burst-suppression pattern. The EEG pattern* consists of bursts of irregular or regular slow waves of very low frequency. They are usually widespread and bisynchronous, but they may be limited to one hemisphere or part of it. Bursts last 1–3 seconds and are separated from each other by low amplitude delta waves or by periods of no activity recognizable at regular gain (Fig. 19.8). Successive bursts may vary in shape. The duration of the intervals between the bursts is often fairly regular in a given recording and ranges from 2 to 10 seconds. The duration increases as the patient's condition worsens. Before death, bursts become shorter, simpler and of lower amplitude; periods of suppression become longer until complete electrocerebral silence supervenes. The complexes are not responsive to stimuli.

*Seizure manifestations* are not associated with this pattern.

*Clinical conditions* causing burst-suppression patterns include a variety of severe disorders of cerebral structure or function. Structural lesions include acute strokes, postanoxic encephalopathy, head injury, Wernicke's disease and encephalitis. Local burst-suppression patterns can be seen over surgically isolated cerebral cortex. Reversible disorders causing this pattern include deep anesthesia and coma due to barbiturates and other CNS depressant drugs, hypothermia and Reye's syndrome.

**19.2.5** *Periodic sharp waves in the temporal areas, often associated with herpes simplex encephalitis. The EEG pattern* consists of single sharp waves with a steep

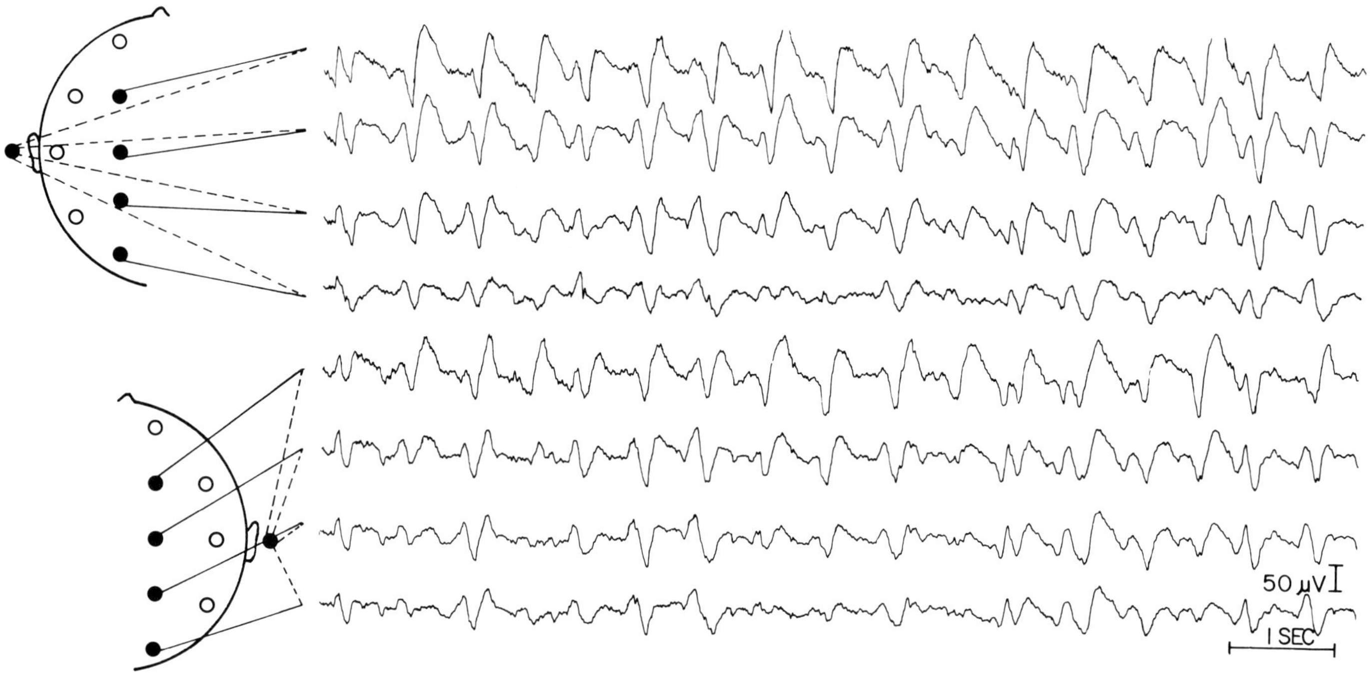


Fig. 19.9. Pattern of triphasic waves at 1–2 Hz with frontal maximum, recorded from a 68-year-old chronic alcoholic in hepatic coma.

rising phase, or of di- and triphasic sharp wave complexes of up to half a second in duration. They are located in one or both temporal regions and recur at intervals of about 1–5 seconds on a background of focal temporal or diffuse slow waves.

*Seizure manifestations* occur in a few patients and consist of rhythmical jerks.

*Clinical conditions* causing this pattern are limited to herpes simplex encephalitis. The complexes begin after the first few days of the disease and persist during the first two weeks.

**19.2.6** *Triphasic waves. The EEG pattern* consists of complexes of a large positive sharp wave preceded and followed by small negative components. These complexes last about 0.15–0.25 seconds and recur about every 0.5 to 2 seconds (Fig. 19.9). They are superimposed on a background of asynchronous and bisynchronous slow waves. Triphasic waves have a wide distribution and may be largest frontally. In some cases they appear up to 150 msec earlier in the frontal areas than in the middle and posterior areas.

*Seizure manifestations* are not directly associated with triphasic waves.

*Clinical conditions* causing triphasic waves are mainly metabolic encephalopathies, especially hepatic, uremic, hypo- and hypernatremic and hypercalcemic encephalopathies. Patterns resembling triphasic waves have occasionally been seen in other conditions, for instance postanoxic encephalopathy, cerebral tumors and infarctions, subdural hematoma, ether anesthesia, intoxication with lithium or penicillin, Binswanger's disease, myoclonus epilepsy of Unverricht-Lundborg and Jakob-Creutzfeldt disease.

## 19.3 ICTAL PATTERNS WITHOUT SPIKES AND SHARP WAVES

The patterns in this section (Table 19.3) are described in the chapters dealing with local and generalized epileptiform activity. They are joined here because they are

TABLE 19.3
Ictal patterns without spikes and sharp waves

| Ictal pattern | Distribution | Interictal patterns | Clinical seizure type |
|---|---|---|---|
| 1. Three hertz rhythmical slow waves | Generalized | 3 Hz spike-and-wave, 3 Hz slow waves, or normal | Absence, absence status, generalized seizures |
| 2. Theta or delta waves | Generalized | Slow spike-and-wave | Tonic seizures |
| 3. Rhythmical 4–6 (2–10) Hz waves | Bilateral or unilateral, temporal or fronto-temporal | Spikes or sharp waves in the temporal area | Partial complex seizures |
| 4. Delta or theta waves in periodic complexes | Generalized | Complexes of SSPE | Myoclonic jerks |
| 5. Periodic or rhythmical slow waves | Localized | None | Epilepsia partialis continua |
| 6. Loss of amplitude ('electro-decremental seizures') | Generalized | Hypsarrhythmia, slow spike-and-wave | Infantile spasms, tonic seizures |
| 7. Paroxysmal low voltage | Temporal, fronto-temporal, bilateral or unilateral | Spikes or sharp waves in the temporal area | Partial complex seizures |
| 8. No change of background | – | Spikes or sharp waves in the temporal area | Partial complex seizures |
| 9. No change of background | – | None | Epilepsia partialis continua |
| 10. Alpha waves | Focal, unilateral | Spikes, sharp waves, abnormal newborn patterns | Neonatal seizures |
| 11. Beta waves | Focal, unilateral | Spikes, sharp waves, abnormal newborn patterns | Neonatal seizures |
| 12. Beta waves | Central | Spikes, polyspikes or normal | Action myoclonus |
| 13. Beta waves (14–20 Hz) | Bilateral or unilateral, maximum temporal or fronto-temporal | Spikes or sharp waves in the temporal area | Partial complex seizures |

related to each other in that they represent ictal activity which (1) has no spikes or sharp waves; (2) usually begins and ends abruptly; and (3) is often recognized only by its association with clinical seizure manifestations. Some of these patterns are local, others are generalized; some occur mainly with one type of interictal pattern or seizure, others occur with many intercatal and seizure types.

**19.3.1** *Generalized ictal slow waves.* *Rhythmical bisynchronous slow waves at 3 Hz* are occasionally seen instead of 3 Hz spike-and-wave discharges in absence attacks, especially in absence status. Similar slow waves may occur as interictal activity in patients with attacks of absences or of other primary generalized seizures.

*Theta or delta waves,* often irregular, asynchronous and arrhythmical, may be associated with tonic seizures which occur especially in patients with slow spike-and-wave discharges.

*Rhythmical 4–6 Hz waves* or, occasionally, 2–10 Hz waves with a maximum in both temporal or fronto-temporal regions are a common ictal pattern of partial complex seizures even in patients who have spike foci in only one temporal lobe.

*Slow waves in periodic complexes* and hypsarrhythmia may be associated with myoclonic jerks, for instance in subacute sclerosing panencephalitis.

**19.3.2** *Local ictal slow waves.* *Rhythmical 4–6 Hz waves,* or 2–10 Hz waves, with a maximum in the temporal or fronto-temporal regions of one hemisphere occur in partial complex seizures.

*Periodic or rhythmical slow waves* are seen instead of periodic lateralizing discharges in some patients with epilepsia partialis continua.

**19.3.3** *Generalized decrease of amplitude.* *Electrodecremental seizures* are associated with sudden reduction of high amplitude background activity such as occurs in hypsarrhythmia and in recordings showing slow spike-and-wave activity;

these patterns are replaced by ictal generalized flattening of the tracing or low amplitude fast activity which lasts for several seconds and is often associated with infantile spasms and tonic seizures. Electrodecremental events also occur in some adults during dystonic seizures.

*The sudden appearance of low voltage activity*, replacing a background which usually does not contain epileptiform activity, is one seizure pattern of partial complex seizures.

*Sudden loss of amplitude* or low voltage fast activity also occurs in attacks of decerebration, often called 'cerebellar fit' (24.6.6).

**19.3.4** *No change of background activity* is a rare accompaniment of partial complex seizures and of epilepsia partialis continua.

**19.3.5** *Alpha waves,* usually unilateral or focal in distribution, can be seen in newborn and very young infants with partial, unilateral and generalized intermittent seizures or status epilepticus; unilateral or bilateral waves of alpha frequency are the ictal pattern of some patients with partial complex seizures.

**19.3.6** *Beta waves* may appear instead of the ictal alpha activity in some newborn infants. Fast waves of 14–20 Hz may appear with a maximum in the temporal or fronto-temporal regions in partial complex seizures at any age after infancy. Central beta rhythm, with or without spikes, may be associated with movement-activated myoclonus in adults, usually as a result of cerebral anoxia (23.7.2).

## 19.4 EPILEPTIFORM PATTERNS WITHOUT PROVEN RELATION TO SEIZURES ('PSEUDO-EPILEPTOGENIC PATTERNS')

These patterns (Table 19.4) are similar to each other in that they (1) consist of epileptiform activity of usually interictal duration, (2) have no corresponding ictal patterns, and (3) are not known to be associated with seizures and neurological diseases except that the first of the patterns listed below may be difficult to distinguish from the interictal activity of some patients with seizures and the second pattern is occasionally seen in hepatic encephalopathies. In the past, claims have been made that the first four patterns below are commonly seen in patients with seizures, in persons with various symptoms referable to the autonomic nervous system, especially dizziness, syncope, nausea, headaches, and in subjects with personality or behavior disorders, but the evidence for these contentions is inconclusive.

**19.4.1** *Six Hz spike-and-slow-wave discharges* ('wave and spike phantom') are of low or medium amplitude, repeat only a few times and rarely last longer than a second (Fig. 19.10). Brief and small bursts of this pattern may be difficult to distinguish from the background. They usually appear bisynchronously, either diffusely or with predominance in some parts, usually the posterior or central regions, but may occur in only one area at a time. They appear mainly in drowsiness and relaxed wakefulness. Discharges in the anterior head regions, especially those containing spikes with high amplitude, tend to show slower frequencies than 6 Hz; some of these discharges may represent interictal generalized epileptiform activity of patients with seizures (Fig. 18.3, Part 2).

Patients showing 6 Hz spike-and-slow waves may also show 14 and 6 Hz positive bursts (see below), and there may be transitions between the two types of discharges. These combinations are common in adolescents whereas 6 Hz spike-and-slow waves alone occur in adults.

TABLE 19.4
Pseudo-epileptogenic patterns

| Pattern name | Wave shape | Duration | Distribution | Age | Vigilance |
|---|---|---|---|---|---|
| 1. Six hertz spike-and-slow-wave ('wave and spike phantom') | Miniature spike-and-wave at 4–7 Hz | Less than 1 sec | Generalized, maximum often posterior | Adults, less often adolescents | Drowsy, awake |
| 2. Fourteen and six hertz positive bursts | Repetitive positive spikes arch-shaped | Less than 1–2 sec | Posterior temporal, parietal, bilaterally independent or synchronous | Adolescents, children; less often adults | Sleep, drowsiness |
| 3. Rhythmical mid-temporal discharge ('RMTD') ('Psychomotor variant') | 6 (4–7) Hz negative sharp waves with notched or flat positive phases | Up to a few seconds | Midtemporal, unilateral, bilateral, independent or bisynchronous | Slightly more in middle-aged females | Sleep |
| 4. Small sharp spikes ('sss'), benign epileptiform transients of sleep ('BETS') | Short spikes, usually small | Less than 50 msec for single phase | Mid- and anterior temporal, often shifting in distribution; unilateral, bilaterally independent or bisynchronous | Adults, adolescents | Sleep |
| 5. Wicket spikes | Often repetitive spikes forming arches | Repeating up to a few seconds | Anterior and middle temporal | Mainly adults | Awake, asleep |
| 6. Occipital spikes and sharp waves of blind persons | Focal spikes and sharp waves | Up to 200 msec | Occipital, unilateral or bilateral | Often children | Awake, asleep |

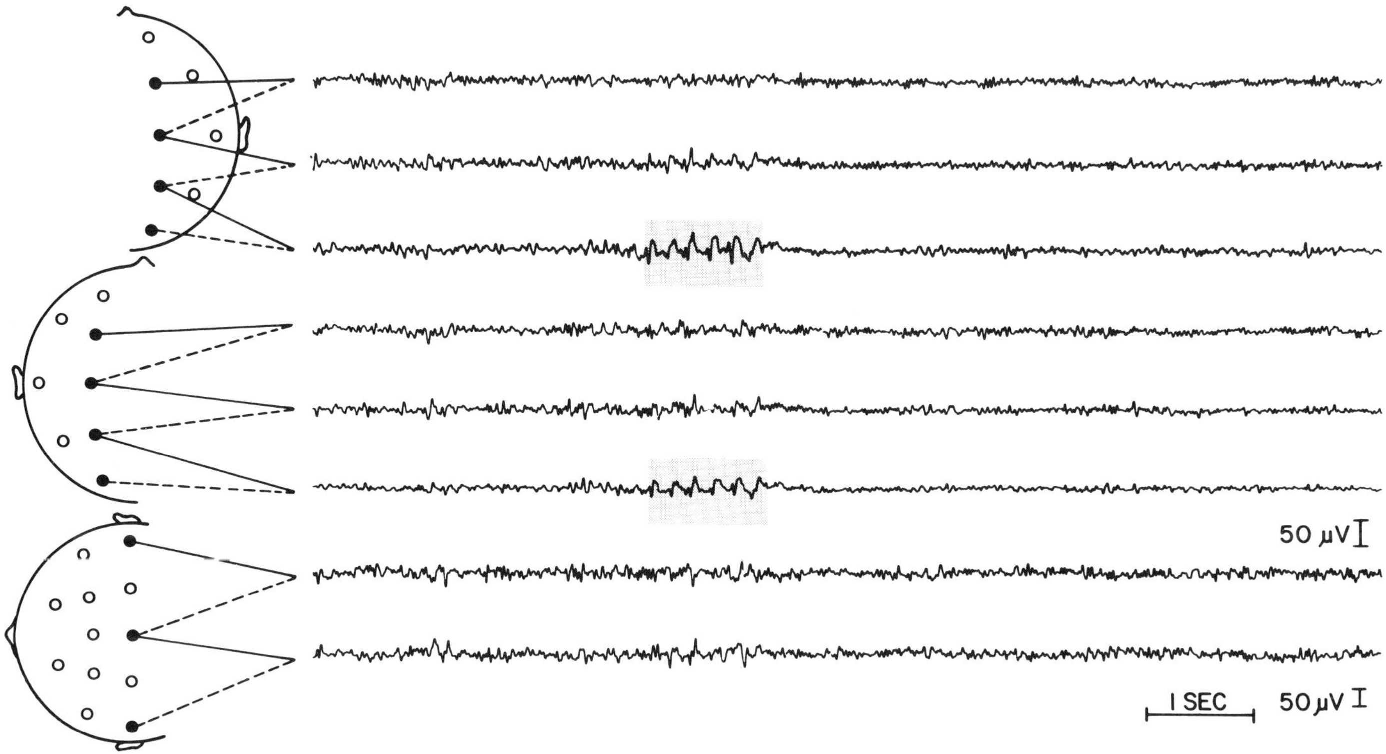


Fig. 19.10. Pattern of 6 Hz spike-and-slow-waves. A brief burst (shaded) appears in the posterior head regions during drowsiness. This 40-year-old woman has a history of headaches, no abnormal findings.

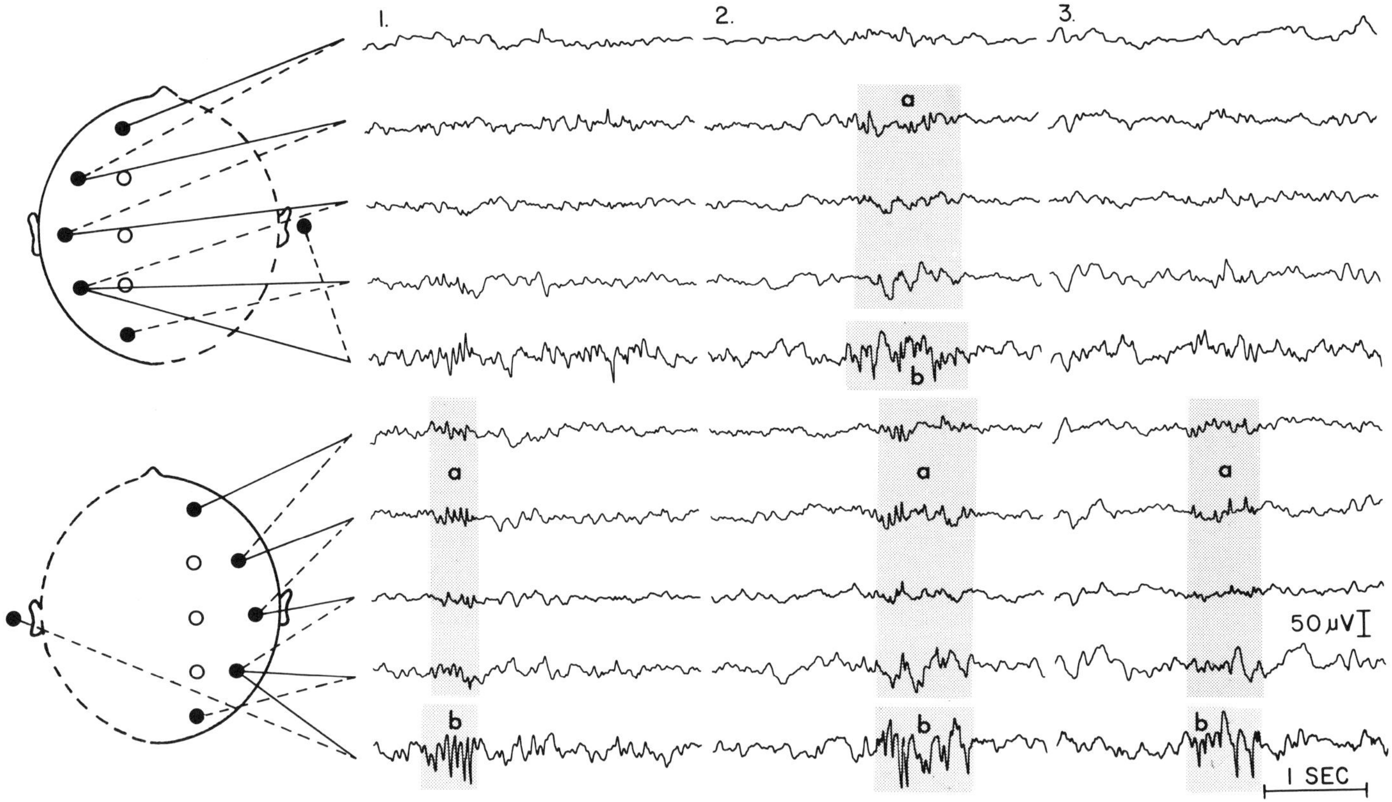


Fig. 19.11. Pattern of 14 and 6 Hz positive bursts. 1, 2 and 3 were recorded within a few minutes of each other during light sleep. Note that the bursts are barely distinguishable in conventional bipolar linkages between adjacent electrodes (a), but are greatly enhanced by the use of long interelectrode distances between posterior temporal electrodes and the opposite ear (b). This 12-year-old girl had a slight concussion 4 days earlier; the neurological examination is normal.

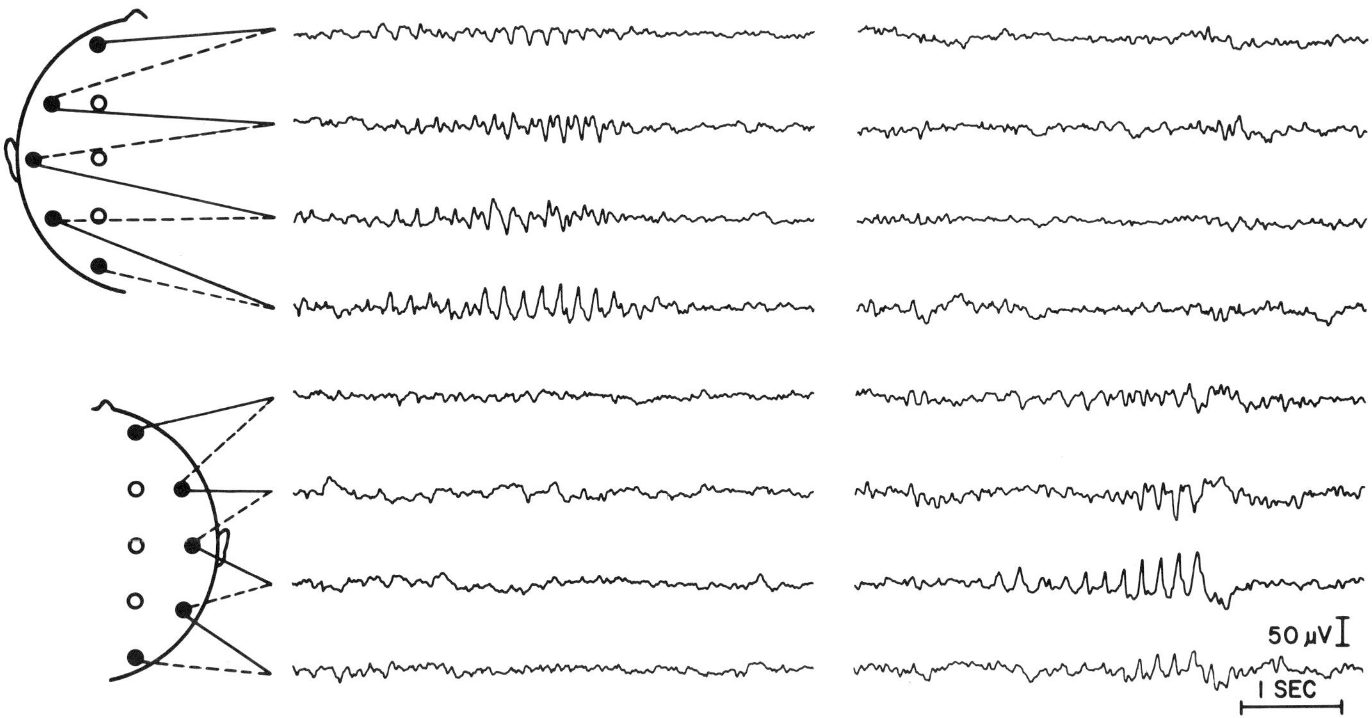


Fig. 19.12. Rhythmical midtemporal discharges (RMTD) at about 6 Hz, occurring independently on either side during light sleep. The patient is a 19-year-old girl with one seizure 5 years earlier, now normal.

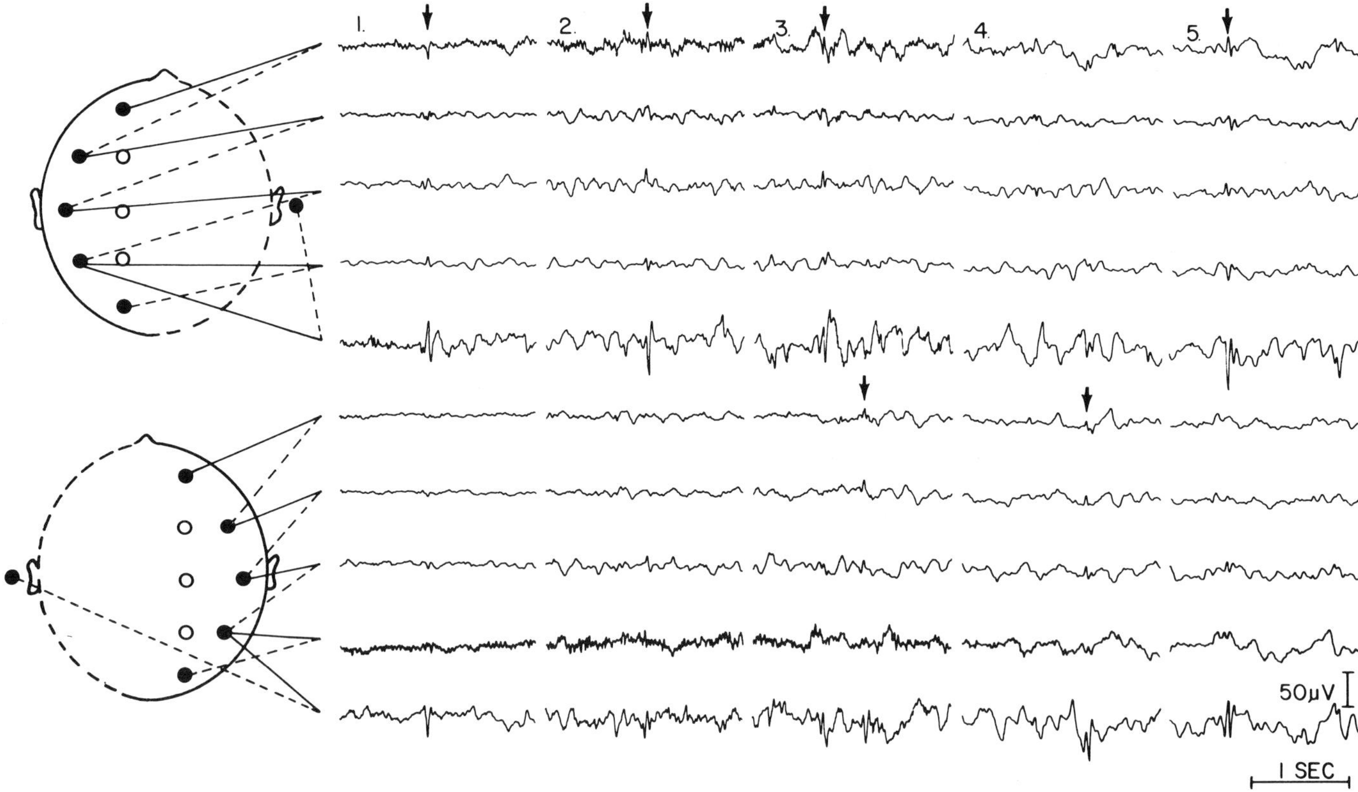


Fig. 19.13. Pattern of small sharp spikes (sss) or benign epileptiform transients of sleep (BETS) occurring independently in the temporal regions during light sleep. 1–5. were recorded within five minutes. Note that the amplitude of the spikes (arrows) is greatly increased in interelectrode linkages from the posterior temporal electrodes to the opposite ears. This 15-year-old girl complains of dizziness which is probably due to hyperventilation.

**19.4.2** *Fourteen and six hertz positive bursts* ('14 and 6 per second positive spikes', 'ctenoids') consist of bursts of brief spikes repeating at 14 Hz or at 6 Hz; spikes of both frequencies may be superimposed (Fig. 19.11). The 14 Hz burst often looks like a sleep spindle with a sharp positive phase. The bursts usually last less than a second and appear bisynchronously or independently in both hemispheres with a maximum in the posterior head regions. They may be difficult to recognize in the usual montages but are brought out by recordings with wide inter-electrode distances. As indicated by their name, the spikes have positive electrical polarity and therefore cause downgoing pen deflections in channels connected through input 1 to electrodes near their origin (3.4.1).

Fourteen and six hertz positive bursts appear during deep sleep in children, during lighter sleep in adolescents and may appear in light sleep or even in wakefulness in adults. They are most common in adolescents where they can be recorded in over one-half of all subjects if the recording time is long enough. In some cases, they show transitions to 6 Hz spike-and-slow wave discharges. An unexplained finding is 14 and 6 Hz positive bursts in comatose patients with acute Reye's syndrome, in severe toxic liver disease, and other metabolic and postanoxic encephalopathies.

**19.4.3** *Rhythmical midtemporal discharges* (formerly also called 'psychomotor variant') are bursts of rhythmical sharp waves at about 6 Hz (range of 4–7 Hz) which often have a top which is flat or notched by a small 12 Hz component (Fig. 19.12). These bursts may last for up to a few seconds. They often begin and end with a gradual increase and decrease of amplitude. They occur in the midtemporal regions, either on one side or on both and then either independently or simultaneously. They are mostly seen in young adults during light sleep. These bursts are distinguished from ictal discharges in patients with interictal temporal lobe spikes in that they do not vary much in duration and wave shape and thus resemble neither the interictal single spikes nor the ictal, sustained and changing discharges of temporal lobe foci.

**19.4.4** *Small sharp spikes* ('sss'), or benign epileptiform transients of sleep ('BETS') have usually low to medium amplitude and a very brief duration of less than 50 msec; they are usually mono- or biphasic (Fig. 19.13). They appear over the temporal regions but shift considerably in distribution. They often occur on both sides, either simultaneously or bisynchronously.

**19.4.5** *Wicket spikes* occur in the anterior or middle temporal areas with a negative polarity and an amplitude of up to more than 200 $\mu$V. They differ from other, abnormal, spikes in that they appear not only intermittently but also repetitively in trains of arch-shaped rhythms resembling mu rhythm.

**19.4.6** *Occipital spikes of blind persons* may occur after lesions of the visual path anterior to the occipital cortex, usually in congenital or long-standing acquired blindness. Associated abnormalities are disorganization of alpha rhythm, loss of photic responses and absence of lambda waves and POSTs. This condition differs from cerebral blindness due to bilateral occipital lesions which may be associated with epileptiform activity and seizures.

## REFERENCES


(*Chapter 19.1*)

Blume, W.T., David, R.B. and Gomez, M.R. (1973) Generalized sharp and slow wave complexes. Brain 96: 289–306.

Blume, W.T. (1978) Clinical and electroencephalographic correlates of the multiple independent spike foci pattern in children. Ann. Neurol. 4: 541–547.

Gastaut, H., Roger, J., Soulayrol, R., Tassinari, C.A., Régis, H. and Dravet, C. (1966) Childhood epileptic encephalopathy with diffuse slow spike-waves (otherwise known as 'petit mal variant') or Lennox syndrome. Epilepsia 7: 139–179.

Gomez, M.R. (1979) Tuberous Sclerosis. Raven Press, New York.

Kellaway, P., Hrachovy, R.A., Frost, J.D. and Zion, T. (1979) Precise characterization and quantification of infantile spasms. Ann. Neurol. 6: 214–218.

Lacy, J.R. and Penry, J.K. (1976) Infantile Spasms. Raven Press, New York.

Markand, O.N. (1977) Slow spike-wave activity in EEG and associated clinical features: Often called 'Lennox' or 'Lennox-Gastaut' syndrome. Neurology 27: 746–757.

Noriega-Sanchez, A. and Markand, O.N. (1976) Clinical and electroencephalographic correlation of independent multifocal spike discharges. Neurology 26: 667–672.

Westmoreland, B.F., Groover, R.V. and Sharbrough, F.W. (1979) Electrographic findings in three types of cerebromacular degeneration. Mayo Clin. Proc. 54: 12–21.

(*Chapter 19.2*)

Celesia, G.G. (1973) Pathophysiology of periodic EEG complexes in subacute sclerosing panencephalitis (SSPE). Electroenceph. clin. Neurophysiol. 35: 293–300.

Charlton, M.H. (1975) Myoclonic Seizures. Excerpta Medica, Amsterdam.

Chatrian, G.E., Shaw, C.M. and Leffman, H. (1964) The significance of periodic lateralized epileptiform discharges in EEG: An electrographic, clinical and pathological study. Electroenceph. clin. Neurophysiol. 17: 177–193.

Ch'ien, L.T., Boehm, R.M., Robinson, H., Liu, C. and Frenkel, L.D. (1977) Characteristic early electroencephalographic changes in herpes simplex encephalitis. Clinical and virologic studies. Arch. Neurol. 34: 361–364.

Chiofalo, N., Fuentes, A. and Gálves, C. (1980) Serial EEG findings in 27 cases of Creutzfeldt-Jakob disease. Arch. Neurol. 37: 143–145.

Cobb, W.A. (1975) Electroencephalographic changes in viral encephalitis. In: Illis, L.S. (Ed.), Viral Diseases of the Central Nervous System. Baillière Tindal, London, pp. 76–89.

Cobb, W.A. (1979) Evidence on the periodic mechanism in herpes simplex encephalitis. Electroenceph. clin. Neurophysiol. 46: 345–350.

Evans, B.M. (1975) Cyclic EEG changes in subacute spongiform and anoxic encephalopathy. Electroenceph. clin. Neurophysiol. 39: 587–598.

Illis, L.S. and Taylor, F.M. (1972) The electroencephalogram in herpes-simplex encephalitis. Lancet 1: 718–721.

Kuroiwa, Y. and Celesia, G.G. (1980) Clinical significance of periodic EEG patterns. Arch. Neurol. 37: 15–20.

MacGillivray, B.B. (1976) Section III. The EEG in liver disease. In: Rémond, A. (Ed.), Handbook of Electroenceph. clin. Neurophysiol., Vol. 15C, Elsevier, Amsterdam, pp. 26–50.

Markand, O.N. and Panszi, J.G. (1975) The electroencephalogram in subacute sclerosing panencephalitis. Arch. Neurol. 32: 719–726.

Schwartz, M.S., Prior, P.F. and Scott, D.F. (1973) The occurrence and evolution in the EEG of a lateralized periodic phenomenon. Brain 96: 613–622.

Shibasaki, H., Yamashita, Y. and Kuroiwa, Y. (1978) Electroencephalographic studies of myoclonus. Myoclonus-related cortical spikes and high amplitude somatosensory evoked potentials. Brain 101: 447–460.

Smith, J.B., Westmoreland, B.F., Reagan, T.J. and Sandok, B.A. (1975) A distinctive clinical EEG profile in herpes simplex encephalitis. Mayo Clin. Proc. 50: 469–474.

Thomas, J.E., Reagan, T.J. and Klass, D.W. (1977) Epilepsia partialis continua. Arch. Neurol. 34: 266–275.

Westmoreland, B.F., Sharbrough, F.W. and Donat, J.R. (1979) Stimulus-induced EEG complexes and motor spasms in subacute sclerosing panencephalitis. Neurology 29: 1154–1157.

(*Chapter 19.4*)

Catani, P., Salzarulo, P. and Findji, F. (1978) Occipital spikes and eye movement activity during paradoxical sleep in visually defective children. Electroenceph. clin. Neurophysiol. 44: 782–784.

Eeg-Olofsson, O. (1971) The development of the electroencephalogram in normal children from the age of 1 through 15 years. 14 and 6 Hz positive spike phenomenon. Neuropaediatrie 2: 405–427.

Harrison, A., Lairy, G.C. and Leger, E.M. (1970) EEG et privation visuelle. Electroenceph. clin. Neurophysiol. 29: 20–37.

Lipman, I.J. and Hughes, J.R. (1969) Rhythmic mid-temporal discharges. An electroclinical study. Electroenceph. clin. Neurophysiol. 27: 43–47.

Maulsby, R.L. (1979) EEG patterns of uncertain diagnostic significance. In: Klass, D.W. and Daly, D.D. (Eds.), Current Practice of Clinical Electroencephalography. Raven Press, New York, pp. 411–419.

Reiher, J. and Lebel, M. (1977) Wicket spikes: Clinical correlates of a previously undescribed EEG pattern. Can. J. Neurol. Sci. 4: 39–47.

Thomas, J.E. and Klass, D.W. (1968) Six-per-second spike-and-wave pattern in the electroencephalogram: A reappraisal of its clinical significance. Neurology 18: 587–593.

White, J.C., Langston, J.W. and Pedley, T.A. (1977) Benign epileptiform transients of sleep. Neurology 27: 1061–1068.

Yamada, T., Young, S. and Kimura, J. (1977) Significance of positive spike bursts in Reye syndrome. Arch. Neurol. 34: 376–380.

# Local slow waves

# 20

SUMMARY

(20.1) *The pattern* of local slow waves consists of waves which have a frequency under 8 Hz and a limited distribution; they are usually restricted to one or a few neighboring electrodes, i.e. to a focus of slow waves; less often, they occupy an entire hemisphere.

(20.2) *The cause* of local slow waves is a circumscribed abnormality located superficially or deeply in a hemisphere. Commonly the abnormality is a structural lesion which has an acute onset or a progressive course. In the case of acute lesions, the slow waves develop at the time of the damage and persist for weeks or months. Slow waves may also occur as a result of transient local abnormalities such as epileptiform activity and ischemia and then outlast the transient event by several hours or a few days.

(20.3) *Other EEG abnormalities* are often associated with focal slow waves and may further clarify the location and type of the underlying lesion.

(20.4) *Grading* of focal slow waves gives an estimate of acuteness and severity of the underlying lesion and is necessary for comparison of successive recordings.

(20.5) *Mechanisms* generating focal slow waves probably include interruption of fiber connections to the cortex and other local derangements.

(20.6) *Specific disorders* associated with focal slow waves include a variety of structural lesions such as tumors, infarcts, hemorrhages, abscesses and several kinds of transient abnormalities such as transient ischemic attacks, migraine, partial seizures and hypertensive encephalopathy.

## 20.1 DESCRIPTION OF PATTERN

Local slow waves consist of waves of less than 8 Hz which commonly appear at only one or a few electrodes, i.e. in a focal distribution (Figs. 20.1; 20.3; 20.4); less common are slow waves which are distributed over an entire hemisphere, i.e. unilateral slow waves (Fig. 20.2). Individual slow waves are often irregular and successive slow waves often are arrhythmical, i.e. composed of different fre-

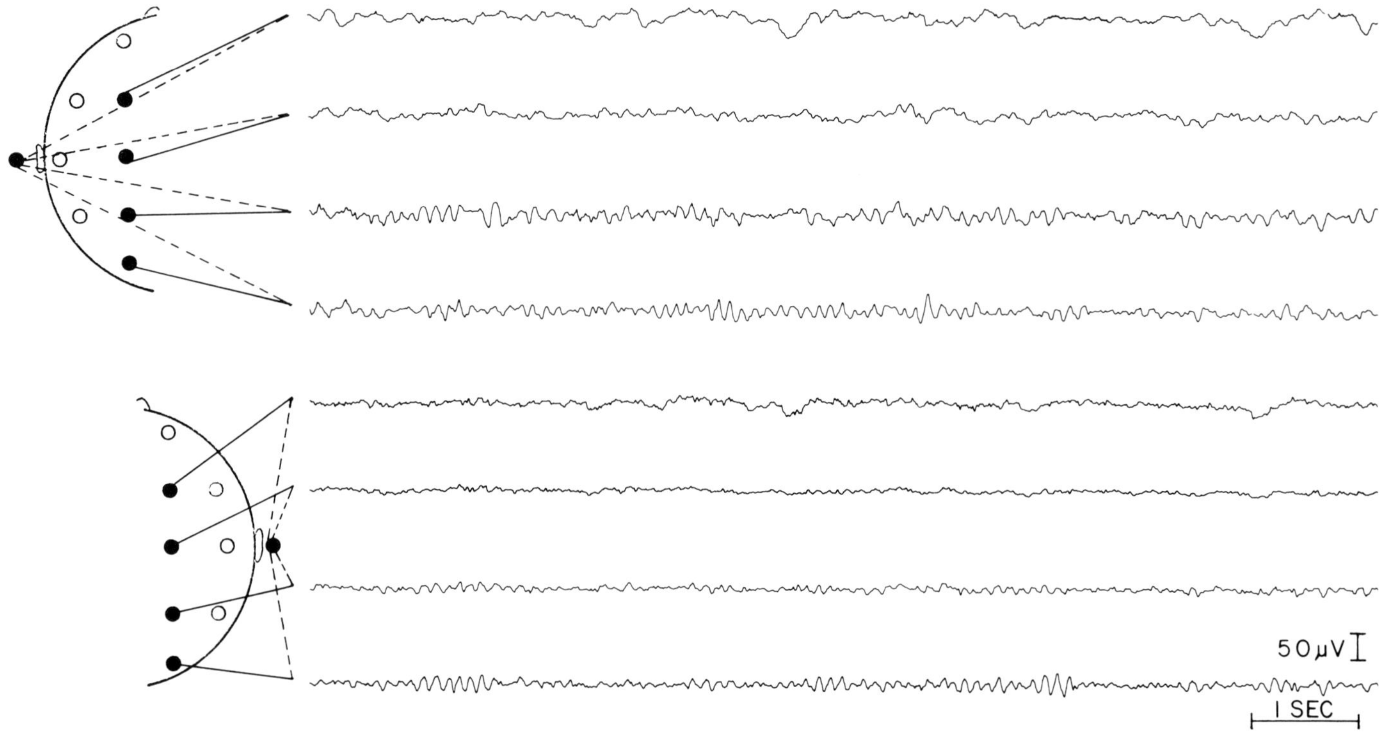


Fig. 20.1. Left fronto-central slow wave focus; the right frontal slow waves are largely due to eye movements. The patient is a 53-year-old man with a 3 year history of partial complex seizures which begin with olfactory hallucinations. A left frontal oligodendroglioma was removed surgically a few days after this EEG recording.

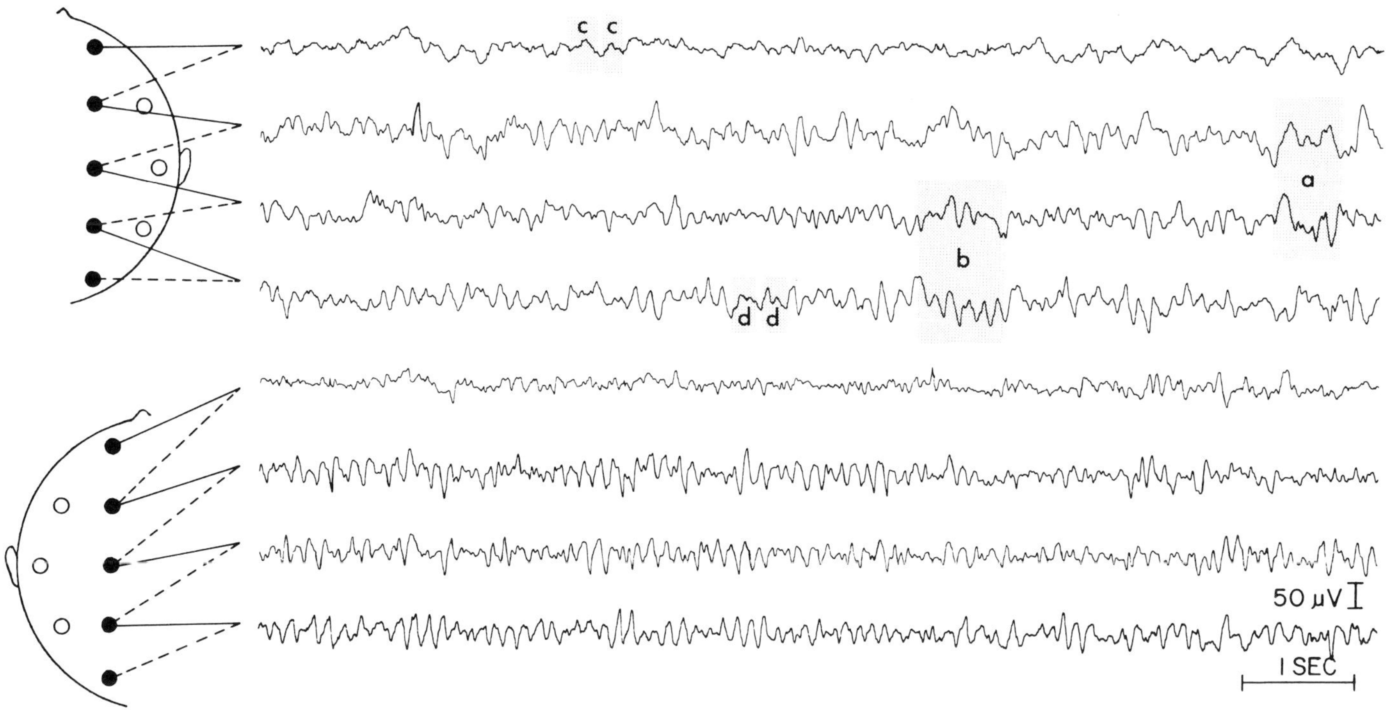


Fig. 20.2. Right centro-parietal slow wave focus. Delta waves have a maximum in the right central (a) and parietal (b) areas; theta waves appear in the right frontal (c) and occipital (d) areas. Occipital alpha rhythm on the right is slower than that on the left. This 76-year-old man had a large cerebral infarct in the distribution of the right middle cerebral artery two days before the EEG.

quencies. Irregular arrhythmical focal slow waves of delta frequency were formerly called 'polymorphic delta waves'.

The slow waves at the center of a focus are usually more persistent and usually of lower frequency than slow waves at the periphery; foci of delta waves are often surrounded by theta waves. The amplitude of slow waves does not always have a maximum at the center; the surrounding slow waves may be larger. Unless excessive, focal slow waves do not entirely replace the background activity but rather mix with it. Focal slow waves of low amplitude may be difficult to distinguish from normal background activity. Arrhythmical focal delta waves generally are not much attentuated by eye opening and alerting nor facilitated by hyperventilation, but surrounding slow waves of theta frequency may show such reactions. Local slow waves are most conspicuous during wakefulness, but may persist into sleep.

## 20.2 CLINICAL SIGNIFICANCE OF FOCAL SLOW WAVES

**20.2.1** *Types of underlying lesions.* *Focal slow waves* indicate a circumscribed lesion which may be due to either lasting structural damage or a transient disturbance in an area of the subcortical white matter or in the thalamic nuclei; however, lesions of the meninges or the subdural space can also cause focal slow waves. Beyond these general characteristics, focal slow waves do not indicate the specific nature of the local lesion and may thus be due to a variety of conditions.

*Lasting structural lesions* which can cause focal slow waves are cerebral infarcts, tumors, contusions, subdural hematoma, local infections, local developmental and degenerative defects. Delta foci surrounded by theta waves suggest acute or progressive superficial lesions; foci of rhythmical activity, especially in the theta range, are more likely due to deeply located or older lesions. However, local damage of any depth and age involving the parietal lobe is likely to produce rhythmical theta waves. Focal slow waves which persist in sleep have been thought to be more likely to indicate superficial or epileptogenic lesions.

Focal slow waves are the most important indicator of local lesions within the cerebral hemispheres of adults and adolescents. Even though some dural and subdural lesions may also cause focal slow waves, lesions which involve the cortex more than the underlying white matter often produce a local decrease of amplitude whereas partial lesions affecting both the cortex and deep midline structures more than the hemispheric white matter and the thalamus are likely to produce bisynchronous slow waves. In infants and young children, lesions similar to those producing focal slow waves in adults are associated with specific epileptiform patterns (19.1).

*Transient cerebral disorders* which can cause episodic focal slow waves are transient ischemic attacks, migraine attacks associated with focal neurological signs, hypertensive and metabolic encephalopathies, some partial seizures, the condition after partial seizures and after mild local head injuries. The slow waves should disappear within hours or a few days of the acute disorder; slow waves which persist longer suggest that lasting damage has occurred.

**20.2.2** *The temporal relation between slow waves and underlying damage* is not perfect. The correlation is best at the beginning: Focal slow waves appear at the onset of sudden structural damage. For instance, focal slow waves are present from the beginning of cerebral infarcts and develop soon after head injuries, giving the EEG a distinct advantage over isotopic and computerized brain scans in the early recognition of these lesions. The correlation between slow waves and the clinical signs of cerebral damage deteriorates with time in that focal slow waves may disappear weeks or months after acute damage even though the clinical signs persist; this discrepancy suggests that further clinical improvement is unlikely. Rarely do slow waves persist after neurological signs have cleared; a persistence of slow waves indicates persistent subclinical cerebral damage.

In many slowly progressive structural lesions, slow waves appear only at or after the onset of clinical signs; however in some cases focal slow waves associated with tumors may be seen at a time when the patient has only few vague symptoms.

**20.2.3** *The spatial relationship between focal slow waves and underlying cerebral lesion varies.* Slow waves in superficial lesions generally are fairly precise indicators of the site of the abnormality. However, in some cases, the slow wave focus may appear in a more lateral and posterior location than that of the cerebral lesion. Rarely do slow wave foci appear far away from the lesion. Lesions which are small and deep, for instance infarcts of the internal capsule, may produce no abnormality in the EEG even though the patient may show considerable neurological abnormalities.

Focal slow waves over an abnormality in one hemisphere may be associated with similar slow waves, usually of lower amplitude, in the opposite hemisphere, particularly in cases of frontal (Fig. 20.1) and occipital lesions. This phenomenon has several possible explanations: (a) an acute infarct or a tumor may produce compression, edema or ischemia in neighboring parts of the opposite hemisphere; (b) impulses from slow wave foci in one hemisphere may travel via commissural fibers to the corresponding area of the other hemisphere to produce slow waves there; (c) the electrical field of a slow wave focus may be conducted through the volume of the interposed tissue to the electrodes over the opposite hemisphere. In the first two instances, bilateral asynchronous frontal or occipital slow wave foci may make it difficult to distinguish between unilateral and bilateral cerebral lesions. In such cases, slight differences in the distribution and timing of slow waves may indicate the area of the primary abnormality. In the case of volume conduction, slow waves in the opposite hemisphere are synchronized, although attenuated, copies of the slow waves of the major focus.

Lesions in the posterior fossa cause focal slow waves only very rarely. Infratentorial lesions may produce arrhythmical slow waves in the occipital regions; these waves are usually bilateral, sometimes asymmetrical and rarely focal. They may be due to pressure on, or ischemia of, the occipital lobes, caused by the infratentorial lesion.

## 20.3 OTHER EEG ABNORMALITIES ASSOCIATED WITH FOCAL SLOW WAVES

In many cases of focal slow waves, the EEG shows other abnormalities which may be helpful in making the clinical diagnosis. In a few instances such abnormalities precede the appearance of focal slow waves and thus become the earliest indication of a local lesion; this is particularly true in cases of cerebral tumors.

**20.3.1** *Widespread asynchronous slow waves* are commonly seen in a hemisphere having a delta focus, or in both hemispheres (Fig. 20.2). They are more common in acute than in chronic lesions and suggest cerebral disturbances due to such possible mechanisms as local distortion of brain tissue, edema, vascular, metabolic or other changes. Widespread slow waves can accompany the reduction of alertness which occurs in some deeply located hemispheric strokes and tumors. The generalized slow waves may become so prominent as to obscure the focal slow waves.

**20.3.2** *Bilaterally synchronous slow waves* usually appear intermittently and in a wider distribution than the more persistent focal slow waves (Fig. 20.3). The bisynchronous slow waves may be larger or more persistent on the side of the focal slow waves but often have a frontal maximum independent of the distribution of the focal slow waves. Bisynchronous slow waves often suggest that the lesion causing

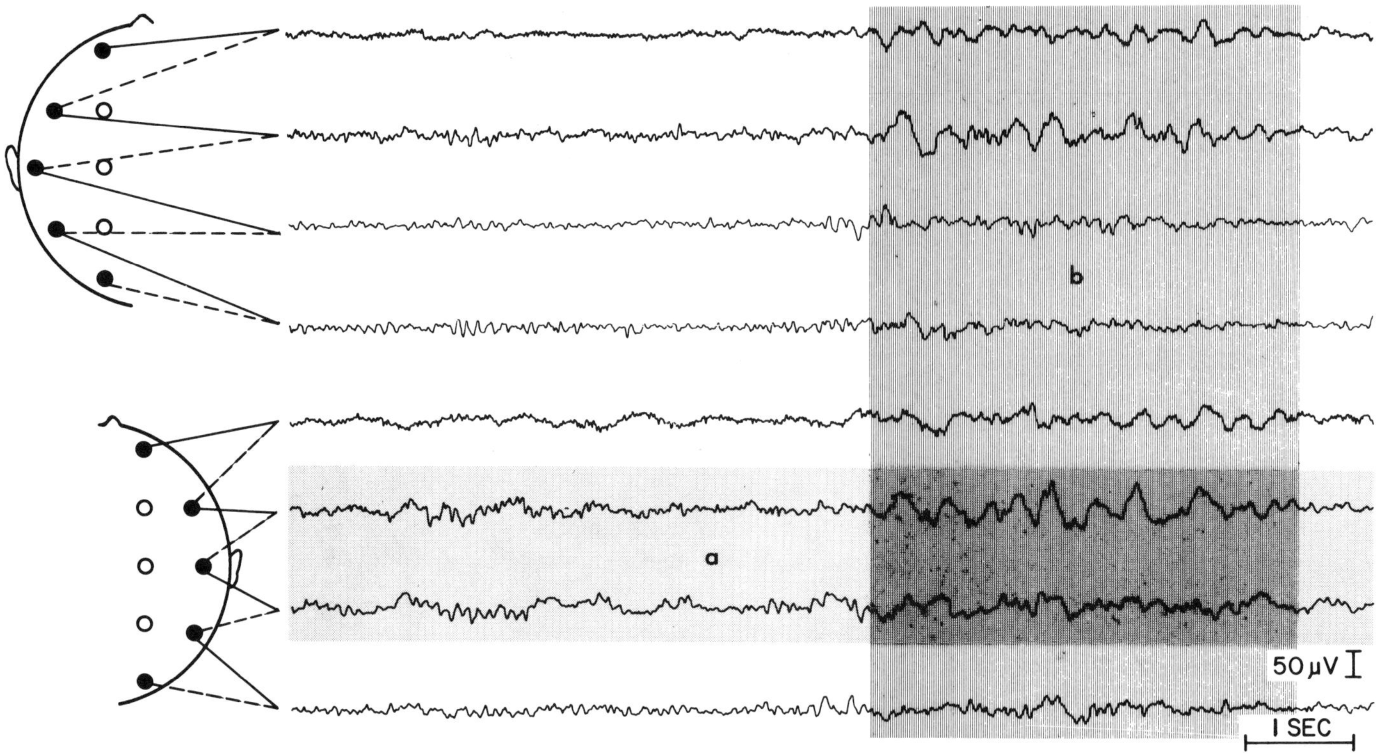


Fig. 20.3. Pattern of combined focal and bisynchronous slow waves. Focal slow waves of 0.5–2 Hz (a) occur continuously in the right temporal area; a burst of bisynchronous slow waves of 2–3 Hz (b) appears with a maximum in the anterior head regions, slightly greater on the right. The patient is a 62-year-old woman with a history of syncope and a decreased left nasolabial fold. Further workup was prompted by the EEG findings and revealed a right sphenoid wing meningioma.

focal slow waves has involved deep midline structures in the anterior, middle or posterior fossa, especially the mesencephalon or diencephalon, by directly invading these structures, by compressing or distorting them, or by rendering them ischemic. Occasionally, bisynchronous slow waves in patients with focal lesions are due to associated toxic or metabolic encephalopathies. Patients with bisynchronous slow waves due to secondary structural or functional involvement of diencephalic or mesencephalic centers often are not fully alert.

**20.3.3** *Focal spikes and sharp waves* may be caused by the same lesion which causes the focal slow waves (Fig. 20.4). On the other hand, slow waves associated with focal spikes or sharp waves may be entirely the result of ongoing epileptiform activity (20.6.6).

**20.3.4** *Asymmetry of alpha rhythm* may result from a reduction of the amplitude and frequency (Fig. 20.2) of alpha rhythm in the hemisphere showing focal slow waves. This happens more often with lesions in the posterior parts of the hemisphere than with anterior lesions, possibly as a result of compression of the posterior structures involved in the production of alpha rhythm. Occasionally, alpha rhythm is reduced on the side opposite to a slow wave focus, perhaps due to compression, or interference with blood supply, of that hemisphere.

**20.3.5** *Asymmetries of beta rhythm, mu rhythm, V waves, K complexes and sleep spindles* may be due to a reduction of the amplitude and incidence of these patterns in the vicinity of a lesion producing a slow wave focus, especially a lesion near the central regions. An isolated depression of beta rhythm, however, is not always a reliable localizing sign because beta rhythm is occasionally increased on the side of a tumor (23.7.2).

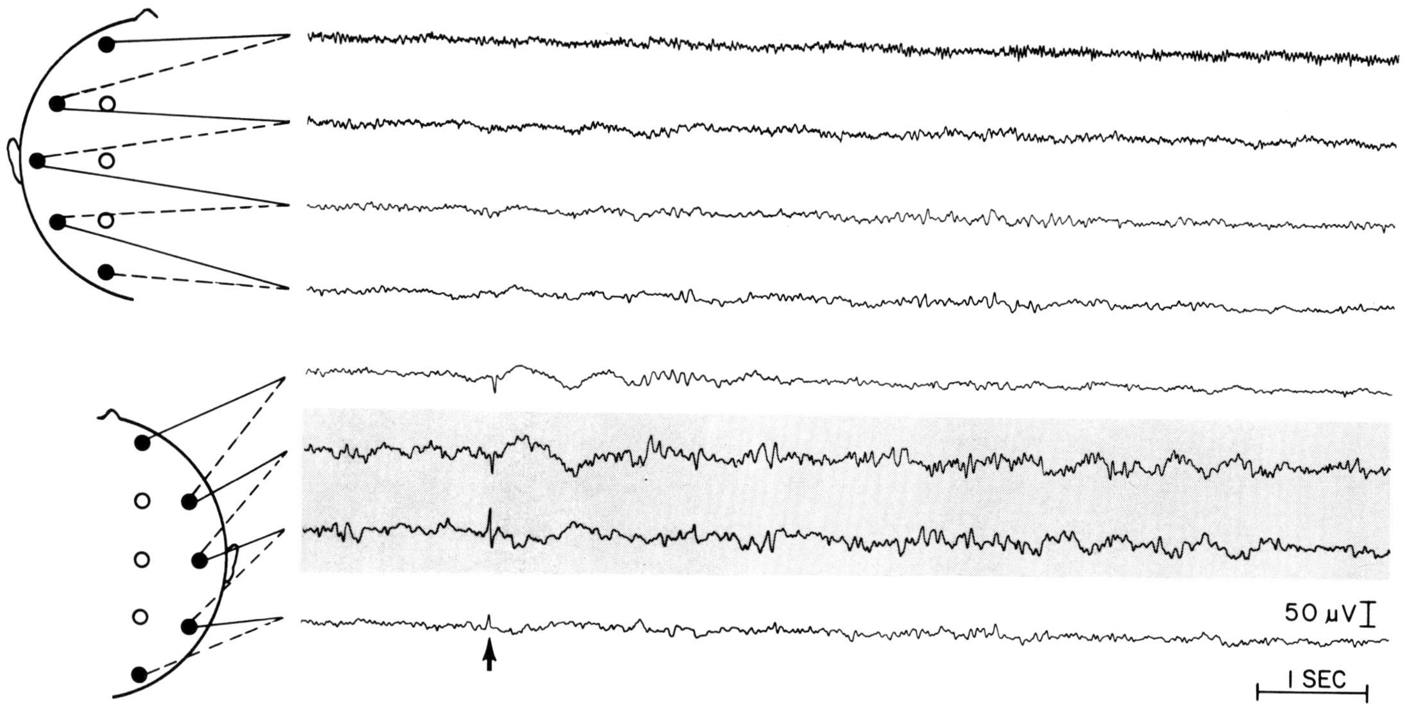


Fig. 20.4. Pattern of combined focal slow waves and focal spikes. Focal slow waves of 1–3 Hz (shaded) appear continuously in the right temporal region; a spike (arrow) appears in the same distribution. The recording was made during drowsiness. The patient is the same as in Fig. 20.3, one year after surgical removal of the meningioma; she had one generalized seizure 10 days before this EEG recording.

## 20.4 GRADING OF FOCAL SLOW WAVES

Grading of focal slow waves is of importance insofar as the degree of abnormality gives an approximate measure of the acuteness and severity of the underlying cerebral damage. A quantitative estimate of focal slow waves may be very important in evaluating improvement or progression of damage in sequential EEG recordings: An increase of slow waves may suggest a tumor; stationary slow waves may suggest a poor prognosis for improvement.

Focal slow waves may be rated as mild, moderate and marked depending on their prominence and frequency. *Mild* slow waves consist of sporadic theta waves which are not much larger than the background and occur on average not more often than once every 10 seconds. *Moderate* slow waves are more persistent or have an amplitude much larger than the background; they often have both theta and delta components. *Marked* slow waves have either high amplitude and persist for most of the time, or they have at least moderate amplitude and persist during the entire recording; they often consist mainly or entirely of delta waves.

## 20.5 MECHANISMS CAUSING FOCAL SLOW WAVES

Since completely destroyed brain tissue and tumors do not generate electrical activity, the focal slow waves caused by such structural lesions must originate from cerebral tissue which is capable of generating electrical activity. A possible mechanism is the interruption of fibers running through the subcortical white matter to the cortex, especially afferents from the brainstem reticular formation which usually suppresses slow wave activity. However, different mechanisms must be operating to produce the focal slow waves seen in association with extracerebral lesions such as subdural hematoma or meningioma; slow waves in these conditions may be due to local cortical ischemia, edema, acidosis or mechanical distortion of nerve cell membranes.

## 20.6 SPECIFIC DISORDERS CAUSING FOCAL SLOW WAVES

**20.6.1** *Degenerative developmental and demyelinating diseases.* Degenerative diseases produce focal slow waves so rarely that the EEG is often used to rule out structural lesions in patients suspected of having degenerative diseases. Exceptions are the temporal slow wave foci which may appear in senile dementia and local slow waves which occur at the beginning of Jakob-Creutzfeldt disease. Developmental diseases cause focal slow waves infrequently even if there is focal cerebral damage. This may be due to the fact that these lesions begin early in life, at a time when local damage produces distortions of background and specific epileptiform patterns (19.1). Later in life, the residual cerebral damage is rarely reflected by discrete focal slow waves.

*Senile and presenile dementia (Alzheimer's disease)* may be associated with an exaggeration of the intermittent focal slow waves which appear in the temporal areas, particularly on the left side, with advancing age (13.4). However, these focal slow waves are a less reliable indicator of dementia than are generalized asynchronous slow waves (21.6.1).

*Jakob-Creutzfeldt disease* may show slow waves locally for a short period before they become generalized, and before periodic complexes appear (19.2.2).

*Normal pressure hydrocephalus* occasionally produces local or generalized asynchronous slow waves (21.6.1).

*Hydrocephalus* in children may be associated with focal slow waves in addition to other abnormalities; focal slow waves are more common at the site of shunt insertions.

*Porencephaly, tuberous sclerosis, and perinatal cerebral damage* may cause residual local slow waves in the EEG after causing generalized abnormalities in infancy (19.1).

*Holoprosencephaly* may cause focal slow waves and focal spikes (17.6.1), emanating from islands of preserved brain tissue.

*Multiple sclerosis and Schilder's disease* cause focal slow waves much less often than they cause widespread slow waves and other abnormalities (21.6.1).

*Bilateral retrobulbar neuritis* in children, causing significant visual loss may lead to occipital slow waves in addition to spikes (17.6.1).

**20.6.2** *Metabolic and toxic encephalopathies.* Focal slow waves are seen in these disorders much less often than are generalized slow waves (22.6.2). Focal slow waves may appear on a background of generalized slow waves during metabolic coma or emerge from generalized slow waves after metabolic coma as a result of local vascular complications, namely transient cerebral ischemia or infarction. Very few metabolic disorders cause focal slow waves without causing generalized slow waves and coma. Focal slow waves may occur in: hypoglycemia, hypoxia and CO poisoning, hyperosmolar coma, for instance in nonketotic hyperglycemia, hyperparathyroidism, porphyria, vitamin B12 deficiency and Wilson's disease. Focal slow waves may occur after myelography with metrizamide.

**20.6.3** *Cerebrovascular diseases.* *Strokes* of the cerebral hemispheres caused by ischemia, embolism or hemorrhage are common causes of focal slow waves. Infarcts in the distribution of the middle cerebral artery often cause local slow waves in the temporal, frontal, central and parietal areas (Fig. 20.2). Occlusion of the anterior cerebral artery, especially at the origin of the artery at the base of the brain, may cause frontal intermittent delta activity (22.6.3), even though this activity is more often due to frontal tumors than to infarctions. A cerebral infarct in the distribution of the posterior cerebral arteries is likely to cause focal slow waves in the occipital and posterior temporal areas. Infarcts of the brainstem rarely produce focal slow waves over the posterior head and are often associated with a normal EEG; they may produce generalized bisynchronous and asynchronous slow waves if they involve the reticular formation in the core of the midbrain (22.6.3) or alpha coma patterns if they involve the pontine reticular formation (25.3.1).

*Multiple infarcts* may be the cause of more than one slow wave focus. Slow wave foci are often acquired in sequence by patients who have successive strokes. The small infarcts responsible for the lacunar state in hypertensive patients often cause no sharply defined slow wave foci but rather result in generalized slow waves (21.6.3). Cerebral air and fat emboli also usually cause generalized rather than focal slow waves (21.6.3).

*Transient ischemic attacks* of the cerebral hemispheres may cause local slow waves or reductions of amplitude (23.6.3). An EEG is rarely recorded during the attack, but slow waves may persist for many hours after the attack, or longer if an infarct has occurred.

*Transient global amnesia,* which is probably due to transient ischemia of the hippocampal part of the temporal lobes, may be associated with intermittent or continuous slow waves or sharp waves during and after attacks.

*Occlusion of the carotid artery* is produced intentionally during surgical repair of a partially occluded artery (carotid endarterectomy). Sudden clamping of the artery may reduce the cerebral blood flow to a level below that needed to prevent infarction. Imminent infarction can be recognized by the appearance of focal or unilateral slow waves within a few minutes after clamping; the slow waves are often followed by loss of amplitude. Lasting cerebral damage can be avoided if a shunt is placed so that blood can bypass the clamped segment of the artery until surgery is completed. Monitoring of the EEG during carotid endarterectomy can thus help to indicate the need for shunting.

*Migraine attacks* can produce local slow waves, especially if the attacks are associated with unilateral neurological abnormalities other than visual symptoms. The slow waves are presumably due to local cerebral ischemia occurring during the attack. If they persist for hours or a few days after the attack, the slow waves may be due to local cerebral edema; if they persist longer, they can be presumed to be due to infarction. Attacks of basilar artery migraine may be associated with focal slow waves in the posterior head regions on one or both sides, or with generalized slow waves; this form of migraine may also produce epileptiform activity in the same distribution. Slow wave foci in patients with headaches unexplained by a recent attack of migraine are sufficiently rare to warrant a workup for mass lesions or vascular malformations.

*Chronic subdural hematoma* commonly causes focal slow waves even though a regional reduction of amplitude is more characteristic (23.6.3). Bilateral subdural hematomas may be associated with any combination of unilateral and bilateral slow waves and asymmetries, including slow waves on one side and amplitude reductions on the other.

*Subarachnoid hemorrhage* produces focal slow waves only occasionally and by one of several possible mechanisms. The hemorrhage may damage the brain locally. Spasm of the bleeding vessel may cause local ischemia or infarction. Bleeding may come from an aneurysm or a vascular malformation which locally compresses the brain. Slow wave foci in the central region suggest bleeding from an aneurysm of the middle cerebral artery; foci in the posterior temporal region have no localizing value. Subarachnoid hemorrhage may cause ipsilateral decrease of amplitude and decrease of alpha frequency; when associated with a lowered level of consciousness, generalized slow waves are practically always present.

**20.6.4** *Cerebral trauma.* *Head injuries* may lead to focal slow waves in addition to the more common initial decrease of amplitude (24.6.4) and subsequent widespread slow waves (21.6.4). In many cases, focal slow waves after head injury are transient, variable in distribution and unassociated with focal neurological signs. They therefore probably do not represent local structural damage but may be explained by temporary local changes of cerebral cirulation or edema. In other instances, they last longer and are due to contusions, intracerebral hemorrhages, acute traumatic subdural or epidural hematoma.

*Progressive traumatic encephalopathy* may produce one or more slow wave foci initially before leading to generalized slow waves (21.6.4).

*Brain surgery* involving the cerebral hemispheres is often followed by focal slow waves. They suggest local brain damage. However, this must be distinguished from the effects of a skull defect which can locally increase the amplitude of generalized slow waves (23.6.4).

*Hemispherectomy* may cause unilateral slow waves in addition to amplitude reductions (23.6.4).

**20.6.5** *Brain tumors.* *Supratentorial brain tumors* are among the most important causes of focal slow waves, and focal slow waves are the most characteristic sign of a supratentorial tumor (Fig. 20.1,3). Focal slow waves of tumors may be associated with other EEG abnormalities such as focal epileptiform activity (Fig. 20.4) and generalized slow waves (Fig. 20.3) which have the implications described earlier (20.3).

Studies of the EEG in patients with brain tumors have revealed several important pieces of clinical information. Frontal tumors tend to produce a considerable amount of focal slow wave activity not only on the side of the tumor but also on the opposite side (Fig. 20.1). Tumors deep in the parietal lobe may cause focal parietal theta rhythm. Multiple metastases occasionally cause more than one slow wave focus. Tumors in older persons are more likely to produce bisynchronous slow waves than are tumors in persons of other ages. Infratentorial tumors, while often causing bisynchronous slow waves, produce local slow waves in the posterior head regions only rarely in adults and slightly more commonly in children. Slow wave foci in the temporal region do not have localizing value.

**20.6.6** *Seizure disorders.* *Postictal* focal slow waves often appear after a seizure of focal onset and may persist for a few days. In a patient who is known to have had a recent seizure but who shows no epileptiform activity in the EEG, focal slow waves can suggest a focal origin of the seizure. Because focal slow waves occasionally appear after primary generalized seizures, the possibility of a focal lesion should be investigated by a repeat EEG done at least one week after a seizure.

*Interictal* focal slow waves raise the suspicion of a local lesion such as a tumor, stroke, injury or malformation which can both damage subcortical tissue, giving rise to the slow waves, and irritate cortical tissue, producing epileptiform activity. However, focal slow waves, mixed with focal spikes or sharp waves, can be seen in stationary epileptogenic lesions as part of the ongoing epileptiform activity.

*Ictal* focal slow waves are rarely the only EEG manifestation of an ongoing seizure; this may be seen in seizures and status epilepticus of partial seizures and in epilepsia partialis continua (19.3.2).

**20.6.7** *Infectious diseases.* *Abscesses* of the cerebral hemispheres are more commonly associated with focal slow waves than with other EEG abnormalities such as unilateral slow waves, focal spikes and sharp waves, periodic lateralizing epileptiform discharges, or local reductions of amplitude. Bisynchronous slow waves are more common with deeply located abscesses. Asynchronous generalized slow waves invariably appear when the level of alertness decreases.

*Meningitis and encephalitis* produce focal slow waves only rarely and when the infection involves one part of the hemispheres more than others. This is usually the case in the acute necrotizing encephalitis of herpes simplex which produces focal slow waves in one or both temporal areas early in the disease (19.2.5).

*Progressive multifocal leukoencephalopathy* may begin locally and be associated with focal slow waves for a while before generalized asynchronous slow waves supervene (21.6.7).

**20.6.8** *Psychiatric diseases. Focal slow waves* have been reported in a great variety of psychiatric disorders. However, this occurrence is so rare and without clear relation to specific diseases that focal slow waves cannot be accepted as manifestation of psychiatric disease and a local cerebral lesion must be excluded by other examinations. This is especially true for patients whose symptoms include dementia where the finding of a slow wave focus in any part of the brain would be strong presumptive evidence for a structural cerebral lesion.

## REFERENCES


Magnus, O., Storm van Leeuwen, W. and Cobb, W.A., eds. (1961) Electroencephalography and cerebral tumours. Electroenceph. clin. Neurophysiol., Suppl. 19: 1–250.

Michel, B., Gastaut, J.L. and Bianchi, L. (1979) Electroencephalographic cranial computerized tomographic correlations in brain abscess. Electroenceph. clin. Neurophysiol. 46: 256–273.

Rodin, E.A., Bickford, R.G. and Svien, H.J. (1953) Electroencephalographic findings associated with subdural hematoma. Arch. Neurol. Psychiat. 69: 743–755.

Roseman, E., Bloor, B.M. and Schmidt, R.P. (1951) The electroencephalogram in intracranial aneurysms. Neurology 1: 25–38.

Sharbrough, F.W., Messick, J.M. and Sundt, T.M. (1973) Correlation of continuous electroencephalograms with cerebral blood flow measurements during carotid endarterectomy. Stroke 4: 674–683.

Shuping, J.R., Rollinson, R.D. and Toole, J.F. (1980) Transient global amnesia. Ann. Neurol. 7: 281–285.

Slatter, K.H. (1968) Some clinical and EEG findings in patients with migraine. Brain 91: 85–98.

van der Drift, J.H.A. and Kok, N.K.D. (1972) Section II. The EEG in cerebrovascular disorders in relation to pathology. In: Rémond, A. (Ed.), Handbook of Electroenceph. clin. Neurophysiol., Vol. 14A, Elsevier, Amsterdam, pp. 12–64.

Vignaendra, V., Ghee, L.T. and Chawla, J. (1975) EEG in brain abscess: Its value in localization compared to other diagnostic tests. Electroenceph. clin. Neurophysiol. 38: 611–622.

# Generalized asynchronous slow waves

# 21


SUMMARY

(21.1) *The pattern* of generalized asynchronous slow waves consists of waves of less than 8 Hz which occur over both hemispheres in such a way that the waves on one side have no constant time relationship with the waves on the other side. Asynchronous slow waves usually vary in frequency and often have irregular shapes. They may be reduced by eye opening and alerting and increased by hyperventilation. They may have a local maximum, i.e. an area of higher amplitude and incidence, in some part of the brain; this pattern differs from a slow wave focus surrounded by generalized slow waves in that focal slow waves have usually a lower frequency and sometimes a lower amplitude than the surrounding slow waves and react less to eye opening, alerting and hyperventilation.

(21.2) *Causes* of generalized asynchronous slow waves include many normal and abnormal conditions. In general, these slow waves are present in all normal subjects during drowsiness and sleep. During wakefulness, slow waves are part of the normal background in subjects of all ages except adults. In adults, a mild to moderate excess of generalized slow waves during wakefulness, although an electrographic abnormality, is found in 10–15% of otherwise normal subjects. A mild or moderate amount of asynchronous generalized slow waves in a wakeful adult can therefore only suggest that a person is somewhat more likely to have a cerebral abnormality. However, a marked amount of these slow waves always indicates a cerebral abnormality. The type of abnormality remains unspecified: Generalized asynchronous slow waves occur in such a great variety of widespread cerebral disorders that they are the most common and least specific EEG abnormality.

(21.3) *Other EEG abnormalities* associated with generalized asynchronous slow waves are usually of greater diagnostic significance.

(21.4) *Grading* of asynchronous slow waves uses the same criteria as used for focal slow waves.

(21.5) *Mechanisms* causing generalized asynchronous slow waves generally interfere with the structure or function of both hemispheres and involve subcortical white matter.

(21.6) *Specific disorders* include a wide variety of cerebral abnormalities.


## 21.1 DESCRIPTION OF PATTERN

Generalized asynchronous slow waves have a frequency under 8 Hz and occur over

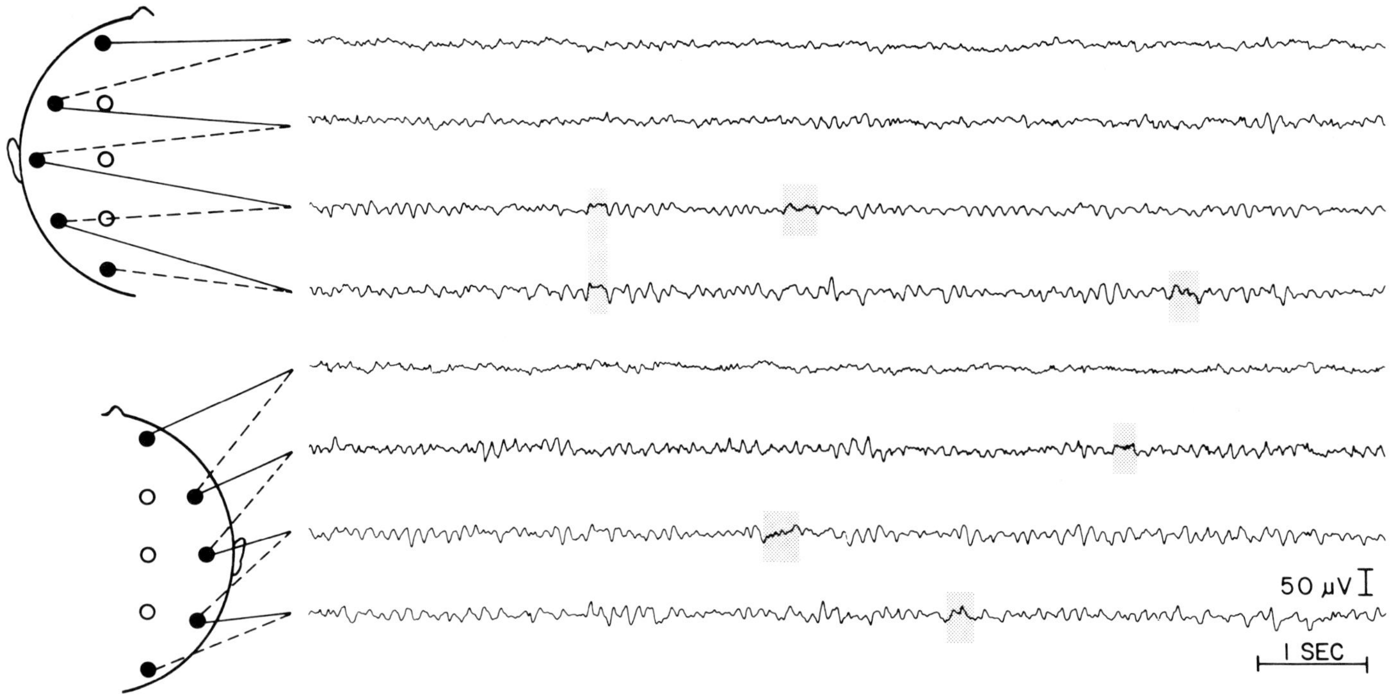


Fig. 21.1. Pattern of generalized asynchronous slow waves with a maximum in the posterior head regions. The slow waves are mainly in the theta range and of low or medium amplitude; a few slow waves are indicated by shading. The slow waves of much lower frequency in the prefrontal regions are eye movement artifacts. The patient is a 53-year-old woman with a schizoid personality disorder and several psychotic episodes, currently treated with 100 mg chlorpromazine every 4 hours.

most or all parts of both hemispheres (Figs. 21.1; 21.2; 21.3). The slow waves in one area have no constant time relationship with slow waves in the corresponding area on the other side. For example, slow waves may appear in some areas when there are no slow waves in other areas; slow waves appearing in different areas at the same time may have different frequency; waves of similar frequency appearing simultaneously in different areas may have varying phase relationship. Even though individual slow waves may often have a fairly regular shape, their rate of repetition usually varies by at least 2–3 Hz, i.e. they are often arrhythmical. The slow waves are reduced by eye opening and alerting, and increased by relaxation and hyperventilation; in some comatose patients, alerting stimuli may paradoxically increase the slow waves (25.4.2). In general, the reactivity of generalized asynchronous slow waves is greater than that of focal slow waves and less pronounced than that of bisynchronous generalized slow waves. Generalized asynchronous slow waves are best recognized during wakefulness because during sleep they are usually obscured by the generalized slow waves of normal sleep patterns.

Although distributed widely, generalized asynchronous slow waves may be more prominent in some areas than in others (Fig. 21.1). They may have a maximum of amplitude and incidence in corresponding parts of both hemispheres or in one area. This local prominence can usually be distinguished from focal slow waves which appear on a background of generalized slow waves since focal waves usually have a lower frequency, and sometimes lower amplitude, than the surrounding slow waves and since they are less reactive to eye opening, alerting and hyperventilation than are generalized asynchronous slow waves.

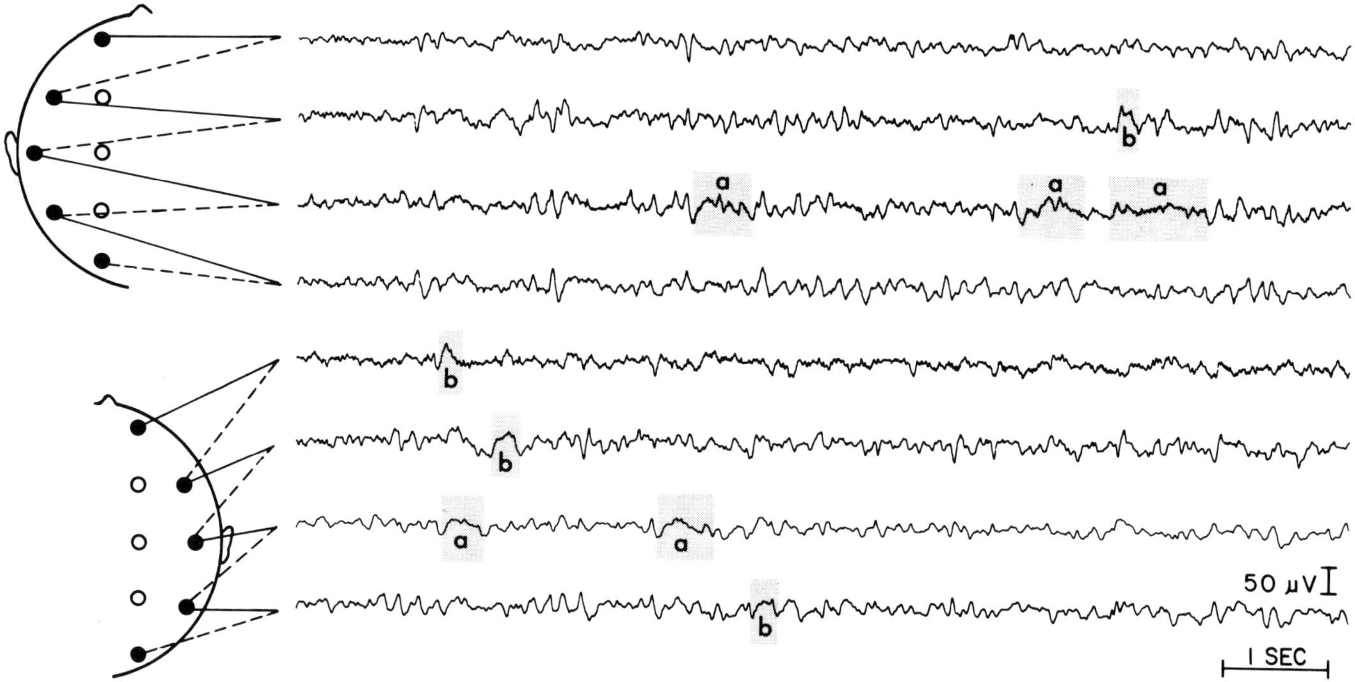


Fig. 21.2. Pattern of generalized asynchronous slow waves of delta (a) and theta (b) frequency and of moderate amplitude. Intermittent rhythmical occipital background activity has a frequency of 5–6 Hz. This 73-year-old man has fairly severe senile dementia.

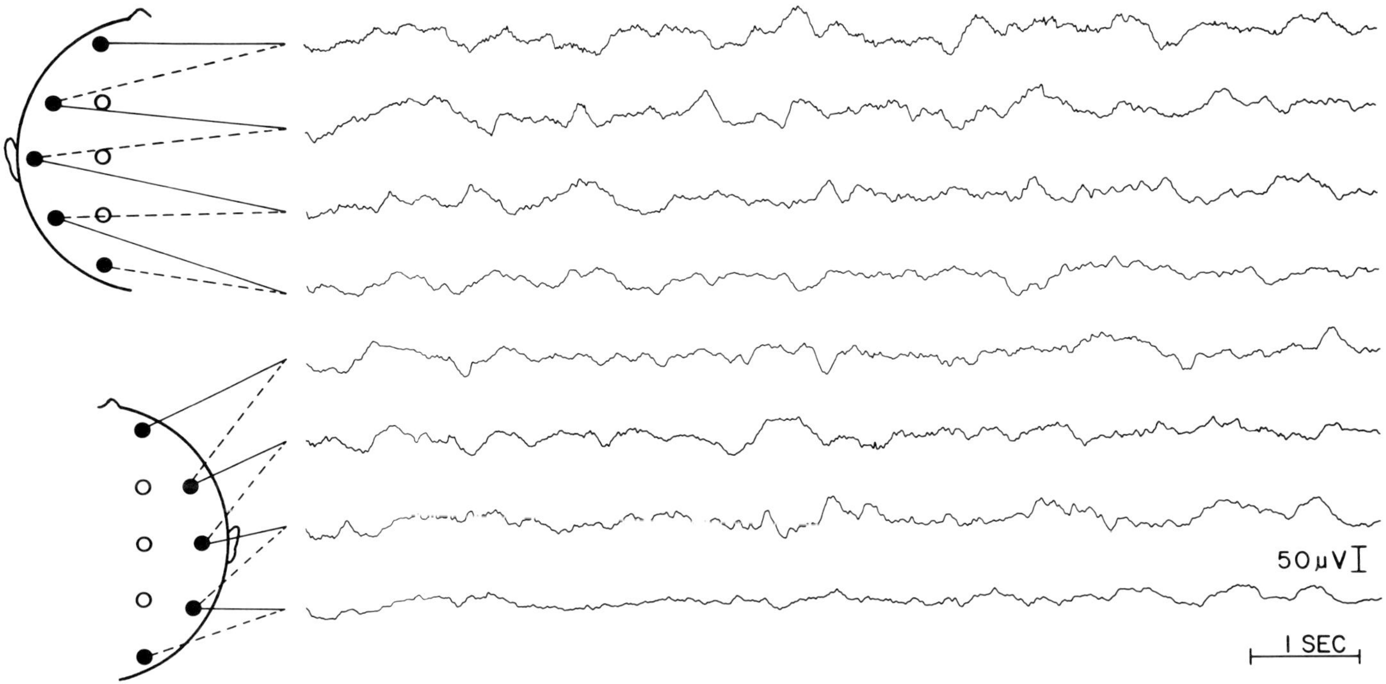


Fig. 21.3. Pattern of generalized asynchronous slow waves of predominantly delta frequency and moderate to high amplitude. This 69-year-old man had a cardiorespiratory arrest, was resuscitated but remained in postanoxic coma for the 2 days before this recording.

## 21.2 GENERAL CLINICAL SIGNIFICANCE OF GENERALIZED ASYNCHRONOUS SLOW WAVES

**21.2.1** *Normal generalized asynchronous slow waves* occur in drowsiness and sleep at all ages. During wakefulness, they are prominent in infants, gradually diminish in children and adolescents, and reach a minimum in adults; slightly greater amounts appear in older persons. The slow waves are therefore abnormal only if they exceed the normal range for the age of the patient.

**21.2.2** *Abnormal amounts of generalized asynchronous slow waves in normal subjects* occur in the waking record of 10–15% of adults and in perhaps even a greater percentage of subjects of other ages; a mild excess is more common than a moderate one. Generalized asynchronous slow waves thus distinguish less sharply between normal and abnormal subjects than do other EEG patterns. This overlap reduces the ability of mild and moderate asynchronous slow wave abnormalities to indicate cerebral abnormalities. Therefore, the finding of this abnormality can only suggest that a patient is more likely to have a cerebral abnormality than a patient with a normal EEG. However, this does not affect the significance of a marked excess of generalized asynchronous slow waves in the waking EEG which indicates a cerebral abnormality in every adult, teenager and child.

**21.2.3** *Abnormal generalized asynchronous slow waves* are due to a wide variety of conditions and are the most common and least specific abnormal EEG pattern. However, an EEG showing only an excess of generalized asynchronous slow waves has a certain negative diagnostic value: The absence of other abnormalities reduces the likelihood of a recent focal brain lesion of the hemispheres considerably, and it reduces the probability of a convulsive disorder slightly.

## 21.3 OTHER EEG ABNORMALITIES ASSOCIATED WITH GENERALIZED ASYNCHRONOUS SLOW WAVES

**21.3.1** *Attenuation, slowing and disorganization of alpha rhythm* often occurs with mild and moderate generalized slow waves (Fig. 20.1). Marked generalized slow waves replace alpha rhythm completely (Fig. 20.3).

**21.3.2** *Bisynchronous slow waves* often appear intermittently in bursts which usually have higher amplitude and restricted distribution and therefore stand out against a background of asynchronous generalized slow waves. Many cerebral abnormalities which eventually lead to bisynchronous slow waves initially cause disorganization of alpha rhythm and mild or moderate asynchronous slow waves, and later produce mixtures of bisynchronous and asynchronous slow waves. The bisynchronous slow waves usually are of greater diagnostic importance than the asynchronous slow waves.

**21.3.3** *Focal slow waves, generalized epileptiform activity, periodic complexes and other abnormal patterns* of greater diagnostic significance than asynchronous generalized slow waves often appear on a background of these slow waves.

## 21.4 GRADING OF GENERALIZED ASYNCHRONOUS SLOW WAVES

*Grading of generalized asynchronous slow waves* depends on their amplitude, incidence and frequency. Mild, moderate and marked abnormalities are distinguished by the same criteria as those given for focal slow waves (20.4).

## 21.5 MECHANISMS CAUSING GENERALIZED ASYNCHRONOUS SLOW WAVES

Generalized asynchronous slow waves may be produced by various mechanisms. Most of them probably interfere with structure or function of both hemispheres and involve subcortical white matter in a wide distribution; rarely are the generalized slow waves an extension of focal slow waves. Widespread interruption or disorganization of cortical input from the brainstem reticular formation may be an important factor in many cases; brainstem lesions cause widespread asynchronous slow waves in some cases although they seem more likely to produce bisynchronous slow waves.

## 21.6 SPECIFIC DISORDERS CAUSING GENERALIZED ASYNCHRONOUS SLOW WAVES

**21.6.1** *Degenerative, developmental and demyelinating diseases.* Most of the degenerative diseases which produce generalized asynchronous slow waves are those which involve the cerebral hemispheres and cause dementia. Degenerative diseases involving the cerebellum, brainstem and spinal cord do not produce EEG abnormalities.

(1) *Senile and presenile dementia (Alzheimer's disease)* is often associated with an exaggeration of age-related EEG changes (13) and thus leads to: (a) excessive generalized asynchronous slow waves; (b) marked slowing, reduction of amplitude and disorganization of alpha rhythm (Fig. 21.2); (c) fairly frequent bursts of focal slow waves, often with sharp contours, appearing in the temporal regions, most often on the left side; (d) the appearance of bilaterally synchronous slow waves. While excessive generalized asynchronous slow waves correlate better with dementia than do the other EEG abnormalities, dementia may become quite obvious before the EEG becomes definitely abnormal.

(2) *Pick's disease* which can usually not be distinguished from Alzheimer's disease on clinical grounds often produces few or no EEG abnormalities even in the presence of rather severe dementia.

(3) *Parkinson's disease* is associated with a mild or moderate amount of generalized asynchronous slow wave activity in less than half of all patients. This is not of great clinical importance because the diagnosis is not based on the EEG; however, it is worth noting that the finding of generalized asynchronous slow waves in a patient with Parkinson's disease should cause no alarm. Cerebral slow waves in the EEG of a patient with Parkinson's disease must be distinguished from artifacts consisting of intermittent or continuous rhythmical 4–6 Hz waves produced by tremor of the head or neck. These slow waves may fall in phase with motor unit action potentials from nearby scalp muscles and generate patterns resembling spike-and-wave discharges.

(4) *Progressive supranuclear palsy* may lead to generalized slow waves in advanced cases, but the initial abnormalities of sleep patterns (24.92) and bisynchronous slow waves in the waking record (22.6.1) are diagnostically more important.

(5) *Huntington's chorea* may be associated with generalized asynchronous slow waves, but the generalized reduction of amplitude is a more important diagnostic feature (24.6.1).

(6) *Jakob-Creutzfeldt disease* is characterized by progressive and widespread slowing of the EEG and by disintegration of alpha rhythm. Moderate or marked slow waves replace all normal background activity in advanced cases. In the end-stage of the disease, the amplitude of all activity may decrease and the EEG may become nearly flat and featureless. Periodic sharp waves, appearing in the early or middle stages of the disease, are the most characteristic abnormal pattern in this disease (19.2.2).

(7) *Normal pressure hydrocephalus* often produces no EEG abnormality but may

be associated with mild or moderate generalized slow waves or with focal slow waves (20.6.1). The generalized slow waves are asynchronous in most cases, in contrast to bisynchronous slow waves which may appear in obstructive hydrocephalus.

(8) *Hydrocephalus in children,* regardless of its cause, may be associated with asynchronous generalized slow waves and other abnormalities including bisynchronous slow waves (22.6.1), focal slow waves (20.6.1), and spike foci (17.6.1).

(9) *Tuberous sclerosis* in adults can cause asynchronous generalized slow waves in addition to bisynchronous slow waves (22.6.1) and focal spikes (17.6.1); infants and young children show different abnormalities (19.1).

(10) *Other degenerative and developmental diseases* may produce generalized asynchronous slow waves as the only abnormality or as one of several abnormalities in some patients; other patients with the same diseases may have normal EEGs. These diseases include: Leber's hereditary optic atrophy, Riley-Day syndrome, Seitelberger's disease, Leigh's disease, microcephaly with or without microgyria, macrogyria or agyria, holoprosencephaly, cerebral palsy, infantile hemiplegia, myotonic dystrophy, Mongolian idiocy.

(11) *Multiple sclerosis* produces generalized asynchronous slow waves, reduction of amplitude (24.6.1) and other abnormalities in approximately one-half of all cases. The incidence of abnormalities varies widely in different groups of patients, probably depending on acuteness, duration and rate of progression of the disease. Longer duration of the disease may account for higher incidences of abnormalities in some studies of benign multiple sclerosis.

(12) *Schilder's disease* also can cause diffuse asynchronous slow waves and other abnormalities.

**21.6.2** *Metabolic and toxic encephalopathies.* Generalized asynchronous slow waves may occur in any of these conditions when they cause significant encephalopathy and therefore do not distinguish these conditions from each other or from other conditions. Mild or moderate slow waves, often associated with a disorganization of the background, are usually the first abnormality in the EEG and marked slow waves may be the only abnormality found in the severest stages. Asynchronous slow waves in these encephalopathies may combine with bisynchronous slow waves and other abnormalities (22.6.2) in adults and children, and with special patterns in infants (19.1).

(1) *Congenital encephalopathies such as phenylketonuria, amaurotic familial idiocy, metachromatic and other leukodystrophies (Krabbe's and Pelizaeus-Merzbacher's diseases* often cause hypsarrhythmia, slow spike-and-waves or multifocal independent spikes (19.1) in infancy and early childhood, but only excessive slow waves at later ages. Thus, the three infantile epileptiform patterns are often found in the infantile (Tay-Sachs) and late infantile (Bielschowski-Jansky) forms of amaurotic familial idiocy but not in the juvenile (Spielmeyer-Vogt) and adult (Kufs) forms which show only asynchronous generalized slow waves and occasional bisynchronous slow waves.

(2) *Wilson's disease* produces generalized asynchronous or focal slow waves in about one-half of all patients, especially those with significant liver disease.

(3) *Acquired metabolic encephalopathies* such as those due to hepatic and renal failure, hypoglycemia, hypoxia and electrolyte imbalances often have an initial phase of generalized asynchronous slow waves and disorganized background followed by combinations of these slow waves with prominent bilaterally synchronous slow waves and other abnormalities. Asynchronous slow waves in these encephalopathies are usually present when the patient begins to become confused and somnolent. Residual slow waves may persist after the end of acute encephalopathies suggesting widespread residual cerebral damage. Metabolic encephalopathies and the corresponding EEG abnormalities are listed in Table 22.1. A few other metabolic encephalopathies produce mainly other EEG abnormalities to

which generalized asynchronous slow waves may be added in some cases. Hypothyroidism leads to a decrease of the frequency of alpha rhythm and a generalized reduction of overall amplitude (24.6.2), hyperthyroidism causes an increase of alpha rhythm frequency (25.1.7) and an excess of fast activity (24.8.2).

(4) *Toxic encephalopathies* commonly produce generalized asynchronous slow waves in acute intoxications, especially those associated with reduced levels of alertness. Common examples are intoxications by alcohol, barbiturates, and other drugs depressing the central nervous system. However, slow waves induced by drugs are not always accompanied by clinical manifestations of encephalopathy: intravenous administration of atropine, chronic intake of sedatives and psychotropic drugs, or myelography with metrizamide can induce generalized slow waves without producing overt mental changes.

*Alcohol.* *Acute alcohol intoxication* may cause generalized asynchronous slow waves, decrease of alpha frequency and increase of central beta activity.

*Chronic alcoholism* itself produces no EEG abnormalities, but asynchronous generalized slow waves may be found when chronic alcoholism is associated with cerebral atrophy in patients over 60 years of age.

*Acute withdrawal syndrome, delirium tremens, and Korsakoff's psychosis* usually induce no more than mild or moderate generalized slow waves; only a few cases of Korsakoff's psychosis show more prominent generalized slow waves similar to those of Wernicke's disease. Beta activity is often prominent and replaces alpha rhythm or is superimposed on it in a harmonic relation to give it a notched appearance. Photic stimulation during the acute withdrawal phase may produce photoconvulsive responses, corresponding with the increased likelihood for withdrawal seizures during this time (25.5.2).

*Wernicke's encephalopathy* usually produces prominent generalized asynchronous slow waves, and often also causes a decrease of alpha rhythm and bisynchronous slow waves.

*Hepatic encephalopathy and subdural hematoma* are indirect results of alcoholism which usually are associated with asynchronous slow waves but often with more characteristic abnormalities: hepatic encephalopathy with bisynchronous slow waves (22.6.2), or triphasic waves (19.2.6), subdural hematoma with focal slow waves (20.6.3) and asymmetries of amplitude (23.6.3).

*Barbiturates* acutely produce prominent central or generalized beta activity and a decrease of alpha rhythm at low or medium blood levels. At higher levels, beta waves and frontal 10–12 Hz waves may persist as generalized asynchronous theta and delta waves emerge and become more prominent until nonreactive delta waves predominate. Then periods of low amplitude activity or of complete electrical silence of a few seconds in duration begin to interrupt the delta waves at short intervals, creating burst-suppression patterns (19.2.4). With deepening coma, the quiet periods increase in duration and the delta waves in the bursts decrease in amplitude and eventually disappear completely. Electrocerebral silence may persist and ultimately indicate cerebral death although the patient and the EEG may recover even after more than 24 hours without recordable EEG.

*Chronic intake of barbiturates* may either cause fast waves or produce no effect on the EEG.

*Barbiturate withdrawal* can produce asynchronous slow waves along with bursts of high amplitude bisynchronous theta waves; photo-convulsive responses (25.5.2) and spontaneous generalized epileptiform activity (18.6.2) may also occur.

*Phenothiazines, haloperidol, rauwolfia derivatives* may produce generalized asynchronous slow waves and slowing of alpha rhythm at moderate doses. Large doses can induce bisynchronous slow waves, prominent beta activity, and bilateral spike-and-wave or polyspike-and-wave patterns.

*Tricyclic antidepressants* may produce generalized asynchronous or bisynchronous slow waves, and bilateral spikes or spike-and-wave discharges.

*Carbon monoxide* and other poisons causing widespread structural brain damage may produce generalized asynchronous slow waves.

*Other toxic agents* of many different types can produce generalized asynchronous slow waves. These include: carbon disulfide, methyl chloride and bromide, organic solvents, manganese, mercury, tin, strontium, lead, arsenic, bismuth, lithium, monoamine oxidase inhibitors, opiates, chloralose. Some of these are associated with a slowing of alpha frequency and bisynchronous slow waves, others with epileptiform activity. Most vitamin deficiencies causing asynchronous slow waves also cause bisynchronous slow waves.

**21.6.3** *Cerebrovascular diseases:*

(1) *Syncope of various causes including Stokes-Adams attacks, transient ischemic attacks of the brainstem,* and other conditions causing transitory reductions of blood flow to the entire brain or to the brainstem produce generalized slow waves only when consciousness fades; bisynchronous slow waves may be added. The slow waves disappear within minutes or hours after recovery from these conditions; persistence of slow waves suggests that structural damage has occurred.

(2) *Postanoxic encephalopathy* is often the direct result of cardiac and respiratory arrest, or the indirect result of metabolic encephalopathy, intracerebral or subarachnoid hemorrhage, or of severe cerebral injury which causes widespread structural cerebral damage and generalized asynchronous slow waves. Depending on the severity of the underlying damage, asynchronous slow waves show higher amplitude and lower frequency (Fig. 21.3) and may be associated with, or replaced by: (a) bursts of bisynchronous slow waves (22.6.3); (b) rhythmical, widespread and unreactive alpha or theta activity (25.3.1); (c) reduced amplitude (24.6.3); (d) spikes or sharp waves (18.6.3, 19.2.2); (e) burst-suppression patterns (19.2.4); (f) electrocerebral silence (24.6.3).

The prognostic value of the EEG in postanoxic encephalopathy is very limited. During the first six hours after the anoxic insult, the EEG has no relation to outcome. Later, the persistence of electrocerebral silence indicates cerebral death (5.4; 24.6.3) whereas the return of a normal EEG has a good prognosis. Between these extremes, the EEG does not clearly predict the outcome. The presence of elements of normal sleep activity and of any EEG response to alerting stimuli suggests less severe damage and a better prognosis (25.4.1; 25.4.2).

(3) *Midbrain strokes* due to thrombosis, embolism or hemorrhage which damage the reticular formation in the central parts of the midbrain reduce the patient's alertness and produce generalized asynchronous slow waves with or without superimposed bisynchronous slow waves. Infarcts in the central parts of the pons may produce coma associated with alpha or theta activity (25.3.1), while infarcts involving the lateral parts of the midbrain or pons usually do not produce alterations of consciousness or EEG abnormalities.

(4) *Multiple cerebral infarcts, lacunar state, fat and air embolism* commonly produce generalized asynchronous slow waves.

(5) *Chronic subdural hematoma* commonly produces generalized asynchronous slow waves, but focal slow waves (20.6.3) and asymmetries (23.6.3) often overshadow this abnormality and always are of greater diagnostic significance.

(6) *Migraine and other headaches* are associated with an abnormally high incidence of generalized asynchronous slow waves and other abnormalities between attacks. Additional abnormalities may appear during migrainous attacks (20.6.3).

**21.6.4** *Cerebral trauma:*

(1) *Mild head injuries* that cause only a brief loss of consciousness or no unconsciousness at all may produce diffuse asynchronous theta and delta waves and a decrease of alpha amplitude and frequency (23.7.1; 25.1.6); the abnormalities usually disappear within hours or days but may persist for weeks even in patients who recover without complications. The abnormalities are generally more severe in children than in adults.

(2) *Severe head injuries* that cause longer periods of unconsciousness are associated with marked generalized asynchronous slow waves and may also be associated with (a) generalized decrease of amplitude (24.6.4), (b) focal decrease of amplitude (23.6.4), (c) focal slow waves (20.6.4), (d) bisynchronous generalized slow waves (22.6.4), (e) early or late focal epileptiform activity (17.6.4), (f) absence of sleep patterns (25.4.1).

(3) *Progressive traumatic encephalopathy* of boxers and other persons exposed to repeated head injuries is often associated with generalized asynchronous and bisynchronous (22.6.4) slow waves; these abnormalities are usually preceded by slowing of alpha rhythm and the appearance of focal slow waves (20.6.4).

**21.6.5** *Brain tumors:*

(1) *Solitary brain tumors* produce asynchronous generalized slow waves only indirectly, namely when they invade or compress midbrain and diencephalic structures so that alertness is reduced. Focal slow waves (20.6.5) or bisynchronous slow waves (22.6.5) may precede this development.

(2) *Multiple metastases* cause asynchronous generalized slow waves as the result of initially discrete slow wave foci or as the result of diencephalic or mesencephalic lesions that reduce alertness.

**21.6.6** *Seizure disorders:*

(1) *Postictal generalized asynchronous slow waves* may persist for up to several days after a generalized seizure; they may remain for a few weeks after electroconvulsive treatment.

(2) *Interictal generalized asynchronous slow waves* are found in a higher percentage of subjects with epilepsy than in the asymptomatic population; the incidence of interictal slow waves is especially high in patients whose seizures are associated with widespread cerebral damage.

(3) *Ictal generalized asynchronous slow waves* are very rare (19.3.1).

**21.6.7** *Infectious diseases:*

(1) *High fever* can lead to generalized asynchronous slow waves and slowing of alpha rhythm in keeping with a reduction of alertness. However, slow waves in patients with only moderate fever may be the expression of a cerebral infection.

(2) *Meningitis* is more likely to produce EEG abnormalities if it extends into the brain; generalized slow waves are more common in children than in adults.

(3) *Encephalitis* of most causes produce generalized asynchronous slow waves as a signal of widespread involvement of cerebral structure or function. Bisynchronous slow waves may be added as the result of toxic or metabolic complications (22.6.2) or of predominant involvement of cortical and subcortical grey matter. Focal slow waves can appear when there is more localized damage, especially that produced by herpes simplex encephalitis and abscesses (20.6.7).

*Subacute sclerosing panencephalitis,* a late complication of measles infection, initially often produces generalized asynchronous slow waves as a background on which the characteristic periodic complexes later develop (19.2.3).

(4) *Progressive multifocal leukoencephalopathy,* a disease of probably viral cause, produces generalized asynchronous slow waves; they may be preceded by a stage of focal slow waves.

(5) *Sydenham's chorea* associated with streptococcal infections, in many cases produces asynchronous generalized slow waves in excess of those of normal children at the same age and in some cases produces bisynchronous slow waves or spikes and sharp waves.

(6) *General paresis* produces asynchronous and, occasionally, bisynchronous slow waves in slightly over one-half of all cases whereas patients with other forms of neurosyphilis usually have a normal EEG.

**21.6.8** *Psychiatric diseases.* The incidence of generalized asynchronous slow waves is slightly higher in patients with various psychiatric diseases than in the general population (Fig. 21.1). This is most evident in schizophrenia where slow waves are seen most often in the catatonic form, least in the paranoid form. However, the slow waves are usually only mild or moderate and therefore do not help in the diagnosis except that (a) the absence of other abnormalities in the EEG may help to exclude gross organic disease and (b) the presence of marked generalized slow waves suggests organic disease.

## REFERENCES


Blom, S. and Hagberg, B. (1967) EEG findings in late infantile metachromatic and globoid cell leucodystrophy. Electroenceph. clin. Neurophysiol. 22: 253–259.

Ch'ien, L.T., Economides, A.N. and Lemmi, H. (1978) Sydenham's chorea and seizures. Clinical and electroencephalographic studies. Arch. Neurol. 35: 382–385.

Courjon, J., ed. (1972) Traumatic disorders. In: Rémond, A. (Ed.), Handbook of Electroenceph. clin. Neurophysiol., Vol. 14B, Elsevier, Amsterdam.

Farrell, D.F. (1969) The EEG in progressive multifocal leukoencephalopathy. Electroenceph. clin. Neurophysiol. 26: 200–205.

Giel, R., De Vlieger, M. and van Vliet, A.G.M. (1966) Headache and the EEG. Electroenceph. clin. Neurophysiol. 21: 492–495.

Haider, I., Matthew, H. and Oswald, I. (1971) Electroencephalographic changes in acute drug poisoning. Electroenceph. clin. Neurophysiol. 30: 23–31.

Hansotia, P., Harris, R. and Kennedy, J. (1969) EEG changes in Wilson's disease. Electroenceph. clin. Neurophysiol. 27: 523–528.

Hockaday, J.M., Potts, F., Epstein, E., Bonazzi, A. and Schwab, R.S. (1965) Electroencephalographic changes in acute cerebral anoxia from cardiac or respiratory arrest. Electroenceph. clin. Neurophysiol. 18: 575–586.

Jóhannesson, G., Brun, A., Gustafson, L. and Ingvar, D.H. (1977) EEG in presenile dementia related to cerebral blood flow and autopsy findings. Acta Neurol. Scand. 56: 89–103.

Jóhannesson, G., Hagberg, B., Gustafson, L. and Ingvar, D.H. (1979) EEG and cognitive impairment in presenile dementia. Acta Neurol. Scand. 59: 225–240.

Kaszniak, A.W., Garron, D.C., Fox, J.H., Bergen, D. and Huckman, M. (1979) Cerebral atrophy, EEG slowing, age, education, and cognitive functioning in suspected dementia. Neurology 29: 1273–1279.

Kurtz, D. (1976) Section VII. The EEG in acute and chronic drug intoxications. In: Rémond, A. (Ed.), Handbook of Electroenceph. clin. Neurophysiol., Vol. 15C, Elsevier, Amsterdam, pp. 88–104.

Lević, Z.M. (1978) Electroencephalographic studies in multiple sclerosis. Specific changes in benign multiple sclerosis. Electroenceph. clin. Neurophysiol. 44: 471–478.

Mellerio, F. and Kubicki, S. (1977) Section VII. B. Encephalopathy due to poisoning. In: Rémond, A. (Ed.), Handbook of Electroenceph. clin. Neurophysiol., Vol. 15A, Elsevier, Amsterdam, pp. 108–135.

Radermecker, F.J., ed. (1977) Infections and inflammatory reactions, allergy and allergic reactions; degenerative diseases. In: Rémond, A. (Ed.), Handbook of Electroenceph. clin. Neurophysiol., Vol. 15A, Elsevier, Amsterdam, pp. 1–108.

Radermecker, F.J. (1977) Degenerative diseases of the nervous system. In: Rémond, A. (Ed.), Handbook of Electroenceph. clin. Neurophysiol., Vol. 15A, Elsevier, Amsterdam, pp. 162–191.

Roberts, M.A., McGeorge, A.P. and Caird, F.I. (1978) Electroencephalography and computerised tomography in vascular and non-vascular dementia in old age. J. Neurol. Neurosurg. Psychiat. 41: 903–906.

Rosadini, G., Rodriguez, G. and Siani, C. (1974) Acute alcohol poisoning in man: An experimental electrophysiological study. Psychopharmacologia 35: 273–285.

Rumpl, E., Lorenzi, E., Hackl, J.M., Gerstenbrand, F. and Hengl, W. (1979) The EEG at different stages of acute secondary traumatic midbrain and bulbar brain syndromes. Electroenceph. clin. Neurophysiol. 46: 487–497.

Silverman, D. (1975) Section VII. The electroencephalogram in anoxic coma. In: Rémond, A. (Ed.), Handbook of Electroenceph. clin. Neurophysiol., Vol. 12, Elsevier, Amsterdam, pp. 81–94.

Stevens, J.R., Sachdev, K. and Milstein, V. (1968) Behavior disorders of childhood and the electroencephalogram. Arch. Neurol. 18: 160–177.

Tarrier, N., Cooke, E.C. and Lader, M.H. (1978) The EEG's of chronic schizophrenic patients in hospital and in the community. Electroenceph. clin. Neurophysiol. 44: 669–673.

Volavka, J. Feldstein, S., Abrams, R., Dornbush, R. and Fink, M. (1972) EEG and clinical change after bilateral and unilateral electroconvulsive therapy. Electroenceph. clin. Neurophysiol. 32: 631–639.

Volavka, J., Matoušek, M. and Roubíček, J. (1966) EEG frequency analysis in schizophrenia. Acta psychiat. scand. 42: 237–245.

# Bilaterally synchronous slow waves

# 22


SUMMARY

(22.1) *The pattern* of bisynchronous slow waves is characterized by waves which have a frequency of less than 8 Hz and occur on both sides of the head so that waves of the same frequency appear at the same time in corresponding areas. These waves may be distributed over the entire head or be limited to one or a few electrodes on each side; in many cases, their distribution shifts from one moment to the next. They usually appear as intermittent trains of waves on a background of lower amplitude. Bisynchronous slow waves commonly are regular and rhythmical in shape, but may be irregular and arrhythmical. These waves are reduced or blocked by eye opening or alerting; they are increased during hyperventilation and drowsiness. A characteristic variety of bisynchronous slow waves is frontal intermittent rhythmical delta activity (FIRDA), also called 'monorhythmic frontal delta' (MFD). This consists of bursts of sinusoidal 2–3 Hz waves of high amplitude and a bifrontal maximum.

(22.2) *The causes* of bisynchronous slow waves include several normal and abnormal conditions. Normal bisynchronous slow waves are seen in infants and children during wakefulness and sleep and in adults during drowsiness and sleep and during and after hyperventilation. Bisynchronous slow waves are abnormal in alert resting adults. Bisynchronous slow waves result from the projection of an abnormality from distant, subcortical structures, especially from the brainstem reticular system and its rostral connections deep at the midline of the posterior, middle and anterior fossa, to the site of EEG production in the cerebral cortex. These abnormalities include (1) diffuse encephalopathies involving subcortical and cortical cerebral grey matter more than cerebral white matter; (2) structural lesions which directly or indirectly involve the mesencephalon, diencephalon, orbital and mesial surfaces of the frontal lobe; and (3) metabolic, toxic and endocrine encephalopathies.

(22.3) *Other EEG abnormalities* include a background of generalized asynchronous slow waves from which bisynchronous slow waves are often difficult to distinguish; however, the special diagnostic implications of bisynchronous slow waves justify the attempt to discriminate between these two varieties of generalized slow waves.

(22.4) *Grading* of bisynchronous slow waves depends on their amplitude and persistence.

(22.5) *Mechanisms* causing bisynchronous slow waves probably involve a central pacemaking system projecting to the cerebral surface.

(22.6) *Specific disorders* include many diseases impairing structure and function of deep midline structures.

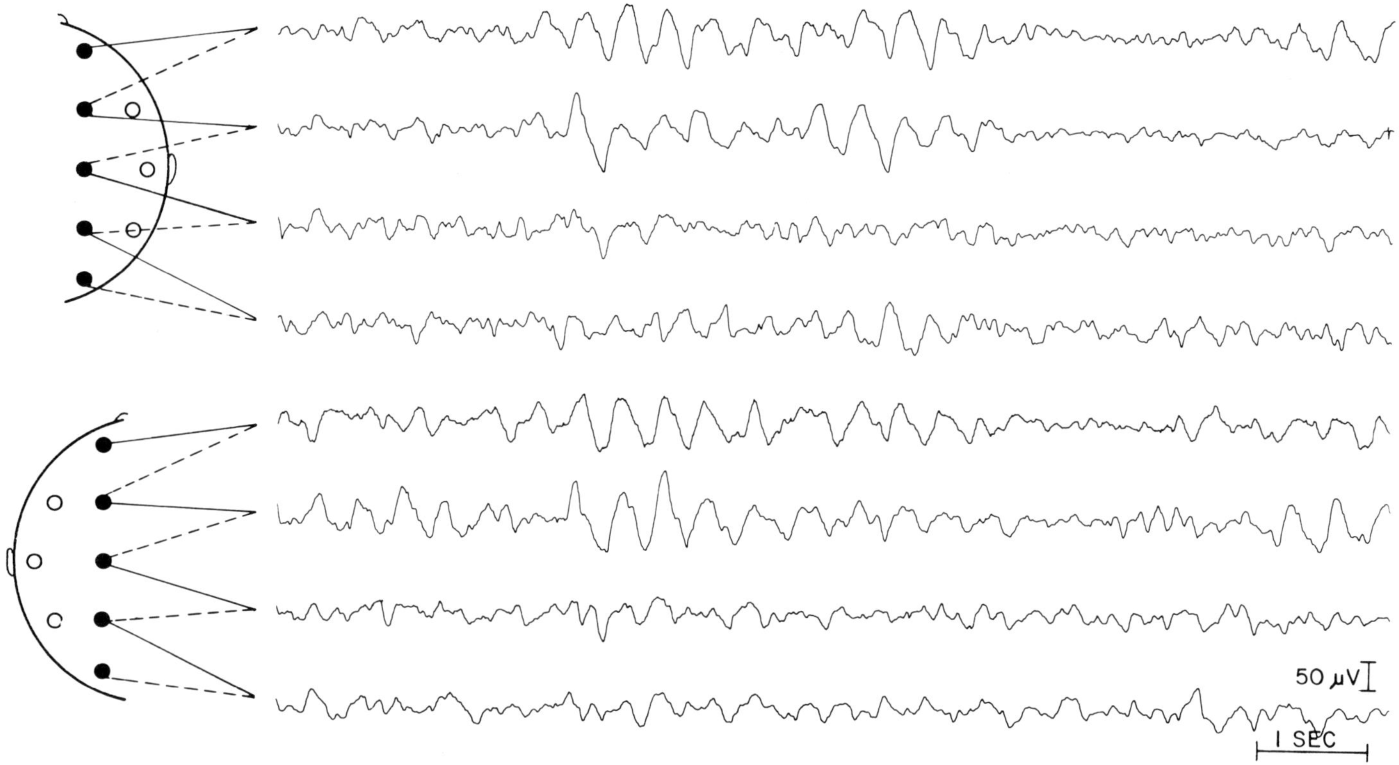


Fig. 22.1. Pattern of frontal intermittent rhythmical delta activity (FIRDA). Trains of bisynchronous slow waves of 2–3 Hz and of high amplitude appear with a maximum in the frontal regions on a background of diffuse slow waves of low to medium amplitude. The patient is an 18-year-old girl who sustained a severe head injury 2 weeks earlier. She had been in coma initially, then was confused and irritated until 2 days before the recording. At the time of the recording, her neurological examination was normal; there were no gross mental symptoms. Followup EEGs 7 weeks and several months later were entirely normal; the patient recovered without deficit. The final diagnosis was brainstem contusion.

*Bisynchronous slow waves* have a frequency of less than 8 Hz and appear simultaneously in corresponding parts of the two hemispheres. Individual waves are commonly sinusoidal or at least regular (Figs. 22.1; 22.2; 22.3). They are usually rhythmical, i.e. they repeat at the same rate and vary by no more than a few hertz over the course of time. They are usually intermittent, lasting for a few seconds and forming trains which begin and end at about the same time on the two sides. The wave peaks in one area do not always coincide with the peaks in another area, but waves of the same frequency in different areas are usually synchronous on the two sides. In contrast to most other slow waves, bisynchronous slow waves of even high amplitude may occur sporadically, separated from each other by periods of entirely normal activity.

Bisynchronous slow waves may be generalized or restricted; they may have a maximum in the same portions of both hemispheres or may be more prominent on one side. Their distribution and prominence, in contrast to that of other slow waves, often varies from moment to moment and may shift from one area to another or from restricted to more generalized. They are abolished or reduced on both sides by eye opening or alerting; they are increased during eye closure, hyperventilation and drowsiness. Abnormal bisynchronous slow waves disappear in the background of normal bisynchronous slow waves during sleep stages I–IV, but may reappear in REM sleep.

Bisynchronous slow waves commonly have delta frequency, medium to high amplitude and are regular and rhythmical (Figs. 22.1; 22.2; 22.3); however, bisynchronous slow waves may have theta frequency, low to medium amplitude and be irregular and arrhythmical (Figs. 22.4; 22.5). Discrete trains of rhythmical delta waves, i.e. intermittent rhythmical delta activity ('IRDA') (Figs. 22.1; 22.2; 22.3) may occur maximally in the frontal areas (frontal intermittent rhythmical delta

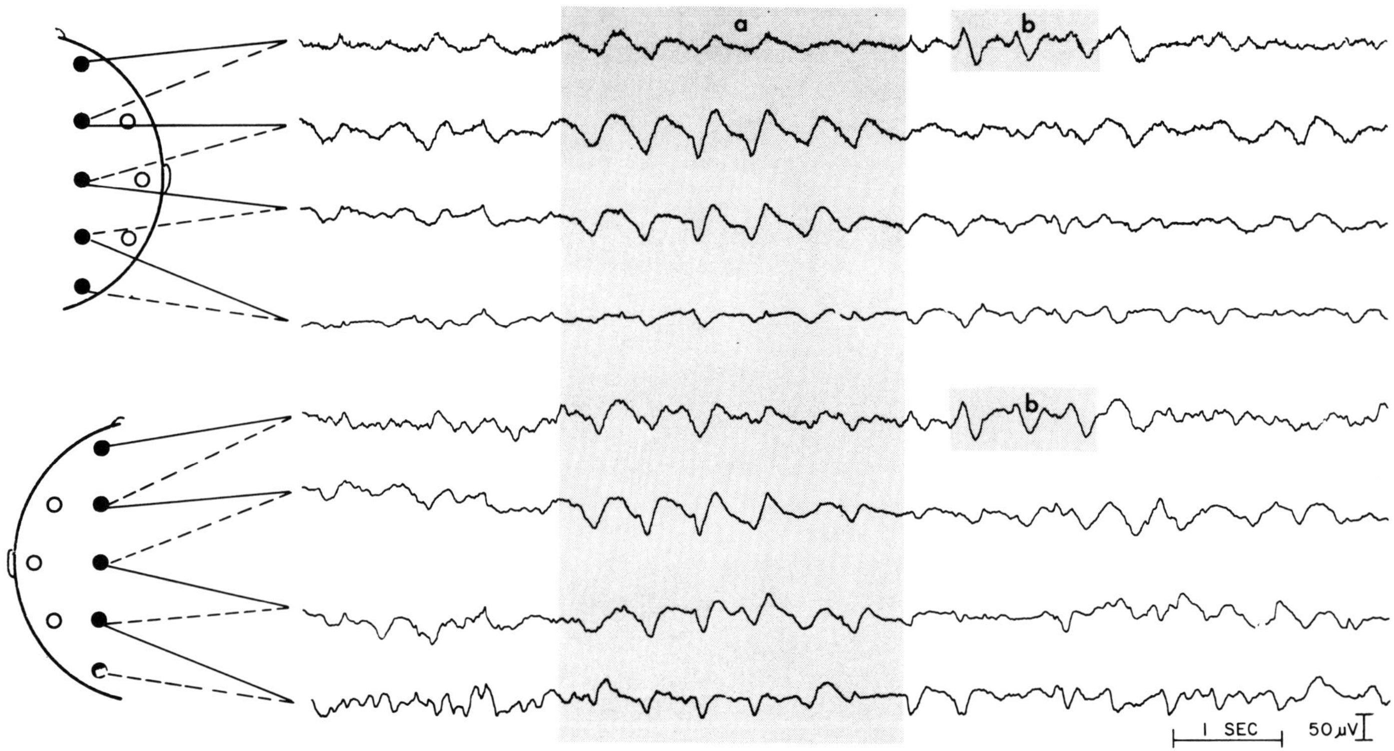


Fig. 22.2. Pattern of bisynchronous slow waves in a wide distribution (a) with interspersed frontal slow waves suggestive of triphasic waves (b). This 54-year-old chronic alcoholic was in hepatic coma at the time of this recording and died a few days later.

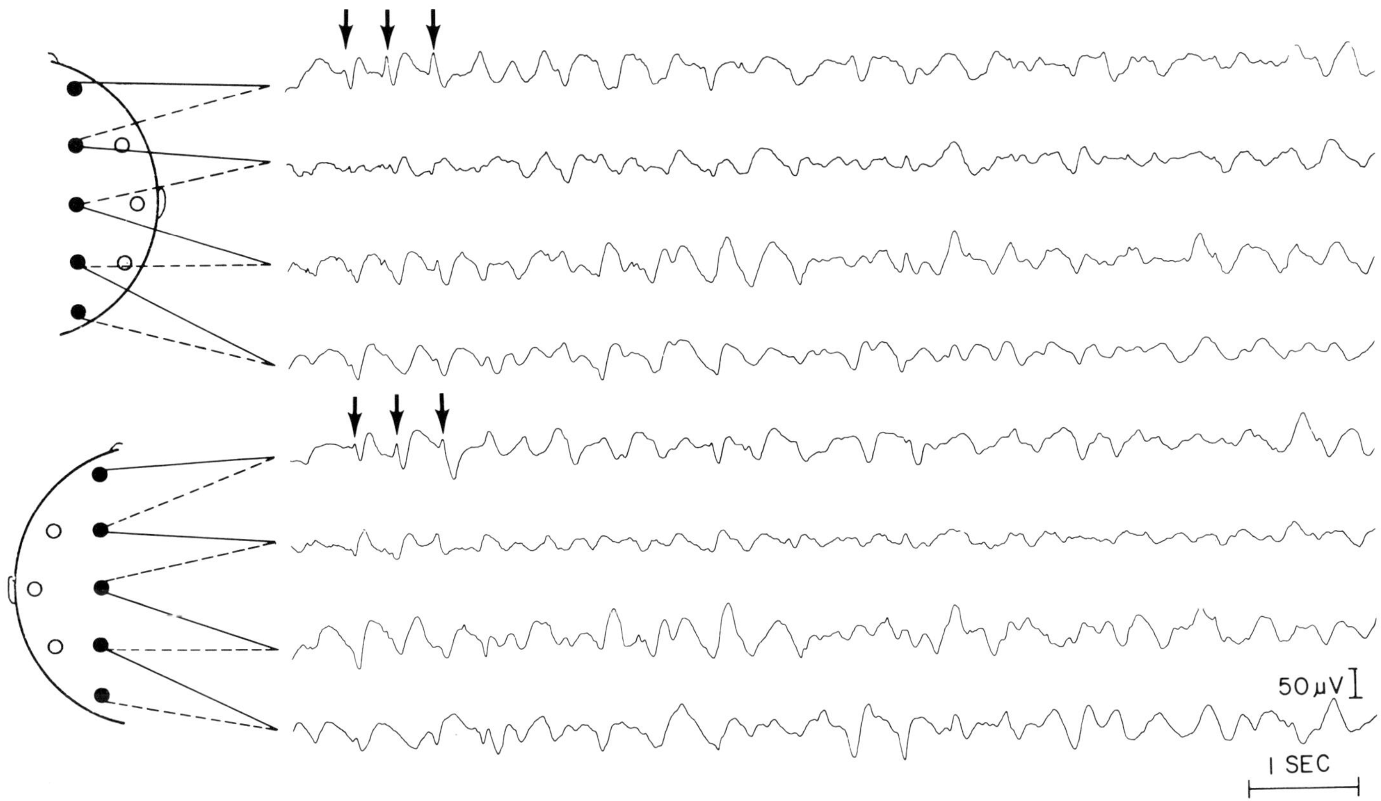


Fig. 22.3. Pattern of continuous bisynchronous slow waves mixed with sharp waves (arrows). This 26-year-old woman was in delirium due to water intoxication with metabolic acidosis and hyponatremia. Her EEG 5 days later was normal; she had completely recovered.

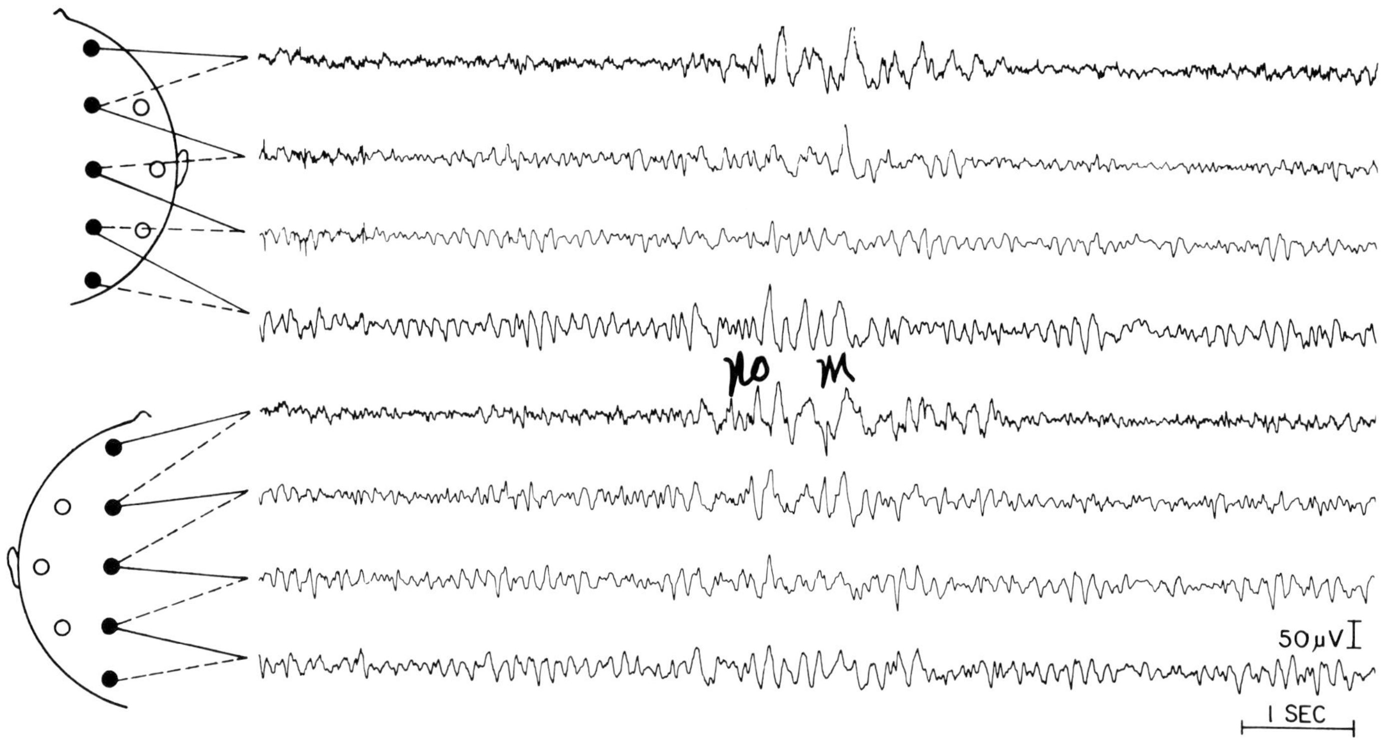


Fig. 22.4. Pattern of paroxysmal bisynchronous slow waves of irregular shape on a normal background. Technician's comment (NO M) means that the patient did not move during this paroxysm. This 58-year-old woman had a parathyroidectomy 18 years earlier. For several weeks before the recording she felt increasingly tired and experienced an episode of nearly fainting. Chvostek and Trousseau signs were positive, serum calcium was decreased at 5.6 mg % and phosphorus was increased at 6.3 mg %.

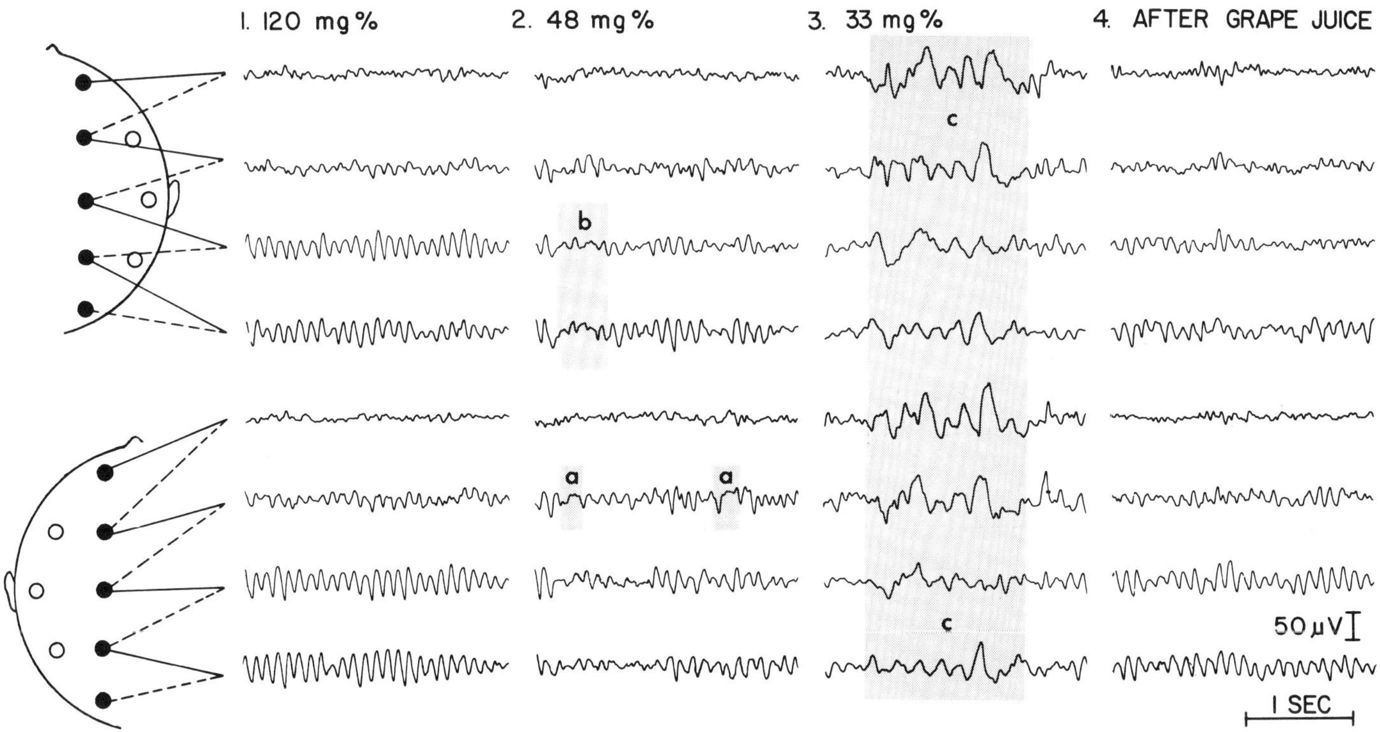


Fig. 22.5. Bisynchronous slow waves induced by hypoglycemia which developed during a glucose tolerance test. 1. Before the beginning of the test, the EEG was normal; 2. At a blood sugar level of 48 mg %, the EEG showed low to medium amplitude diffuse theta (a) and delta (b) waves of low to medium amplitude; 3. At a blood sugar level of 33 mg %, bursts of high amplitude bisynchronous delta and theta waves appeared with a maximum in the frontal regions (c); 4. After the patient drank some grapefruit-juice, the EEG returned almost completely to normal. This recording is of an 18-year-old boy with two episodes of nearly fainting several hours after the last meal.

activity, 'FIRDA', Fig. 22.1) or in the occipital areas (occipital intermittent rhythmical delta activity, 'OIRDA'). Because these waves usually are of only a single frequency, they have been called 'monorhythmic frontal delta' (MFD) activity. Other names, implicating their origin, are 'rhythmes à distance' or 'projected slow waves'.

## 22.2 CLINICAL SIGNIFICANCE OF BISYNCHRONOUS SLOW WAVES

**22.2.1** *Normal bisynchronous slow waves* are seen (1) during drowsiness and sleep at any age; (2) during wakefulness in subjects under the age of 20 years; (3) in response to hyperventilation at any age, especially childhood; (4) in adults having the rare patterns of slow alpha variant and of posterior slow waves (11.7).

**22.2.2** *Abnormal bisynchronous slow waves* are those occurring under conditions other than the ones listed above and usually reflect abnormalities located deeply in the brain and at some distance from the recording site. These abnormalities may be diffuse or circumscribed structural lesions, or disorders of cerebral function.

*Diffuse structural damage* may produce bisynchronous slow waves if it involves grey matter of subcortical structures alone or in combination with cortical grey matter, especially when the grey matter is damaged more than the hemispheric white matter. This is the presumed cause of bisynchronous slow waves in some degenerative encephalopathies.

*Circumscribed structural lesions* may cause bisynchronous slow waves either directly or indirectly. Lesions which are located near the midline at the base of the brain may directly involve the brainstem, diencephalon or the orbital and mesial surfaces of the frontal lobes (Fig. 22.1); lesions located near these structures may secondarily invade, compress, or distort them or render them ischemic or edematous

(Fig. 20.3). While increased intracranial pressure by itself does not alter the EEG until it reaches the range of the arterial blood pressure, it can produce herniation of the uncus of the temporal lobe which distorts the brainstem and thereby induces bisynchronous slow waves.

*Disorders of cerebral function* include mainly encephalopathies of toxic and metabolic etiology (Figs. 22.2; 22.3; 22.4; 22.5). The bisynchronous slow waves in these encephalopathies may disappear when the underlying abnormality is reversed. Transient bisynchronous slow waves may also be seen during and after generalized seizures, in attacks of vertebral-basilar migraine or of vertebral-basilar ischemia, in syncope and in transient global amnesia.

## 22.3 OTHER EEG ABNORMALITIES ASSOCIATED WITH BISYNCHRONOUS SLOW WAVES

**22.3.1** *Reduction, slowing and disorganization of alpha rhythm* may occur with mild or moderate bisynchronous slow waves (Fig. 22.5).

**22.3.2** *Generalized asynchronous slow waves* may be so prominent as to obscure bisynchronous slow waves. They usually are not seen in cases of uncomplicated deep circumscribed lesions.

**22.3.3** *Generalized epileptiform activity* may be superimposed on bisynchronous slow waves; if they fall in phase with the slow waves, they may form patterns similar to spike-and-wave complexes (Fig. 22.3). The mixture of bisynchronous slow waves and generalized epileptiform activity is characteristically seen in metabolic encephalopathies.

**22.3.4** *Focal slow waves, local reduction of amplitude or focal epileptiform* *activity* suggest either a local lesion which primarily produces focal EEG abnormalities and secondarily involves subcortical structures producing bisynchronous slow waves (Fig. 20.3), or a metabolic or toxic encephalopathy which primarily produces bisynchronous slow waves and secondarily causes local cerebral damage producing focal EEG abnormalities.

## 22.4 GRADING OF BISYNCHRONOUS SLOW WAVES

*Grading* of bisynchronous slow wave abnormalities depends on their persistence and amplitude. *Mild* bisynchronous slow waves are those which appear only a few times during an entire resting record; they usually have no more than medium amplitude. *Moderate* bisynchronous slow waves consist of more frequent and longer bursts of slow waves, usually of medium or high amplitude. *Marked* bisynchronous slow waves occupy at least half of the recording time; they often have high amplitude.

## 22.5 MECHANISMS CAUSING BISYNCHRONOUS SLOW WAVES

The bilaterally synchronous appearance of slow waves, like that of bilaterally synchronous epileptiform activity, is commonly thought to be due to the faulty action of a central pacemaker which projects abnormal impulses diffusely to the cerebral cortex causing slow waves to be generated synchronously on both sides (1.2). The system responsible for the synchronization of the two hemispheres is unknown but is probably located in the brainstem and diencephalon and may be identical with part or all of the reticular formation. This hypothesis could explain why three very different types of basic cerebral pathology, namely diffuse damage to subcortical and cortical grey matter, local lesions near deep midline structures, and metabolic and toxic encephalopathies, all cause bisynchronous slow waves. Diffuse damage to subcortical and cortical grey matter may cause bisynchronous slow waves by damaging both the subcortical and cortical components of the reticulocortical system implicated in the production of this abnormality. Local damage to deep midline structures may directly or indirectly interfere with the reticular formation and its rostral projections to the cerebral cortex. Metabolic and toxic encephalopathies are known to preferentially affect the function of mesencephalic and diencephalic centers, especially those responsible for alertness.

## 22.6 SPECIFIC DISORDERS CAUSING BILATERALLY SYNCHRONOUS SLOW WAVES

**22.6.1** *Degenerative, developmental and demyelinating diseases:*

(1) *Presenile and senile dementia (Alzheimer's disease)* is in some cases associated with bifrontal synchronous slow waves bus asynchronous slow waves (21.6.1) and other abnormalities are generally more common.

(2) *Parkinson's disease* is rarely associated with bisynchronous slow waves; asynchronous slow waves are more common (21.6.1).

(3) *Progressive supranuclear palsy* may produce bisynchronous slow waves, usually after the sleep EEG has become abnormal (24.92).

(4) *Other diseases* may induce bisynchronous slow waves in some cases: Leber's hereditary optic atrophy, Ramsey-Hunt's cerebellar myoclonic dyssynergia, myotonic dystrophy, tuberous sclerosis, hydrocephalus, and others.

(5) *Multiple sclerosis* causes bisynchronous slow waves in some patients, often in combination with asynchronous slow waves (21.6.1).

**22.6.2** *Metabolic and toxic encephalopathies.* *Bisynchronous slow waves* occur in the mild or moderate stages of many of these disorders (Table 22.1 and Figs. 22.3;

Table 22.1

| | Decreased alpha frequency | Generalized asynchronous slow waves | Focal slow waves | Triphasic waves | Spikes |
|---|---|---|---|---|---|
| ACTH, cortisone Rx | + | + | | | (+) |
| Acute anoxia, pulmonary insufficiency | + | + | | | |
| Addison's disease | + | + | | | (+) |
| Cerebromacular degenerations | | ++ | | | |
| CO poisoning | | + | | | |
| Dialysis encephalopathy | + | + | (+) | | + |
| Hepatic encephalopathy (Fig. 22.2) | + | + | | + | |
| Hydration (Hyponatremia, Fig. 22.3) | | + | | | + |
| Hyperglycemia without ketoacidosis | | | | | + |
| Hyperparathyroidism (Hypercalcemia) | + | + | (+) | + | |
| Hypoglycemia | + | + | + | | + |
| Hypokalemia (alkalosis) | + | + | | | |
| Hypoparathyroidism pseudohypo-parathyroidism (Hypocalcemia, Fig. 22.4) | + | + | | | + |
| Hypopituitarism | | + | | | |
| Porphyria | + | + | + | | + |
| Renal encephalopathy | | + | + | + | + |
| Thyrotoxicosis | | + | | | + |
| Vitamin B-12 deficiency | + | + | + | | |
| Wernicke's encephalopathy | + | + | | | |
| Wilson's disease | | + | + | (+) | |

22.4) and are commonly associated with other abnormalities, namely slowing of alpha rhythm and generalized asynchronous slow waves, and less often with focal slow waves, triphasic waves, and generalized or focal spikes and sharp waves.

In acute encephalopathies, EEG abnormalities appear in a sequence which roughly parallels the severity of the disorder. At the mildest stage, bisynchronous slow waves do not appear spontaneously but may be induced by hyperventilation; at this stage, photic stimulation may produce an increased or abnormal response. Alpha rhythm decreases in frequency and may decrease in prominence (Fig. 22.5, Part 2). Spontaneous bisynchronous slow waves appear first in short bursts (Fig. 22.5, Part 3, Fig. 22.4), later in long trains or continuously (Figs. 22.2; 22.3). Asynchronous generalized slow waves may appear as soon as alpha rhythm becomes disorganized; these slow waves become prominent and replace alpha rhythm when alertness becomes impaired. Other abnormalities which may appear at this stage are focal slow waves and focal, unilateral or generalized spikes or sharp waves. With increasing severity, generalized asynchronous slow waves obscure all other abnormalities; the patient then is usually in deep coma. Death is often preceded by activity of low amplitude which may be interrupted by bursts of slow waves to form burst-suppression patterns. If the underlying metabolic or toxic abnormality is reversed at any point, the EEG abnormalities may regress in reverse sequence except that generalized slow waves may persist to indicate that widespread cerebral damage has resulted, or focal slow waves may appear while generalized slow waves are present or as they disappear to indicate that local structural damage has occurred.

Most chronic metabolic encephalopathies produce bisynchronous slow waves, slowing of alpha rhythm and generalized asynchronous slow waves. One or more of these abnormalities are seen in vitamin B12 deficiency, Wilson's disease, metachromatic leukodystrophy, Krabbe's disease, Wernicke's encephalopathy and dialysis encephalopathy; dialysis encephalopathy may also produce repetitive bisynchronous spike-and-wave complexes. However, a few metabolic encephalopathies produce bisynchronous slow waves only rarely and are characterized mainly by other abnormalities: Hypothyroidism decreases the frequency (25.1.6) and amplitude (24.7.3) of alpha rhythm, hyperthyroidism increases alpha frequency (25.1.7), the lipidoses and other metabolic derangements, when seen in infants and young children, produce hypsarrhythmia, slow spike-and-waves and multifocal independent spikes (19.1).

**22.6.3** *Cerebrovascular diseases:*

(1) *Transient ischemia* of the brain in general and of the brainstem in particular, as seen in syncope, in attacks of transient brainstem ischemia and of basilar artery migraine, can lead to bisynchronous slow waves which appear when consciousness begins to fade and abate when consciousness is regained. If they do not completely disappear in a few days, lasting damage is likely to have occurred.

(2) *Strokes* due to thrombosis, embolism or hemorrhage involving the central parts of the upper midbrain and diencephalon can lead to bisynchronous slow waves, often associated with asynchronous slow waves (21.6.3). Large hemispheric strokes, especially hypertensive hemorrhages, may lead to edema and to compression of the brainstem and thereby produce bisynchronous slow waves mixed with focal and asynchronous generalized slow waves. Even strokes in the distribution of the anterior cerebral artery, causing damage to deep parts of the frontal lobe, are capable of producing bisynchronous intermittent frontal delta activity.

(3) *Postanoxic encephalopathy* may be associated with bisynchronous slow waves as one of many abnormalities (21.6.3) and indicate involvement of deep structures of the brain.

(4) *Chronic subdural hematoma* may produce intermittent bisynchronous slow waves, especially in cases with fluctuating levels of consciousness; focal slow waves (20.6.3) and amplitude changes (23.6.3) are more common and more characteristic of subdural hematoma.

(5) *Subarachnoid hemorrhage* may be associated with bisynchronous slow waves in addition to asynchronous slow waves in patients with impaired consciousness; focal slow waves may be present and reflect local damage (20.6.3).

(6) *Moyamoya disease in children* may be associated with bisynchronous posterior slow waves.

**22.6.4** *Cerebral trauma:*

(1) *Head injury* may produce bisynchronous slow waves either at the onset of unconsciousness when the EEG shows reduction of amplitude (23.6.4, 24.6.4), or as patients emerge from deep coma when the EEG shows asynchronous slow waves and other abnormalities (21.6.4) due to local or widespread cerebral damage. Bisynchronous slow waves indicate a relatively light stage of post-traumatic coma. Intermittent bisynchronous slow waves may persist for days or weeks not only after severe (Fig. 22.1) but also after fairly mild head injuries.

(2) *Epidural and acute subdural hematoma* may initially produce bisynchronous slow waves; focal delta waves (20.6.4) and reduction of amplitude (23.6.4) follow.

(3) *Psychosurgery,* for instance coagulation of the anterior parts of the internal capsule or of the thalamus and internal globus pallidus may produce bisynchronous frontal intermittent delta activity, presumably by interrupting subcortical connections to the frontal cortex.

(4) *Progressive traumatic encephalopathy* may produce bisynchronous slow waves in addition to asynchronous slow waves (21.6.4).

**22.6.5** *Brain tumors:*

(1) *Infratentorial tumors* may cause bisynchronous slow waves if they invade or compress the midbrain or distort the diencephalon. These slow waves are thus often produced by tumors which arise within or near the central structures of the midbrain, for instance ependymomas and pineal tumors. In contrast, tumors located at

some distance from these structures, for instance cerebellar tumors and meningiomas of the posterior fossa, may grow to considerable size without compressing the brainstem and producing bisynchronous slow waves. Tumors of the lower brainstem, such as pontine gliomas, do not usually cause EEG abnormalities.

(2) *Supratentorial tumors* are likely to cause bisynchronous slow waves if they are located in or near the diencephalon or the mesial and orbital parts of the frontal lobe. Tumors in other locations may cause bisynchronous slow waves by secondarily involving the deep midline structures. Other associated EEG abnormalities are described above (22.3). Combinations of bisynchronous slow waves with focal slow waves (Fig. 20.3) and focal epileptiform activity are particularly suggestive of deeply located supratentorial tumors. Bisynchronous slow waves as a manifestation of supratentorial tumor are more likely to be found in old persons than in young adults.

(3) *Pseudotumor cerebri* or benign intracranial hypertension shares with cerebral tumors only the name but not the pathology or EEG abnormalities. In contrast to obstructive hydrocephalus (21.6.1), it produces no EEG abnormality in most patients, but mild or moderate bisynchronous slow waves may occasionally be seen.

**22.6.6** *Seizure disorders:*

(1) *Interictal* bisynchronous slow waves appear in some patients with primary generalized seizures. In particular, patients with absence attacks often show interictal bisynchronous rhythmical waves of 3 Hz. Interictal slow waves may be only indirectly related to seizures: They may be the manifestation of diseases causing seizures, for instance metabolic encephalopathies or myoclonus epilepsy, or they may be the result of disorders caused by seizures, for instance subdural hematomas or brainstem contusions.

(2) *Ictal* bisynchronous slow waves are rarely the only manifestation of a seizure (19.3.1). Bisynchronous slow waves in combination with generalized spikes or sharp

waves form part of spike-and-waves of many epileptiform patterns.

(3) *Postictal* bisynchronous slow waves may occur in addition to asynchronous postictal slow waves (21.6.6).

**22.6.7** *Infectious diseases:*

(1) *Fever, reduced alertness, metabolic abnormalities* and electrolyte imbalances associated with infections may cause bisynchronous slow waves even if the brain is not infected.

(2) *Meningitis and encephalitis* may cause bisynchronous slow waves in conditions in which they cause asynchronous slow waves (21.6.7).

(3) *Sydenham's chorea* causes bisynchronous slow waves in many cases; asynchronous slow waves may also appear (21.6.7).

**22.6.8** *Psychiatric diseases:*

(1) *Personality disorders, behavior disturbances and schizophrenia* are occasionally associated with bisynchronous slow waves. However, this abnormality, like other abnormal EEG patterns, is not very common in psychiatric diseases. Therefore, organic causes for this abnormality have to be excluded, particularly treatable conditions such as metabolic and toxic encephalopathies, frontal, hypothalamic and pituitary tumors which all may cause psychiatric symptoms.

(2) *Kleine-Levin syndrome* during attacks may be associated with bursts of bisynchronous slow waves on a background of asynchronous slow waves; these abnormalities are not entirely explained by drowsiness and sleep.

## REFERENCES


Allen, E.M., Singer, F.R. and Melamed, D. (1970) Electroencephalographic abnormalities in hypercalcemia. Neurology 20: 15–22.

Bingley, T. and Persson, A. (1978) EEG studies on patients with chronic obsessive-compulsive neurosis before and after psychosurgery (stereotaxic bilateral anterior capsulotomy). Electroenceph. clin. Neurophysiol. 44: 691–696.

Dow, R.S. (1961) The electroencephalographic findings in acute intermittent porphyria. Electroenceph. clin. Neurophysiol. 13: 425–437.

Gastaut, H. and Fischer-Williams, M. (1957) Electro-encephalographic study of syncope. Its differentiation from epilepsy. Lancet 2: 1018–1025.

Glaser, G.H., ed. (1976) Metabolic, endocrine and toxic diseases. In: Rémond, A. (Ed.), Handbook of Electroenceph. clin. Neurophysiol., Vol. 15C, Elsevier, Amsterdam.

Gloor, P., Kalaby, O. and Giard, N. (1968) The electroencephalogram in diffuse encephalopathies: Electroencephalographic correlates of grey and white matter lesions. Brain 91: 779–802.

Gloor, P. (1976) Section IV. Generalized and widespread bilateral paroxysmal activities. In: Rémond, A. (Ed.), Handbook of Electroenceph. clin. Neurophysiol., Vol. 11B, Elsevier, Amsterdam, pp. 52–87.

Harner, R.N. and Katz, R.I. (1975) Section IV. Electroencephalography in metabolic coma. In: Rémond, A. (Ed.), Handbook of Electroenceph. clin. Neurophysiol., Vol. 12, Elsevier, Amsterdam, pp. 47–62.

Hasegawa, K. and Aird, R.B. (1963) An EEG study of deep-seated cerebral and subtentorial lesions in comparison with cortical lesions. Electroenceph. clin. Neurophysiol. 15: 934–946.

Heller, G.L. and Kooi, K.A. (1962) The electroencephalogram in hepato-lenticular degeneration (Wilson's disease). Electroenceph. clin. Neurophysiol. 14: 520–526.

Jóhannesson, G., Brun, A., Gustafson, L. and Ingvar, D.H. (1977) EEG in presenile dementia related to cerebral blood flow and autopsy findings. Acta Neurol. Scand. 56: 89–103.

Martinius, J., Matthes, A. and Lombroso, C.T. (1968) Electroencephalographic features in posterior fossa tumors in children. Electroenceph. clin. Neurophysiol. 25: 128–139.

Sidell, A.D. and Daly, D.D. (1961) The electroencephalogram in cases of benign intracranial hypertension. Neurology 11: 413–417.

Su, P.C. and Goldensohn, E.S. (1973) Progressive supranuclear palsy. Arch. Neurol. 29: 183–186.

van der Drift, J.H.A. and Magnus, O. (1962) The EEG with space occupying intracranial lesions in old patients. Electroenceph. clin. Neurophysiol. 14: 664–673.

Wallace, P.W. and Westmoreland, B.F. (1976) The electroencephalogram in pernicious anemia. Mayo Clin. Proc. 51: 281–285.

Wilkus, R.J. and Chiles, J.A. (1975) Electrophysiological changes during episodes of the Kleine-Levin syndrome. J. Neurol. Neurosurg. Psychiat. 38: 1225–1231.

# Localized and lateralized changes of amplitude: Asymmetries

# 23

SUMMARY

(23.1) *The pattern* of asymmetry is characterized by differences in amplitude of the EEG recorded from the two sides of the head. Differences in amplitude may involve the entire background or only some background patterns. Local reduction of the amplitude of alpha rhythm in some cases is associated with reduction of alpha frequency.

(23.2) *Causes* of asymmetry are unilateral lesions, most of which are superficial. The amplitude is usually reduced on the side of the lesion, rarely increased. Amplitude may be reduced by local cortical damage, for instance by superficial infarctions, tumors and head injuries, or by transient disturbances of cerebral function, for instance by attacks of transient ischemia and migraine. Extracerebral lesions can also change EEG amplitude: Subdural hematomas may reduce it and skull defects may increase it. Alpha rhythm may be reduced by lesions of thalamocortical connections, i.e. lesions not located at the cortex of the posterior head regions where alpha rhythm is produced. In some instances, alpha rhythm is reduced by lesions in the anterior head regions.

(23.3) *Other EEG abnormalities,* if limited to one side, may further help to indicate the side of the underlying cerebral abnormality.

(23.4) *Grading* of asymmetries depends on degree and persistence of amplitude differences.

(23.5) *Mechanisms* of asymmetries involve either changes of cortical EEG production as in the case of structural or functional cortical lesions, or alterations of the media between cortex and recording electrodes such as fluid collections or skull defects.

(23.6) *Specific disorders* causing asymmetries include many clinically important diseases.

(23.7) *Asymmetries of alpha, beta, mu and other rhythms* are seen in a small variety of clinical conditions.

## 23.1 DESCRIPTION OF PATTERN

Asymmetry consists of a difference in the amplitude of activity recorded from corresponding areas on the two sides of the head (Figs. 23.1; 23.2; 23.3). Asymmetries usually affect all types of background activity during wakefulness and sleep

(Fig. 23.1); occasionally they involve only the alpha rhythm, beta rhythm, mu rhythm, responses to photic stimulation and hyperventilation, or sleep patterns. A local decrease in the amplitude of alpha rhythm is often associated with a decrease of alpha frequency. Lesions which cause an asymmetry of normal background activity may also cause an asymmetry of abnormal activity. This can produce difficulties in identifying the side of the abnormality. For instance, a superficial lesion reducing the amplitude of the EEG on the same side may also cause bilateral abnormalities such as slow waves or epileptiform activity. This combination makes the abnormal activity appear with a higher amplitude on the uninvolved side and falsely suggests that the uninvolved side is the abnormal one (Fig. 23.2). To correctly identify the involved side in these cases, the EEG reader must carefully search (a) for normal patterns which should be reduced in amplitude on the

TABLE 23.1
Asymmetries

| Abnormal patterns | Causes | Mechanisms | Examples of diseases |
|---|---|---|---|
| Decreased amplitude of all types of activity | Local cortical damage | Decreased cortical EEG production | Cortical infarct, Sturge-Weber syndrome |
| | Local disorder of cortical function | As above | Local cortical ischemia |
| | Unilateral increase of media between cortex and recording electrodes | Decreased electrical impedance within the conducting media | Subdural hematoma |
| | | Increased electrical impedance between cortex and recording electrodes | Skull hyperostosis |
| Of alpha, beta, mu rhythm, sleep patterns | Defect may be distant, at presumed site of pacemaker | Decreased rhythmical input to cortex | Cerebral infarcts, tumors, injuries, without reliable relation to location of rhythm |
| Increased amplitude | Skull defects | Decreased electrical impedance between cortex and electrodes | Postoperative skull defect |

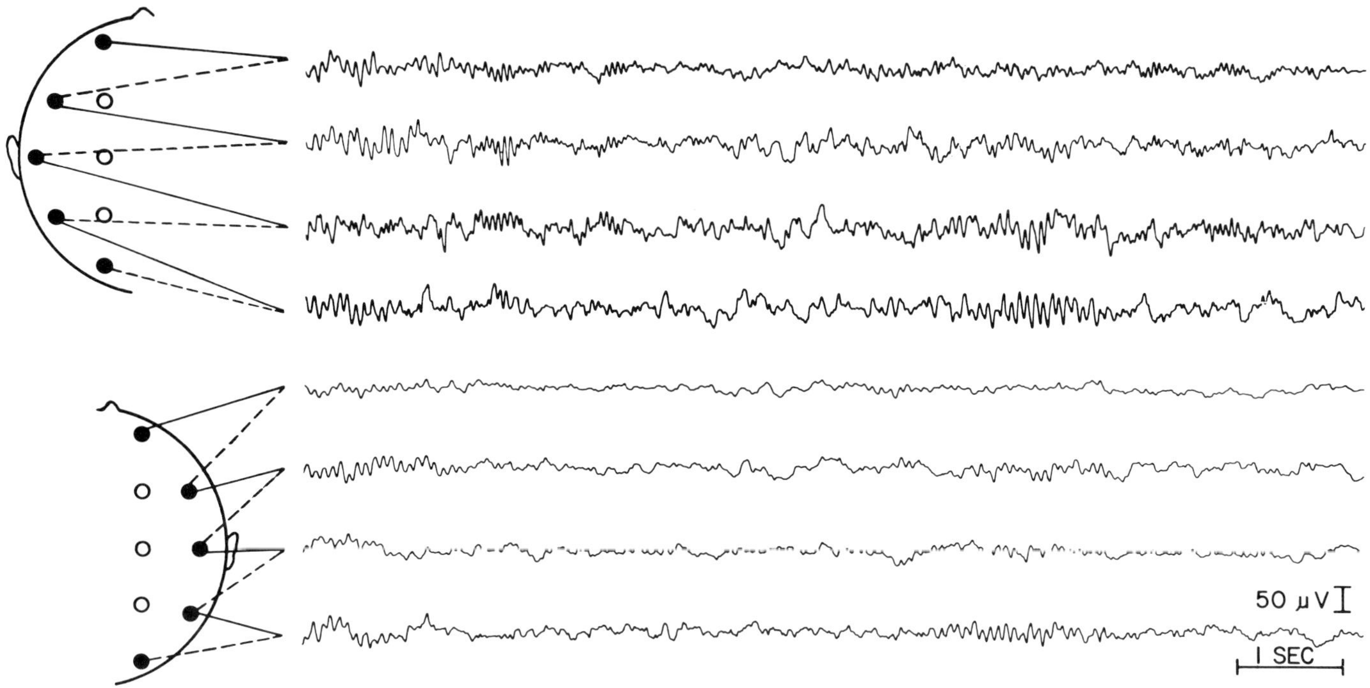


Fig. 23.1. Pattern of asymmetry of normal background activity. Sleep spindles and slow waves of sleep are attenuated over the right side. This 7-year-old boy has signs characteristic of Sturge-Weber syndrome: a right facial naevus, cerebral calcifications extending into the parietal and temporal areas, and left-sided and generalized motor seizures.

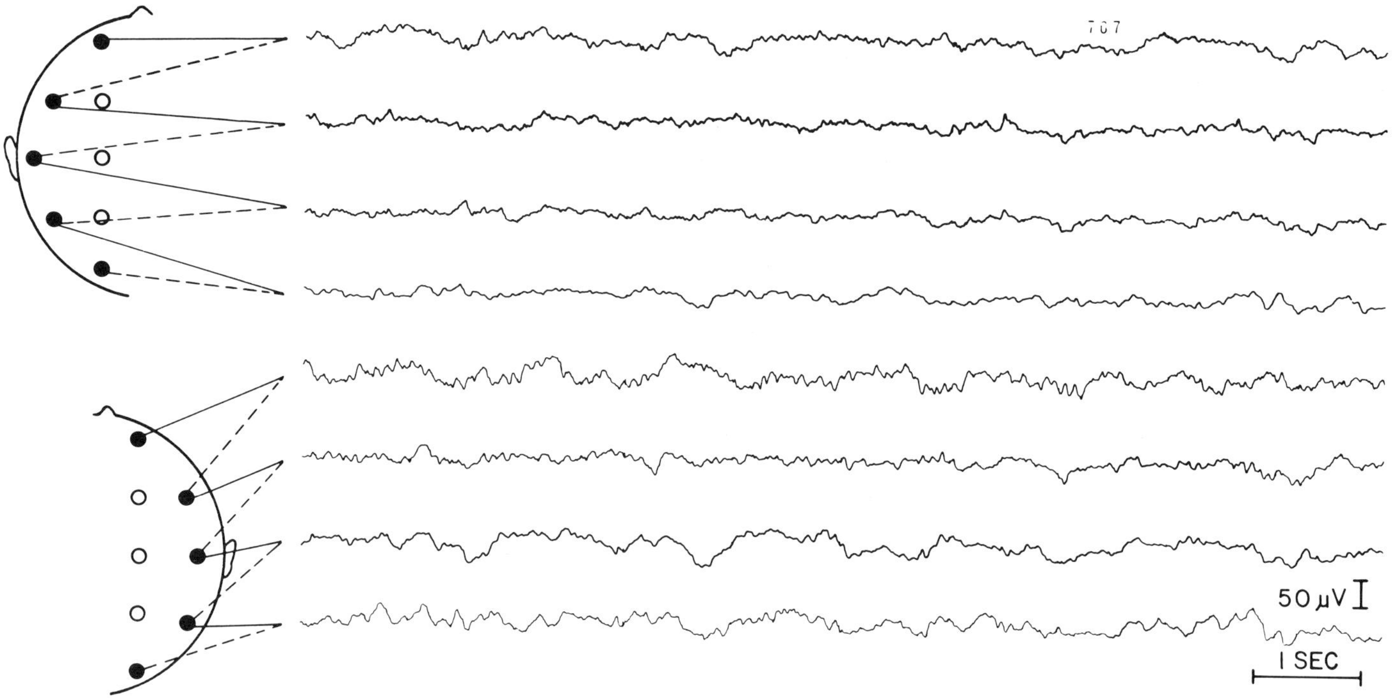


Fig. 23.2. Pattern of asymmetry combined with generalized asynchronous slow waves. The reduction of amplitude on the left side attenuates the generalized slow waves on that side and thereby makes them appear with higher amplitude on the right side, falsely suggesting a right-sided cerebral abnormality. The correct localization of an abnormality on the left side is suggested by the circumstance that the faster frontal rhythms are also reduced on the left side. The patient is a 37-year-old chronic alcoholic in coma. A large chronic subdural hematoma on the left side was evacuated a few hours after this EEG recording.

abnormal side (Fig. 23.1) and (b) for additional abnormalities that may be limited to the abnormal side.

Asymmetries of activity in large parts of the hemispheres can be recognized with referential recordings. However, asymmetries between small areas are better detected with bipolar linkages between closely spaced electrodes. Alternating montages make the detection of slight asymmetries easier than do block montages (4.2.3). Asymmetry of amplitude can be accepted as having a cerebral cause only if asymmetries in electrode placement, gross asymmetries of electrode impedance, and differences of gain and filter settings have been excluded.

## 23.2 CLINICAL SIGNIFICANCE OF ASYMMETRIES

**23.2.1** *Normal asymmetries* are those described earlier for alpha rhythm and for photic driving (11.1.5; 14.3.3). Mu rhythm occurs independently on the two sides but should be symmetrical on average.

**23.2.2** *Abnormal asymmetries* are usually due to a decrease of amplitude on the side of the cerebral abnormality. Only rarely is the amplitude increased on the involved side causing activity of lower amplitude to appear on the normal side. However, in the absence of associated localizing abnormalities, or in the presence of bilateral abnormal EEG activity, it may be difficult to decide which side is abnormal (see above).

*Asymmetries of all background activity.* *A decrease of amplitude of all types of activity* in one area is due either to a reduction of cortical EEG production or to an increase of the media separating the cortex from the recording electrodes. Reductions of cortical electrogenesis may be long-lasting and due to structural lesions such as cortical strokes, tumors and injuries; transient reductions may follow focal seizures or be due to reversible conditions such as transient local ischemia or migraine. An increase of material between cortex and recording electrodes explains reduction of amplitude seen in many cases of subdural hematoma.

*An increase of amplitude of all types of activity* in one area is much rarer than a decrease of amplitude. It is usually due to a local skull defect.

*Asymmetry of alpha rhythm* has little localizing value. A local decrease of the amplitude in the posterior head regions may be due (a) to a lesion of the underlying cortex; (b) to a lesion of the thalamus or its connections to the underlying cortex; or (c) to a lesion in the frontal and central regions.

*Asymmetry of beta rhythm* may be the earliest and most sensitive indicator of a local lesion: An increase may be seen as the first sign of a superficial brain tumor, a decrease may be the last evidence of a long-standing atrophic scar.

*Asymmetry of other rhythms* are increases and decreases of mu rhythm, hyperventilation responses and sleep activity. They may occur in isolated fashion but are usually associated with asymmetries of other patterns and raise the suspicion of a lesion on the side of the lower amplitude.

## 23.3 OTHER ABNORMALITIES ASSOCIATED WITH ASYMMETRIES

**23.3.1** *Focal slow waves* may appear in an area of reduced amplitude suggesting that white matter under the cortex is involved as well as the cortex itself and that the cortical function is not completely abolished. The center of the lesion may show waves of the slowest frequencies and of the lowest amplitude.

**23.3.2** *Focal epileptiform activity* may appear in or near the area of depressed amplitude suggesting local irritation of the cortex. The combination of focal epileptiform activity and reduced amplitude may be the manifestation of a cortical epileptogenic lesion or the result of a very recent focal seizure.

**23.3.3** *Generalized asynchronous and bisynchronous slow waves and generalized epileptiform activity* may be attenuated on the side of a lesion causing a reduction of amplitude and thus falsely suggest a lesion on the opposite side (see above).

## 23.4 GRADING OF ASYMMETRIES

*Grading of asymmetries* depends on the degree and persistence of amplitude differences between the two sides. An asymmetry of activity other than alpha rhythm is rated *mild* if the amplitude in one area is intermittently but consistently reduced to about two-thirds of that on the other side. A *moderate* asymmetry consists of a persistent reduction of amplitude up to about one-half of that on the other side. An asymmetry is rated *marked* if the amplitude is reduced to less than one-half of that on the opposite side. Because alpha rhythm may be asymmetrical in normal subjects (11.1.5), asymmetries of this rhythm have to be greater than those of other activity to be rated mild, moderate and marked.

## 23.5 MECHANISMS CAUSING LOCAL CHANGES OF AMPLITUDE

**23.5.1** *Decreases of amplitude* are due to mechanisms which vary with the type of underlying lesion:

(1) *Reduction of cortical EEG production* may be due to structural damage reducing the total area of functioning membrane of cortical nerve cells, particularly of the large pyramidal neurons which are the major generators of the EEG (1.1). A temporary reduction of electrocortical potential changes may be due to a transient decrease of regional cerebral blood flow resulting in local hypoxia and hypoglycemia. These conditions may completely depolarize cortical neurons and make their membrane incapable of responding to excitatory and inhibitory input.

(2) *Interposition of material* between the cortical generators and the recording electrodes can attenuate the EEG by one of two mechanisms; the effect depends on the electrical properties of the interposed material. Substances of high impedance such as thickened skull or greasy scalp act as insulators and partly isolate the electrocortical potentials from the recording electrodes. Substances of low impedance such as subdural blood or spinal fluid act as conductors within the volume under the electrodes and shunt the potential differences before they reach the electrodes.

(3) *Selective decreases of alpha rhythm* may be due to derangements of thalamocortical networks producing the impulses which synchronize the potential changes in cortical neurons in the posterior head regions (1.2). The mechanisms whereby frontal and central lesions reduce posterior alpha rhythm is unknown but may be related to the production of ischemia in structures engaged in the production of this rhythm.

**23.5.2** *Increases of amplitude* are commonly seen after craniotomy and are partly due to reduced impedance between the EEG generator and the recording electrodes; in addition, local cortical irritation may produce local increases of cortical output.

## 23.6 SPECIFIC DISORDERS CAUSING ASYMMETRIES OF AMPLITUDE

**23.6.1** *Developmental, degenerative and demyelinating diseases:*

(1) *Porencephaly, holoprosencephaly and other defects* due to developmental malformation, perinatal injury or disease may show reduced EEG amplitude in addition to focal slow waves (20.6.1) and focal epileptiform activity over areas of atrophic brain defects.

(2) *Sturge-Weber syndrome* is commonly associated with a decrease of amplitude on the side of the naevus (Fig. 23.1). This decrease may be found in infancy before

cortical calcium deposits develop. The EEG may also show focal slow waves and focal epileptiform activity (17.6.1) in the same area; bilateral synchronous slow waves and widespread epileptiform activity (19.1) may be present.

(3) *Paget's disease* may cause a local increase in the thickness of the skull and thereby decrease the amplitude of the EEG over the involved area.

(4) *Multiple sclerosis* may produce a local decrease of EEG amplitude with or without other abnormalities (21.6.1).

**23.6.2** *Metabolic and toxic encephalopathies.* A local or unilateral decrease of amplitude is not a direct result of these diseases but may occur as the result of complications, especially of cortical infarcts in renal, hypertensive, hypoglycemic and anoxic encephalopathy, and of subdural hematoma in hepatic and Wernicke's encephalopathy.

**23.6.3** *Cerebrovascular diseases:*

(1) *Attacks of transient ischemia* involving the cortex of parts of the cerebral hemispheres may cause a local decrease of amplitude. The effects of acute local ischemia can be observed when EEG monitoring is used during carotid endarterectomies: A local reduction of amplitude, usually preceded by slow waves (20.6.3), may occur after clamping of the internal carotid artery.

(2) *Strokes* involving the cortex may cause a prolonged reduction of amplitude over the infarcted area. Focal slow waves may be present in the same area or in the surrounding parts during the acute stage but a reduction of amplitude may outlast other EEG abnormalities in the chronic stage.

(3) *Chronic subdural hematoma* causes a unilateral or focal decrease of background amplitude in about one-half of all cases; alpha rhythm may be depressed more than other background activity. Focal slow waves (20.6.3) are even more common than a decrease of amplitude in chronic subdural hematoma (Fig. 23.2),

but the decrease of amplitude is an important signal of a superficial lesion and should always raise the suspicion of a subdural hematoma.

(4) *Subarachnoid hemorrhage* may produce amplitude asymmetry especially if there is local cortical damage or significant vasospasm.

(5) *Migraine* may cause unilateral reduction of amplitude during attacks. Between attacks, patients with migraine may show persistent reductions of background amplitude, especially of alpha rhythm, possibly representing residuals of vascular damage incurred during an attack.

**23.6.4** *Cerebral trauma:*

(1) *Head injuries* that are mild may lead to an immediate and transient decrease of amplitude which does not indicate definite cerebral damage. Severe head injuries can cause various EEG abnormalities initially (21.6.4) and may later be followed by a long-lasting decrease of amplitude indicating residual structural damage due to contusions, intracerebral hemorrhage, epidural and acute subdural hematomas. Traumatic hemorrhages of newborn infants may be characterized by large areas of depressed amplitude.

(2) *Subgaleal hematoma,* a collection of blood between skull and scalp occurring mainly in infants with linear skull fractures, acts like a subdural or epidural hematoma in that it attenuates the amplitude of the EEG locally.

(3) *Scalp edema,* often caused by infiltration of intravenous fluids given through scalp veins to newborn infants, is a possible source of local attenuation of EEG amplitude.

(4) *Cranial defects* such as burrholes or larger defects remaining after neurosurgical operations are characterized by a local increase of background amplitude. These asymmetries appear not only in recordings from electrodes placed over the defect but also in recordings from electrodes on bone near the edges of the defect. Alpha rhythm of higher amplitude may be recorded on the side of bony defects near

the posterior head regions. Beta rhythm may be found near bone defects in any part of the head; contralateral beta rhythm may be either absent or of lower amplitude. Bone defects near the central regions are often associated with a mu-like rhythm, local slow waves and sharp waves, all of which block like mu rhythm (11.3); mu rhythm of lower amplitude is not always present on the other side (Fig. 23.3). The appearance of these unilateral rhythms near a bone defect raises the question whether they are due only to the bone defect which may cause a fairly selective reduction of electrical impedance for fast EEG rhythms or to a change in the electrical activity produced by underlying cortex. A cerebral abnormality is more likely if (a) the activity on the two sides differs not only in amplitude but also in wave form and frequency, (b) recording from electrodes at some distance from the edge of the bone defect also shows abnormalities, and (c) differences of amplitude develop gradually after removal of the bone. While the disappearance of an asymmetry after replacement of the bone (Fig. 23.3) suggests that the asymmetry was due to the bone defect, its persistence does not necessarily indicate that it is due to a cerebral abnormality because persisting gaps between skull and replacement may cause persistent asymmetries of impedance. Moreover, even if asymmetries are due to a cerebral abnormality, the abnormality may consist of no more than local meningo-cortical adhesions and cortical gliosis; only in the case of clearcut focal slow waves and spikes would one suspect the recurrence of an underlying cerebral lesion such as a tumor or a subdural hematoma, or the development of an epileptogenic focus.

(5) *Hemispherectomy,* i.e. the partial or complete removal of a hemisphere reduces the amplitude of the EEG on the operated side in most cases but causes little change in some. The EEG on the operated side is probably generated by the opposite hemisphere and by deep remnants of the operated hemisphere and conducted electrotonically to the recording electrodes on the operated side. The electrotonically conducted EEG is attenuated by the electrical shunting effect of

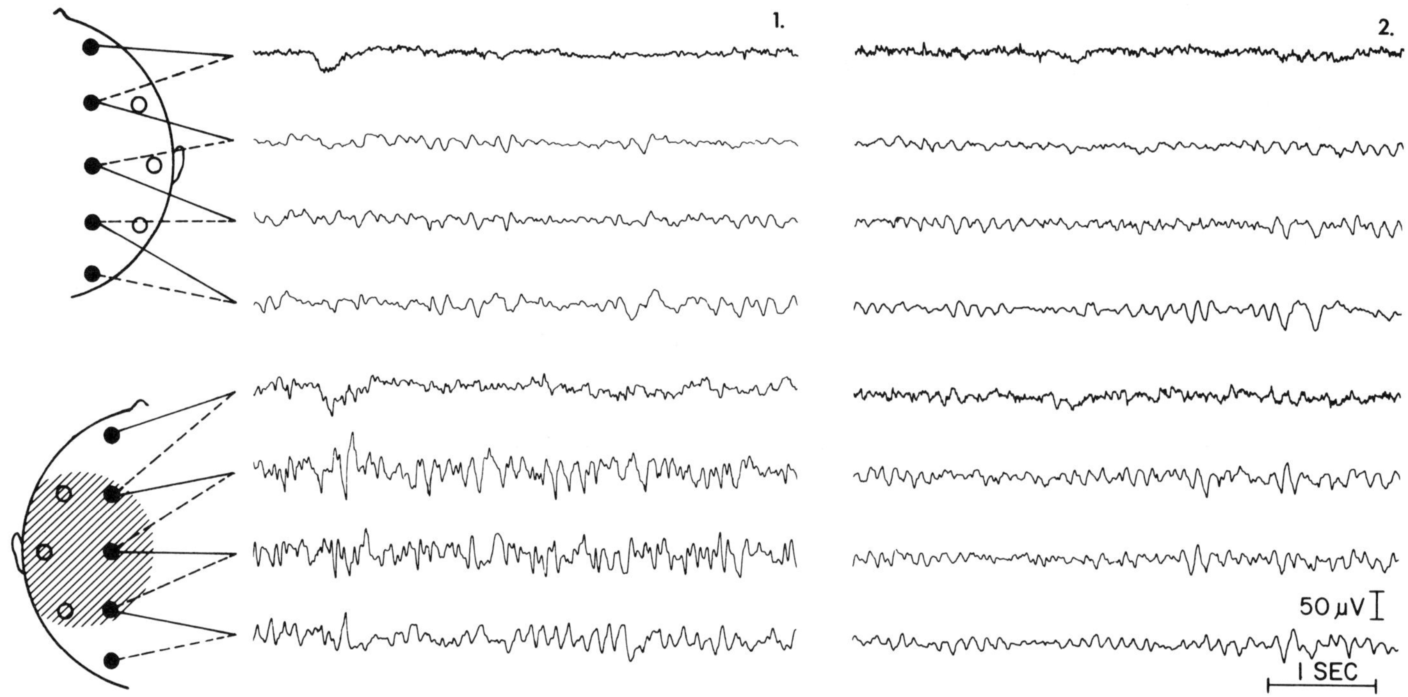


Fig. 23.3. Pattern of local amplitude changes due to a skull defect. 1. Theta waves resembling mu rhythm appear at the left central electrode which is located over a skull defect indicated by the hatched area in the diagram on the left. Frontal beta rhythm and occipital alpha rhythm are also larger on the left than on the right side. 2. After repair of the skull defect, both sides show symmetrical activity. This 48-year-old woman had an acute traumatic subdural hematoma evacuated 2 months before the recording in part 1; part 2 was recorded 3 months after repair of the skull defect. She had no neurological abnormalities at the time of either recording.

cerebrospinal fluid which usually accumulates in the operated space.

**23.6.5** *Brain tumors.* *Primary and metastatic brain tumors* sometimes, although rarely, first manifest by an asymmetry of amplitude in general or of alpha, beta or mu rhythm in particular (23.7.2).

**23.6.6** *Seizure disorders:*

(1) *Postictal* local reduction of amplitude commonly appears immediately and only for a few minutes after a focal seizure discharge.

(2) *Interictal asymmetry* is usually due to the lesion causing the seizures, for instance an old cerebral infarct, residual damage after a head injury, Sturge-Weber syndrome or porencephaly.

(3) *Ictal* decreases of amplitude are usually bilateral (19.3.3), even in partial complex seizures (17.1.3). However, a local reduction of amplitude often briefly precedes focal seizure discharges.

**23.6.7** *Infectious diseases:*

(1) *Encephalitis* of any etiology can produce a local reduction of amplitude in the area of maximum involvement. A lasting reduction may indicate residual local damage.

(2) *Abscesses* can decrease the amplitude of all background activity or of alpha, beta or mu rhythm only.

(3) *Progressive multifocal leukoencephalitis* in its early stages may reduce the amplitude of background activity locally before causing generalized asynchronous slow waves (21.6.7).

(4) *Thrombophlebitis* of the cerebral venous sinuses may reduce the amplitude of all activity locally or unilaterally, especially in the acute phase when unilateral seizure discharges or status epilepticus are also likely to occur.

**23.6.8** *Psychiatric diseases* without gross organic abnormalities are not associated with localized or lateralized reductions of EEG amplitude. Therefore, the finding of an asymmetry in a patient with psychiatric disease should raise the suspicion of an organic cerebral lesion.

## 23.7 ASYMMETRIES OF ALPHA, BETA, MU AND OTHER RHYTHMS

A decrease of the amplitude of one of these rhythms is usually part of an amplitude reduction involving all types of activity in one area. However, in a few conditions, the amplitude of one of these rhythms is reduced on one side or in one area while the amplitude of other activity remains symmetrical or is not reduced to the same extent. To be abnormal, an asymmetry of these rhythms must exceed their normal range of asymmetry. A selective asymmetry of one of these rhythms, without other associated abnormalities, may represent either a decrease of amplitude on one side or an increase of amplitude on the other and therefore does not indicate the abnormal side. However, a selective decrease of amplitude of a rhythm is often associated with a decrease of the frequency of that rhythm, or with other unilateral or focal EEG abnormalities which help to lateralize the underlying lesion correctly. In many instances, asymmetry of alpha rhythm is due to a posterior lesion and asymmetries of central beta and of mu rhythm are due to anterior lesions, but these rules have many exceptions.

**23.7.1** *Asymmetries of alpha rhythm:*

(1) *Chronic subdural hematoma* may show a preferential depression of alpha rhythm. This is seen more commonly with posterior than with anterior hematomas.

(2) *Hemispheric infarcts* may reduce the amplitude of alpha rhythm more than that of other activity; a decrease of alpha activity may be the last residual ab-

normality of old infarcts.

(3) *Migraine* may reduce alpha rhythm unilaterally acutely during the attack; alpha rhythm may be found to be asymmetrical in the interval between attacks without other evidence for infarction.

(4) *Head injuries* can lead to a unilateral decrease of the amplitude of alpha rhythm acutely. Asymmetry of alpha rhythm may be present while other EEG abnormalities due to the injury are also present; the alpha asymmetry may persist and be the last residual of severe head injuries or the only effect of mild head injuries.

(5) *Brain tumors and abscesses* involving the hemispheres, the thalamus or the floor of the third ventricle may selectively decrease alpha amplitude.

**23.7.2** *Asymmetries of beta and mu rhythm:*

(1) *Developmental lesions* reduce beta rhythm if they lead to cortical defects such as those in porencephaly or local atrophy.

(2) *Degenerative diseases* may produce an asymmetrical reduction of beta and mu rhythm before producing generalized reductions of amplitude.

(3) *Vascular diseases* may cause atrophic lesions producing selective reductions of beta and mu rhythm; central fast activity activated by movement may be seen in postanoxic action myoclonus.

(4) *Cerebral trauma, and brain operations* leading to skull defects, are followed by a local increase of fast activity or mu rhythm, often associated with other abnormalities (23.6.4).

(5) *Brain tumors and abscesses* may cause a reduction or an increase of beta and mu rhythm as the earliest EEG abnormality.

(6) *Ictal and interictal* beta activity may be produced by epileptogenic foci (19.3.6).

**23.7.3** *Asymmetry* of photic responses is abnormal only if it clearly exceeds the wide normal range of asymmetry (14.3.3). A selective asymmetry of the photic response may be due to a lesion involving the posterior part of the central visual path on the side of the lower amplitude (25.5.1). However, similar asymmetries are often found in patients without other evidence for circumscribed damage, for instance in patients with migraine or with a history of mild head injuries.

**23.7.4** *Asymmetry of sleep activity* may be normal in infants; asynchrony of sleep spindles may be found up to the age of about 4–5 years. Asymmetry and asynchrony may persist in infants and children with perinatal cerebral lesions, especially hydrocephalus. Asymmetry of sleep spindles can occur at any age as the result of hemispheric tumors, infarcts, Sturge-Weber's syndrome, leucotomy and other conditions.

## REFERENCES

Chatrian, G.E., Somasundaram, M. and Foltz, E.L. (1969) EEG changes in subgaleal hematomas. Electroenceph. clin. Neurophysiol. 26: 524–527.

Cobb, W. and Sears, T.A. (1960) A study of the transmission of potentials after hemispherectomy. Electroenceph. clin. Neurophysiol. 12: 371–383.

Cobb, W.A., Guiloff, R.J. and Cast, J. (1979) Breach rhythm: The EEG related to skull defects. Electroenceph. clin. Neurophysiol. 47: 251–271.

Goldensohn, E.S., O'Brien, J.L. and Ransohoff, J. (1961) Electrical activity of the brain. In patients treated with hemispherectomy or extensive decortication. Arch. Neurol. 5: 210–220.

Green, R.L. and Wilson, W.P. (1961) Asymmetries of beta activity in epilepsy, brain tumor, and cerebrovascular disease. Electroenceph. clin. Neurophysiol. 13: 75–78.

Fukuyama, Y. and Tsuchiya, S. (1979) A study on Sturge-Weber syndrome. Report of a case associated with infantile spasms and electroencephalographic evolution in five cases. Eur. Neurol. 18: 194–204.

Jaffe, R. and Jacobs, L. (1972) The beta focus: Its nature and significance. Acta Neurol. Scand. 48: 191–203.

Kelly, J.J., Sharbrough, F.W. and Westmoreland, B.F. (1978) Movement-activated central fast rhythms: An EEG finding in action myoclonus. Neurology 28: 1037–1040.

Marshall, C. and Walker, A.E. (1950) The electroencephalographic changes after hemispherectomy in man. Electroenceph. clin. Neurophysiol. 2: 147–156.

Nealis, J.G.T. and Duffy, F.H. (1978) Paroxysmal beta activity in the pediatric electroencephalogram. Ann. Neurol. 4: 112–116.

# Generalized changes of amplitude: Symmetrically high and low amplitude

# 24

SUMMARY

(24.1) *The patterns* of generalized changes of amplitude consist of a bilateral symmetrical decrease or increase of amplitude of all types of normal activity or of specific patterns only. Such changes of amplitude are best recognized by comparison with previous recordings from the same subject because the amplitude of normal patterns differs widely in the general population. While abnormally low amplitude can be defined by voltage criteria, there is practically no upper limit for the amplitude of normal patterns except that an abnormal increase of beta activity is characterized by an increase of amplitude above its normal low level in addition to an increase of its persistence.

(24.2) *Causes* of bilateral abnormally low amplitude are similar to those producing unilateral reductions of amplitude, namely bilateral superficial lesions which reduce cortical function transiently or in a lasting manner or which change the media between cortex and recording electrodes. Bilateral reductions of amplitude may also be due to widespread cerebral diseases such as Huntington's chorea, postanoxic encephalopathy and other generalized damage leading to cerebral death and to changes of cortical function caused by toxic and metabolic diseases.

(24.3) *Other EEG abnormalities* include generalized asynchronous slow waves and periodic complexes.

(24.4) *Grading* of low amplitude is best done by indicating upper voltage levels of prevailing EEG activity.

(24.5) *Mechanisms* causing bilateral reductions of all types of background activity include reductions of cortical EEG production and alterations of the electrical impedance of the media between cortex and recording electrodes. Selective changes of the amplitude of specific rhythms are probably due to selective involvement of distant structures controlling the production of these rhythms by the cortex.

(24.6) *Specific disorders* reducing overall amplitude include a wide variety of structural and functional abnormalities.

(24.7) *Bilateral decrease of alpha rhythm* may result from some toxic and metabolic conditions and from anxiety.

(24.8) *Generalized increase of beta rhythm* is seen mainly as a result of tranquilizers and sedatives and of some metabolic disorders.

(24.9) *Sleep patterns* may be changed in amplitude by drugs and metabolic disorders.

Table 24.1
Generalized changes of amplitude

| Abnormal patterns | Causes | Mechanisms | Examples of diseases |
|---|---|---|---|
| Decreased amplitude of all types of activity | Bilateral cortical damage | Decreased cortical EEG production | Bilateral cortical infarcts, postanoxic encephalopathy |
| | Widespread cerebral damage, involving cortex and subcortex | Decreased cortical EEG production, decreased rhythmical input to cortex | Huntington's chorea, Jakob-Creutzfeldt disease, postanoxic encephalopathy |
| | Widespread disturbance of cortical function | Same as above | Anoxia, hypothermia, hypothyroidism, preterminal toxic-metabolic encephalopathies, head injury, postictal coma, anxiety |
| | Bilateral increase of media between cortex and recording electrodes | Decreased electrical impedance within the conducting media | Bilateral subdural hematomas |
| | | Increased electrical impedance between cortex and recording electrodes | Dry scalp, Paget's disease |
| of alpha rhythm | Mild metabolic disturbances | Decreased cortical EEG production | Early hepatic, hypothyroid, hypoparathyroid encephalopathy |
| | Functional subcortical disturbance | Decreased rhythmical input to cortex | Anxiety |
| of sleep patterns | Structural brainstem damage | As above | Progressive supranuclear palsy, pontine lesions |
| | Functional brainstem disturbance | As above | Phenylketonuria, hypothyroidism, uremia |
| Increased amplitude | | | |
| of all types of activity | No known pathological cause | | |
| of beta rhythm | Functional disturbance | Unknown | Sedatives and tranquilizers, hyperthyroidism, anxiety |
| of sleep patterns | As above | Increased input to cortex | Tricyclic antidepressants, flurazepam |

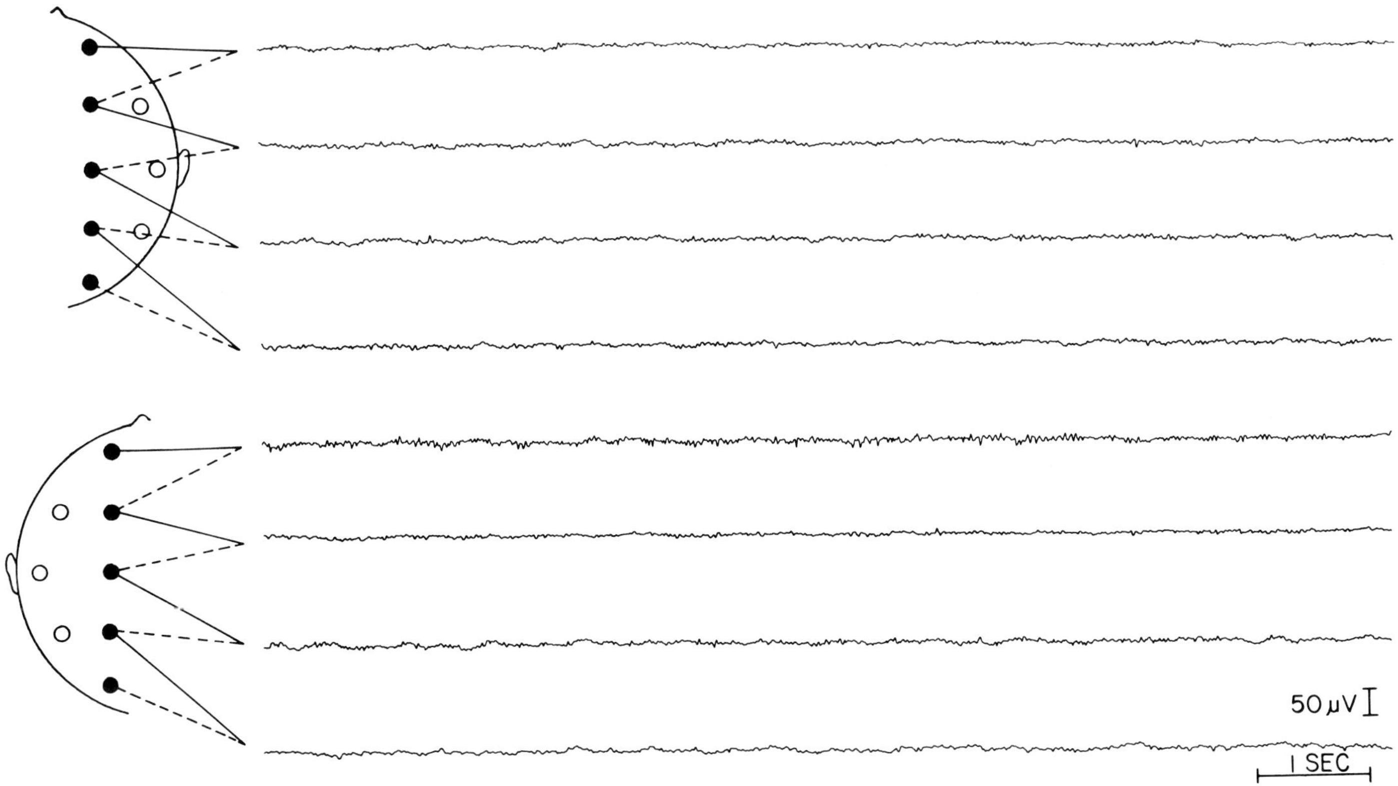


Fig. 24.1. Pattern of very low amplitude. There is no activity over 10 $\mu$V. The patient is a 66-year-old woman with a family history of Huntington's disease who has had progressive chorea and dementia for over 12 years.

## 24.1 DESCRIPTION OF PATTERNS

**24.1.1** *Abnormally low amplitude in general* consists of activity not exceeding 20 $\mu$V in any channel during relaxed wakefulness while the eyes are closed (Figs. 24.1; 24.2). The low amplitude must be sustained: Transient reductions of amplitude due to transient anxiety, mental effort, eye opening or intermittent increase or decrease of alertness are not abnormal. Because amplitude increases with interelectrode distances up to about 10 cm, the diagnosis of abnormally low amplitude requires the use of such long interelectrode distances. Correct gain settings, calibration signals and electrode impedances are essential to make the diagnosis of low amplitude. Special recording methods are needed to establish the absence of all electrocerebral activity (5.4).

**24.1.2** *Abnormally low amplitude of specific patterns* can be diagnosed only by comparison with previous recordings from the same subject because of the great variability of the amplitude of normal patterns between subjects. Complete absence of alpha rhythm in teenagers and young adults and absence of sleep spindles after the first weeks of life suggests an abnormality.

**24.1.3** *Abnormally high amplitude* of all types of activity cannot be well defined. Even though activity of over 100 $\mu$V is uncommon in wakeful adults, it is usually abnormal not because of its amplitude but because of its wave shape and is then classified according to this aspect of its abnormality.

**24.1.4** *Abnormally high amplitude of specific patterns* can be diagnosed only by comparison with previous records from the same individual. One exception is that of persistent beta activity of medium amplitude which is abnormal since beta activity is usually intermittent and of low amplitude in normal individuals.

## 24.2 CLINICAL SIGNIFICANCE OF HIGH AND LOW AMPLITUDE

**24.2.1** *Normal* high amplitude occurs in the waking record up to teenage and in deep stages of sleep at any age. Normal low amplitude of under 20 $\mu$V occurs transiently as a result of eye opening, mental effort, anxiety, alerting or drowsiness.

**24.2.2** *Abnormally low amplitude of all activity. Abnormally low amplitude in normal subjects* can be seen in about 5–10% of adults but is not acceptable as normal in younger persons. The reduction of amplitude is usually mild in degree, i.e. the waking record contains some activity of 10–20 $\mu$V. Such low voltage patterns (11.8) in adults are similar to slight excesses of generalized asynchronous slow waves in that they do not sharply distinguish between normal and abnormal subjects. This does not affect the significance of a moderate and marked reduction of overall amplitude which is abnormal at any age.

*Abnormally low amplitude in abnormal conditions* may be either transient and due to acute anoxic, toxic and metabolic factors, head injury, postictal state, or permanent and due to lasting damage resulting from these conditions or from other diseases significantly involving the cortex, such as Huntington's chorea. An increase of the material between cortex and recording electrodes such as that caused by bilateral subdural hematoma may produce a bilateral reduction of amplitude.

**24.2.3** *Abnormal decreases of specific patterns* are presumably due to abnormalities involving the afferents to the cortex which are responsible for the production of these patterns. For instance, interruption of thalamocortical connections may reduce alpha rhythm while disturbances of brainstem function may decrease sleep spindles.

**24.2.4** *Abnormal increases of specific patterns* of clinical importance are the increases of beta rhythms produced by toxic and metabolic conditions, especially by barbiturates and other sedatives, tranquilizers and by hyperthyroidism.

### 24.3 OTHER EEG ABNORMALITIES ASSOCIATED WITH HIGH AND LOW AMPLITUDE

**24.3.1** *Generalized asynchronous slow waves* are often produced by the same conditions which reduce amplitude in general.

**24.3.2** *Bursts of periodic sharp waves and slow waves* may alternate with activity of low amplitude in burst-suppression and other special patterns (19.2).

### 24.4 GRADING OF AMPLITUDE CHANGES

**24.4.1** *'Low amplitude'* describes a record which contains activity over 10 μV but no activity over 20 μV. *'Very low amplitude'* indicates the presence of activity of no more than 10 μV. *'Electrocerebral silence'* or *'electrocerebral inactivity'* denotes the absence of activity over 2 μV (5.4).

**24.4.2** *High amplitude,* not being abnormal per se, is usually described in terms of its absolute amplitude or of its amplitude relative to that of the background.

### 24.5 MECHANISMS CAUSING GENERALIZED CHANGES OF AMPLITUDE

**24.5.1** *Reduction of cortical potentials* and

**24.5.2** *Increased distance between cortex and recording electrodes* are caused by mechanisms similar to those causing local decreases of amplitude (23.5.1) if these mechanisms involve both sides of the head.

**24.5.3** *Selective decreases of amplitude of patterns* over both sides of the head must be assumed to be due to interference with distant structures which control the production of these patterns in the cortex. Thus, bilateral reduction of alpha rhythm may be due to bilateral interruption of the input from thalamic nuclei which probably induces alpha rhythm in the cortex or to an increase in the activity of diencephalic and mesencephalic structures which normally abolishes alpha rhythm under conditions of increased and decreased alertness. A reduction of sleep spindles may be due to a decreased efficiency of impulses from the lower brainstem areas which are thought to be responsible for the production of this pattern.

The terms 'desynchronization', 'arousal' or 'alerting' are sometimes used to describe replacement of widespread activity of medium or high amplitude, for instance alpha rhythm or slow waves, by activity of low amplitude. It is thought that the disappearance of these patterns, which often occurs in response to alerting stimuli, may be due to a failure in the synchronization of the underlying neuronal potentials (1.2). However, because the mechanisms reducing the amplitude of the EEG are not precisely known, the reduction of amplitude is best described in terms which do not make any implications regarding an underlying mechanism.

**24.5.4** *High amplitude of all types of activity* may, in some cases, be due to relatively short distances between cortex and recording electrodes or to thin skull. Other causes for high amplitude of normal activity in adults are unknown. While abnormally low cerebral metabolism causes low amplitude and normal metabolism is required for maintenance of normal amplitude, an increase of metabolism does not increase amplitude but rather causes waves of abnormal frequency.

**24.5.5** *High amplitude of beta rhythm* seen in some toxic and metabolic conditions remains unexplained.

## 24.6 SPECIFIC DISORDERS CAUSING A GENERALIZED DECREASE OF AMPLITUDE OF ALL TYPES OF ACTIVITY

**24.6.1** *Degenerative, developmental and demyelinating diseases:*

(1) *Huntington's chorea* is characterized by activity of very low amplitude which correlates with the cortical atrophy observed in this disease (Fig. 24.1). In the early stages of the disease when background features are still distinguishable, alpha rhythm becomes disorganized, asynchronous generalized slow waves appear, and sleep spindles and K complexes disappear. The EEG of family members at risk does not predict later development of the disease.

(2) *Jakob-Creutzfeldt disease* leads to a decrease of overall amplitude in the advanced stages, i.e. after generalized asynchronous slow waves have vanished. Activity of very low amplitude is also present during the intervals between periodic generalized sharp waves (19.2.2).

(3) *Senile and presenile dementia (Alzheimer's disease)* is associated with a decrease of background amplitude in some cases; alpha and beta rhythm are usually affected most. Generalized slow waves (21.6.1) are a more reliable indicator of dementia.

(4) *Microcephaly* may cause low amplitude of the EEG in addition to other abnormalities (21.6.1).

(5) *Multiple sclerosis* in malignant, progressive cases may be associated with a generalized reduction of amplitude although generalized asynchronous slow waves (21.6.1) are a more common abnormality in this disease.

**24.6.2** *Metabolic and toxic encephalopathies.* Many of these encephalopathies reduce the amplitude of the EEG by reducing cerebral blood flow, oxygen supply and metabolism. Hypo- or hyperthermia can also decrease EEG amplitude.

(1) *Acute cerebral anoxia* leads first to asynchronous (21.6.3) and bilaterally synchronous slow waves which may be followed by a generalized decrease of amplitude and electrocerebral silence (24.6.3) if anoxia persists.

(2) *Hypothermia* leads to a decrease of EEG amplitude and frequency beginning at about 25 °C. Electrocerebral activity disappears completely at 10–20 °C. Because reduction of amplitude even after long periods of hypothermia is reversible, hypothermia must be excluded as a cause or contributing factor in cases of electrocerebral silence in the determination of cerebral death (24.6.3). Currently accepted guidelines require that EEGs for this purpose be made at body temperatures of 90 °F (32.2 °C) or more (5.4).

(3) *Hyperthermia* of over 42 °C reduces the amplitude of the EEG. Moderate hyperthermia can increase the amplitude of background activity; slow waves appear when consciousness becomes clouded.

(4) *Hypothyroidism* usually reduces the frequency (25.1.6) and organization of alpha rhythm and characteristically leads to an overall reduction of amplitude. Generalized asynchronous slow waves may also be present and sleep spindles are often reduced or absent.

(5) *Hypoparathyroidism and pseudohypoparathyroidism* may lead to a reduction of amplitude in general and of alpha rhythm in particular as one of several abnormalities (22.6.2).

(6) *Renal and hepatic encephalopathy* may reduce the amplitude of all activity or of alpha rhythm in the milder stages; in advanced hepatic encephalopathy, a sudden decrease of amplitude is often associated with sudden clinical deterioration. Bisynchronous slow waves (22.6.2) and other abnormalities are most common in the intermediate stages.

(7) *Intoxication with barbiturates and other drugs* depressing the central nervous

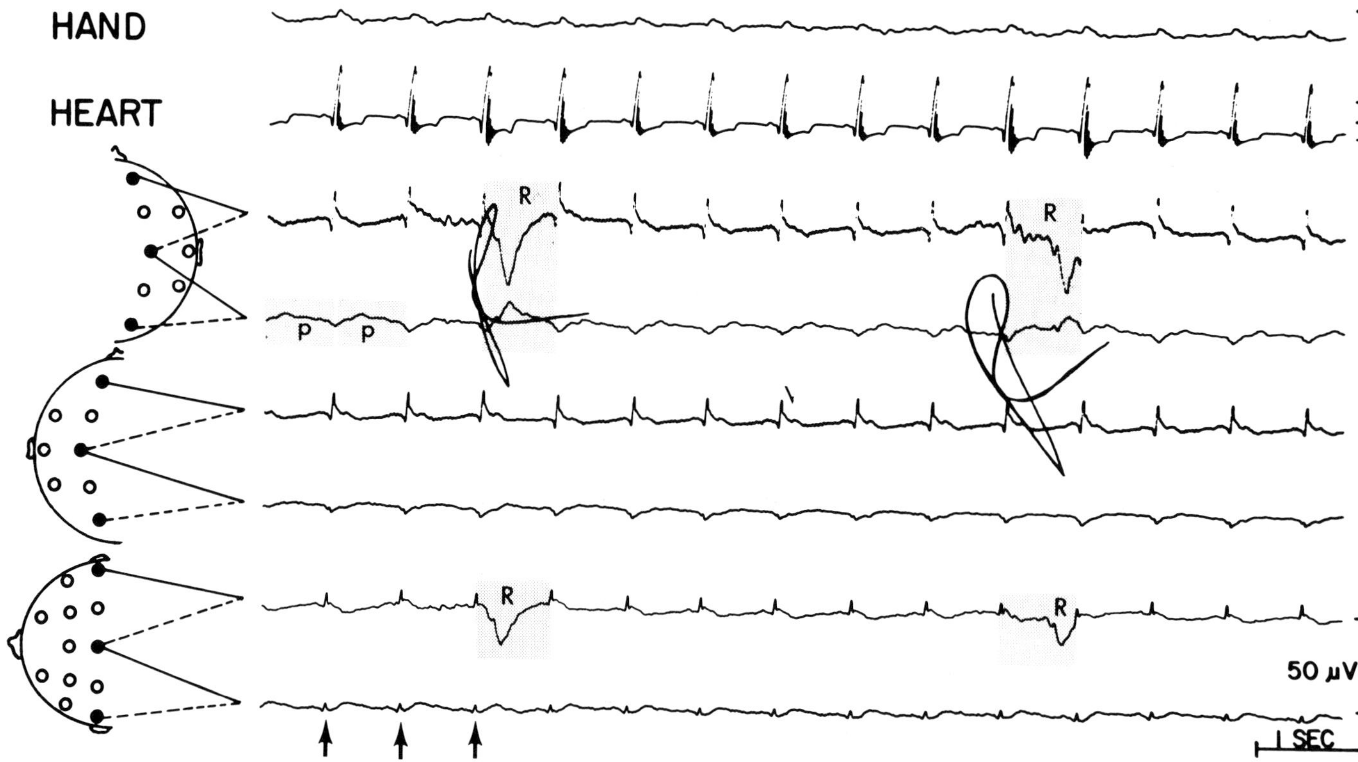


Fig. 24.2. Pattern of electrocerebral silence. The recording is made with widely spaced electrodes and high sensitivity. The artifacts commonly seen in this type of recording are due to heart beat (arrows), pulse waves (p) and movement by artificial respiration (R). This recording is from a 65-year-old woman who had a cardiac arrest 3 days earlier and was in postanoxic coma without spontaneous respiration and brainstem mediated reflexes since then. EEG and clinical condition did not change over the next 24 hours and she was pronounced cerebrally dead.

system leads to loss of amplitude preterminally. However, electrocerebral silence may develop fairly long before cerebral death (5.4): Partial or complete recovery of EEG and cerebral function is possible even after more than 24 hours of electrocerebral silence. Intoxication with barbiturates and other central nervous system depressant drugs must therefore be excluded in the evaluation of electrocerebral silence as an indicator of cerebral death.

**24.6.3** *Cerebrovascular diseases:*

(1) *Syncope,* Stokes-Adams attacks and other conditions producing a generalized reduction of cerebral blood flow, like acute anoxia from other causes, produce first generalized slow waves (21.6.3) and then a generalized decrease of amplitude.

(2) *Postanoxic encephalopathy* causes generalized asynchronous slow waves (21.6.3) and other EEG abnormalities. Low amplitude may occur either early, i.e. during the first few hours or days, or late, i.e. as a residual after other EEG abnormalities have abated. If low amplitude of early onset persists, the prognosis is poor.

(3) *Cerebral death* is often the immediate result of cerebral anoxia which is most often caused by cardiac or respiratory arrest; toxic, metabolic and traumatic disorders can cause cerebral death directly or through cardiorespiratory arrest and anoxia. To fulfill the criteria required for the diagnosis of cerebral death, the EEG must show no electrocerebral activity over 2 $\mu$V in two successive recordings made with special precautions and in the absence of hypothermia and poisoning with drugs depressing central nervous function (5.4); when recorded with proper techniques, the EEG demonstrating electrocerebral silence usually contains much artifact (Fig. 24.2).

(4) *Bilateral subdural hematomas* may reduce the amplitude of the EEG over wide parts of both hemispheres and are often associated with focal slow waves (20.6.3).

(5) *Vertebro-basilar insufficiency* seems to be associated with an increase in the

incidence of low voltage EEG patterns between attacks.

(6) *Air embolism* may suddenly reduce the amplitude of the EEG or induce generalized slow waves (21.6.3), usually more on the right side than on the left.

**24.6.4** *Cerebral trauma.* *Head injury,* if mild, may produce a brief decrease of amplitude with or without loss of consciousness. Severe head injuries that lead to coma may be associated with prolonged or progressive reduction of amplitude which carries a poor prognosis. An apparent decrease of amplitude occurs in comatose patients with generalized slow waves of high amplitude (21.6.4) during recovery.

**24.6.5** *Brain tumors.* Tumors do not reduce overall amplitude directly; pituitary tumors may cause low amplitude by producing hypothyroid encephalopathy.

**24.6.6** *Seizure disorders:*

(1) *Ictal decreases of amplitude* may occur at the beginning of a generalized seizure. A reduction of amplitude may be the only ictal manifestation in some forms of seizures (19.3.3). Flattening of the EEG, or low amplitude fast activity, also occurs during 'cerebellar fits' which, despite their name and paroxysmal character, are not seizures but attacks of intermittent decerebration; the underlying mechanisms are not yet fully understood but probably involve a sudden increase of intracranial pressure, generalized cortical ischemia, or an abrupt change of the function of the brainstem reticular formation.

(2) *Postictal depression* of amplitude appears immediately after most generalized seizures and lasts a few minutes until slow waves supervene.

**24.6.7** *Infectious diseases:*

(1) *Encephalitis and meningitis* can reduce overall EEG amplitude during the

acute phase of the disease. Persistence of reduced amplitude indicates residual widespread cerebral damage.

(2) *Progressive multifocal leukoencephalopathy* may reduce amplitude widely or induce generalized asynchronous slow waves (21.6.7).

**24.6.8** *Psychiatric diseases.* Anxiety reduces overall amplitude mainly by reducing alpha rhythm (24.7.2).

## 24.7 GENERALIZED DECREASE OR ABSENCE OF ALPHA RHYTHM

**24.7.1** *Normal attenuation of alpha rhythm* occurs with eye opening, alerting, mental effort, anxiety, and decrease of alertness to the level of drowsiness. A slight degree of anxiety is a normal reaction of many subjects to their first EEG recording and usually disappears during the course of the recording. The transient nature of these normal patterns of alpha attenuation distinguishes them from the low voltage patterns and from the effects of pathological anxiety.

**24.7.2** *Acute and chronic anxiety reactions* of psychiatric relevance produce commonly a persistent reduction of alpha rhythm and often an enhancement of beta rhythm. In the absence of beta rhythm, the results of anxiety reactions may be identical with the low voltage pattern.

**24.7.3** *Hypothyroidism* in mild cases may reduce alpha rhythm preferentially in addition to reducing alpha frequency; more severe cases usually show a reduction of all types of activity.

**24.7.4** *Hypoparathyroidism and pseudohypoparathyroidism* may lead to a selective reduction of alpha rhythm in addition to other abnormalities (22.6.2).

**24.7.5** *Hepatic encephalopathy* in its earliest stages may be associated with a selective decrease of alpha rhythm and an increase of beta rhythm.

**24.7.6** *Cushing's disease* often shows a paucity of alpha rhythm and an increase of beta rhythm in an otherwise normal EEG.

## 24.8 GENERALIZED INCREASE OF BETA RHYTHM

**24.8.1** *Normal* prominence of beta rhythm varies widely; beta rhythm is very prominent in some normal subjects and absent in others. However, the persistence of beta rhythm of more than low amplitude during most of the recording time may suggest an abnormality.

**24.8.2** *Hyperthyroidism* produces prominent fast activity either in the central regions or in a wide distribution. This activity mixes with, or replaces alpha rhythm. The frequency of alpha rhythm is often increased (25.1.7).

**24.8.3** *Barbiturates, benzodiazepines, other sedatives and tranquilizers* acutely induce widespread fast activity with a maximum in the central and frontal regions. This persists during wakefulness until stage I or II of sleep and becomes more conspicuous when alpha rhythm disappears. Barbiturates in doses producing coma cause nonreactive frontal 10–12 Hz rhythms. Many patients chronically taking barbiturates lose this fast activity.

**24.8.4** *Acute and chronic anxiety* are usually associated with an increase of fast activity in addition to the reduction of alpha activity.

**24.8.5** *Hepatic coma* may be associated with an increase of fast activity in the early stages when alpha rhythm disappears and before generalized slow waves start.

**24.8.6** *Cushing's disease* may be associated with an increase of beta activity.

**24.8.7** *Diabetes insipidus* may produce an increase of fast activity but no other EEG abnormality unless it is caused by a structural cerebral lesion.

**24.8.8** *Metachromatic leukodystrophy* may be associated with increased beta activity before the onset of slow waves.

## 24.9 CHANGES OF AMPLITUDE OF SLEEP PATTERNS

**24.9.1** *Phenylketonuria* may be associated with absent, jagged or sharp spindles and K complexes during sleep while the waking record may show hypsarrhythmia, multifocal independent spikes or slow spike-and-waves (19.1).

**24.9.2** *Progressive supranuclear palsy* may cause reduction of sleep spindles, V waves and K complexes and disturbances of sleep cycles (25.4.5) even before the waking record shows abnormalities.

**24.9.3** *Hypothyroidism, hypoparathyroidism, uremia and chlorpromazine intake* are among other conditions which reduce sleep spindles more than overall amplitude.

**24.9.4** *Tricyclic antidepressants and hypnotics,* notably flurazepam, increase sleep spindles.

## REFERENCES

American Neurological Association (1976) Statement regarding method for determining that the brain is dead. Trans. Am. Neurol. Ass. 101: 322–323.

Arfel, G., Casanova, C., Naquet, R., Passelecq, J. and Dubost, C. (1967) Étude électro-clinique de l'embolie gazeuse cérébrale en chirurgie cardiaque. Electroenceph. clin. Neurophysiol. 23: 101–122.

Beecher, H.K. (1968) A definition of irreversible coma. JAMA 205: 337–340.

Cabral, R., Prior, P.F., Scott, D.F. and Brierley, J.B. (1977) Reversible profound depression of cerebral electrical activity in hyperthermia. Electroenceph. clin. Neurophysiol. 42: 697–701.

Celesia, G.G. and Andermann, F. (1964) Some observations on the electrographic correlates of the decerebrate attack. Electroenceph. clin. Neurophysiol. 16: 295–300.

Jørgensen, E.O. (1974) EEG without detectable cortical activity and cranial nerve areflexia as parameters of brain death. Electroenceph. clin. Neurophysiol. 36: 70–75.

Niedermeyer, E. (1963) The electroencephalogram and vertebrobasilar artery insufficiency. Neurology 13: 412–422.

Schultz, M.A., Schulte, F.J., Akiyama, Y. and Parmalee, A.H. (1968) Development of electroencephalographic sleep phenomena in hypothyroid infants. Electroenceph. clin. Neurophysiol. 25: 351–358.

Scott, D.F., Heathfield, K.W.G., Toone, B. and Margerison, J.H. (1972) The EEG in Huntington's chorea: A clinical and neuropathological study. J. Neurol. Neurosurg. Psychiat. 35: 97–102.

Sishta, S.K., Troupe, A., Marszalek, K.S. and Kremer, L.M. (1974) Huntington's chorea: An electroencephalographic and psychometric study. Electroenceph. clin. Neurophysiol. 36: 387–393.

Trewby, P.N., Casemore, C. and Willians, R. (1978) Continuous bipolar recording of the EEG in patients with fulminant hepatic failure. Electroenceph. clin. Neurophysiol. 45: 107–110.

# 25

# Deviations from normal patterns

SUMMARY
Several patterns are abnormal due to features other than those described in the preceding chapters. These patterns include: (1) *abnormal frequency of alpha rhythm;* (2) *abnormal reactivity of alpha rhythm;* (3) *activity of alpha frequency in coma and seizures;* (4) *abnormal timing and incidence of sleep patterns;* (5) *abnormal photic responses; (6) immature patterns.*

## 25.1 ABNORMAL FREQUENCY OF ALPHA RHYTHM

**25.1.1** *Description of patterns.* *Unilateral increase or decrease of alpha frequency* is abnormal if it results in frequency differences of over 1 Hz. The underlying abnormality is much more likely to be located on the side of the lower alpha frequency, but this cannot be determined with certainty unless other lateralizing EEG abnormalities are present.

*Bilateral increase or decrease of alpha frequency* can be diagnosed with certainty only by comparing two records from the same patient and by taking into account any changes of age and differences in alertness. To qualify as abnormal, a difference of alpha frequency should consistently equal or exceed 2 Hz between recordings made at intervals of less than one year and at apparently similar levels of alertness. In the interpretation of a single record, the finding of a frequency of less than 8 Hz in adults, or of less than the normal range in younger persons, is abnormal. It is obvious that many significant reductions of alpha frequency will escape detection by this criterion if no control recordings are available because significant reductions may occur without exceeding the lower normal value of 8 Hz.

A bilateral increase of the frequency of alpha rhythm beyond the upper limit of 13 Hz transforms alpha rhythm into fast alpha variant, i.e. beta rhythm which has similar distribution and blocking as alpha rhythm and which is abnormal only if it represents a significant increase in comparison with a recent control recording from the same subject.

TABLE 25.1
Deviations from normal patterns

| Abnormal patterns | Causes | Examples of diseases |
|---|---|---|
| 1. Bilateral decrease of alpha frequency | Generalized disturbance of cerebral function: | |
| | Metabolic disorders | Hypothyroidism, hepatic and renal encephalopathy |
| | Change of rhythmical input to cortex | Reduced alertness |
| | Bilateral structural damage to occipital cortex or its thalamic input | Alzheimer's disease, multiple infarcts, subdural hematoma |
| 2. Unilateral decrease of alpha frequency | Unilateral disturbance of function of occipital cortex or its thalamic input | Transient ischemic attack, condition after mild head injury |
| | Unilateral structural damage to occipital cortex or its thalamic input | Unilateral chronic subdural hematoma, condition after severe head injury, cerebral infarct |
| 3. Bilateral increase of alpha frequency | Metabolic disorders | Hyperthyroidism, fever |
| 4. Unilateral failure of alpha blocking | Parietal or temporal lobe lesions | Tumors, infarcts |
| 5. Bilateral failure of alpha blocking on monocular input | Disorders of one eye or optic nerve | Monocular blindness |
| 6. Absence of alpha rhythm, presence of occipital spikes (Table 19.4) | Long-standing diseases of both eyes or central visual path | Congenital or early acquired binocular blindness |
| 7. Alpha frequency coma | Central pontine lesions | Infarcts, head injuries |
| | Widespread cerebral damage | Postanoxic encephalopathy |
| 8. Ictal activity of alpha or beta frequency (Table 19.3) | Local or widespread cerebral damage in newborns | Infantile partial or generalized seizures or status epilepticus |
| | Irritative temporal lobe lesions | Partial complex seizure activity |

**25.1.2** *Clinical significance of frequency changes of alpha rhythm.* *Bilateral decrease of alpha frequency* is often due to conditions which slow the metabolism of the brain. Many of these conditions are associated with a decrease of alertness, memory, awareness and orientation. Some of these conditions are transient, for instance toxic or metabolic encephalopathies; others are associated with long-standing damage, for instance cerebral atrophy or bilateral subdural hematomas. Generalized slowing of alpha rhythm may be an early signal of various types of abnormalities which later produce other, more specific, abnormalities.

*Unilateral decrease of alpha frequency* occurs in conditions which also cause a unilateral decrease of the amplitude of alpha rhythm. Such decreases may be the only residual EEG abnormality in mild or old vascular or traumatic lesions of the posterior head regions, but they occasionally appear early in expanding tumors and in lesions of the central and frontal areas.

*Bilateral increase of alpha frequency* occurs in some conditions of increased cerebral metabolism.

*Unilateral increase of alpha frequency* is very rare.

**25.1.3** *Other EEG abnormalities associated with abnormal frequency of alpha rhythm.* *Abnormal amplitude of alpha rhythm* may appear in the same distribution as abnormal frequency of alpha rhythm, especially in unilateral changes.

*Bisynchronous and asynchronous generalized slow waves* often appear on a background of slow alpha frequency.

**25.1.4** *Grading of abnormal frequency of alpha rhythm* is best carried out by indicating actual frequencies.

**25.1.5** *Mechanisms causing abnormal frequency of alpha rhythm* are probably similar to mechanisms causing changes of amplitude of alpha rhythm (23.5.1; 24.5.3).

**25.1.6** *Specific disorders causing unilateral or bilateral decrease of alpha frequency:*

(1) *Degenerative, developmental and demyelinating diseases. Senile and presenile dementia (Alzheimer's disease)* causes abnormal slowing of alpha rhythm which is of less diagnostic importance than are asynchronous generalized slow waves (21.6.1).

*Myotonic dystrophy* may cause slowing of alpha rhythm; this is probably due to the endocrine disturbances characteristic of this disease.

(2) *Metabolic and toxic encephalopathies.* Many of these encephalopathies produce early slowing of alpha frequency before causing other abnormalities (Table 22.1) and disappearance of alpha rhythm. The most important encephalopathies in this group are due to acute anoxia, Vitamin B12 deficiency, hypoglycemia, hepatic and renal failure, porphyria, Addison's disease, hyper- and hypoparathyroidism, Wernicke's disease, acute intoxication with barbiturates, alcohol, antipsychotics, amphetamines, lithium, marihuana and other psychotropic drugs. Hypothyroidism may cause slowing of apha rhythm often followed by reduction of amplitude without other abnormalities.

(3) *Cerebrovascular diseases.* Local or generalized slowing of alpha rhythm occurs temporarily in transient local or generalized cerebral ischemia. Persistent slowing of alpha rhythm may be seen in bilateral or multiple cerebral infarcts, lacunar state of hypertensives, unilateral and bilateral subdural hematomas, thalamic infarcts, mesencephalic infarcts, postanoxic encephalopathy, subarachnoid hemorrhage with obtundation.

(4) *Cerebral trauma. Head injuries* of mild intensity may produce no more EEG abnormalities than a slowing of alpha rhythm, with or without a reduction of its amplitude. Patients recovering from more severe head injuries may show a decrease of alpha frequency, amplitude, or both as the last residual EEG abnormality. Repeated head injuries, for instance those of boxers, may produce lasting and

progressive reduction of the frequency of alpha rhythm in addition to generalized slow waves (21.6.4).

(5) *Brain tumors.* *Infratentorial tumors* may reduce alpha frequency and amplitude on both sides in addition to producing bisynchronous slow waves and other abnormalities (22.6.5).

*Supratentorial tumors,* especially those in the posterior head regions and the thalamus, may decrease alpha frequency and amplitude on the side of the tumor in addition to producing focal or lateralized slow waves (20.6.5).

(6) *Seizure disorders.* *Ictal discharges* sometimes consist of rhythmical waves of alpha or slower frequency (19.3) which are usually easily distinguished from alpha rhythm.

*Postictal slowing of alpha frequency* may persist longer than other postictal changes (20.6.6; 21.6.6).

(7) *Infectious diseases.* *Non-specific slowing of alpha rhythm* may occur in many infectious diseases including those not directly involving the brain; this slowing is commonly associated with fever and a reduction of the level of consciousness.

*Cerebral infections* causing widespread cerebral damage may produce slowing of alpha rhythm in addition to other abnormalities (21.6.7).

(8) *Psychiatric diseases.* *Endogenous depression* is associated with a decrease of the mean frequency of alpha rhythm in some patients who have no manic cycles. Schizophrenia is associated with a wider scatter of alpha frequency between patients than seen between normal persons; the mean frequency of alpha rhythm is reduced in patients with chronic schizophrenia.

**25.1.7** *Specific disorders causing unilateral or bilateral increase of alpha frequency:*

(1) *Hyperthyroidism,* including that induced by treatment, is commonly associated with an increase of alpha frequency; the absolute amount of alpha rhythm may

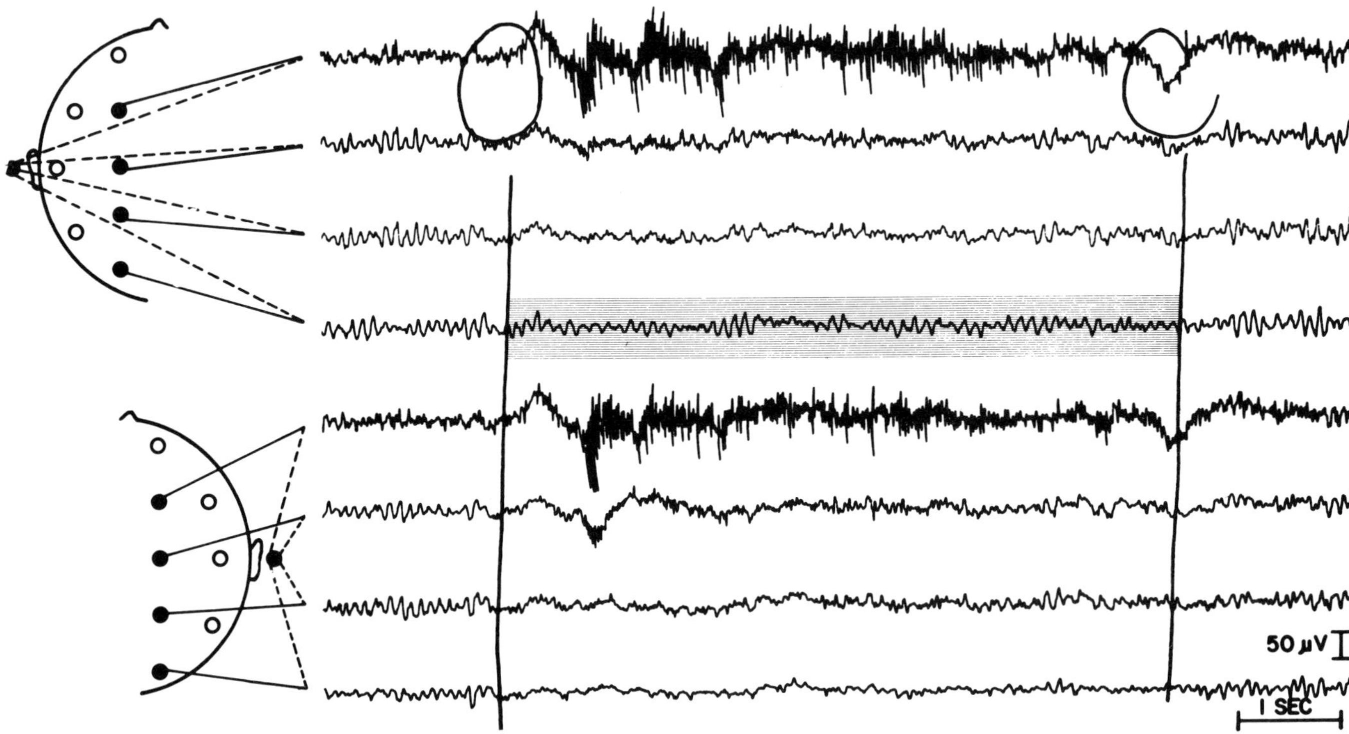


Fig. 25.1. Unilateral failure of blocking of alpha rhythm. Before eye opening (O) and after eye closing (C), alpha rhythm is present and symmetrical on the two sides. While the eyes are open, alpha rhythm is blocked normally on the right side but persists on the left (shaded). This 32-year old woman sustained a head injury without loss of consciousness 9 days before the EEG recording and had some receptive aphasia which cleared gradually.

be reduced. Other abnormalities are often present. Many patients show beta rhythm, some have diffuse spikes and sharp waves, and a few have prominent generalized asynchronous slow waves. Treatment of the hyperthyroidism gradually reverses all abnormalities except for the asynchronous slow waves.

(2) *Fever* may increase alpha frequency unless it is associated with decreasing awareness which can lead to a decrease of alpha frequency.

## 25.2 ABNORMAL REACTIVITY OF ALPHA RHYTHM

**25.2.1** *Unilateral failure of alpha blocking* on eye opening may occur with lesions of the parietal and temporal lobe on the side which fails to block (Fig. 25.1). This sign may be present in the absence of any other EEG abnormality and therefore may be the most sensitive and earliest indicator of lesions in those areas.

**25.2.2** *Bilateral failure of alpha blocking:*

(1) *Normal subjects* show great variability of alpha blocking and may have only very brief reductions of alpha amplitude in response to eye opening and alerting.

(2) *Unilateral cerebral lesions* which cause confusion may abolish the blocking of alpha rhythm before they produce other EEG abnormalities. In general, these are lesions in regions other than the specific sensory receiving area, for instance frontal and temporal lesions, or parietal lesions of the type producing unilateral failure of alpha blocking when not associated with confusion.

(3) *Binocular blindness* when acquired after the development of alpha leads to a loss of the reactivity of alpha rhythm to eye opening. Alpha rhythm in this condition may have a central or unusually wide distribution. Like congenitally blind persons, persons with acquired blindness may have no alpha rhythm and may develop occipital spikes even in the absence of occipital lesions (19.4.6).

(4) *Monocular blindness* or loss of discriminative vision can cause failure of alpha blocking in both hemispheres when the blind eye is opened; opening of the seeing eye produces normal bilateral alpha blocking.

## 25.3 ACTIVITY OF ALPHA FREQUENCY IN COMA AND SEIZURES

**25.3.1** *Alpha frequency coma* or *alpha pattern coma* denotes a pattern of rhythmical waves which have alpha or theta frequency but differ from true alpha rhythm in that they occur in comatose patients, are not restricted to the posterior head regions, and do not block in the usual fashion. In some cases, these waves show little variation in frequency and are the only activity present; in other cases, their frequency varies by several hertz, and generalized slow waves may be added. Two groups of patterns may be distinguished which loosely correspond with two types of lesions; however, there is much overlap between these groups.

(1) *Predominantly posterior alpha activity* shows either no reaction to alerting stimuli or a variable attenuation of the alpha activity. This pattern can be seen in patients with lesions in the central parts of the pons, most commonly in patients with pontine infarcts (Fig. 25.2). The appearance of sleep patterns in these patients is associated with a relatively good prognosis (25.4.1).

(2) *Generalized or predominantly frontal alpha activity* without reaction to alerting stimuli can be seen in patients with widespread cerebral damage, especially that following cardiac or respiratory arrest, prolonged hypoglycemia or bilateral damage to midline thalamic nuclei (Fig. 25.3). This form of alpha activity is generally less regular than that seen in pontine lesions. Focal or generalized slow waves or amplitude abnormalities may also be present. The alpha pattern is usually seen for up to four days after the insult and is later replaced by other abnormalities. Sleep patterns occur rarely in these patients. Their prognosis for survival and recovery is poor.

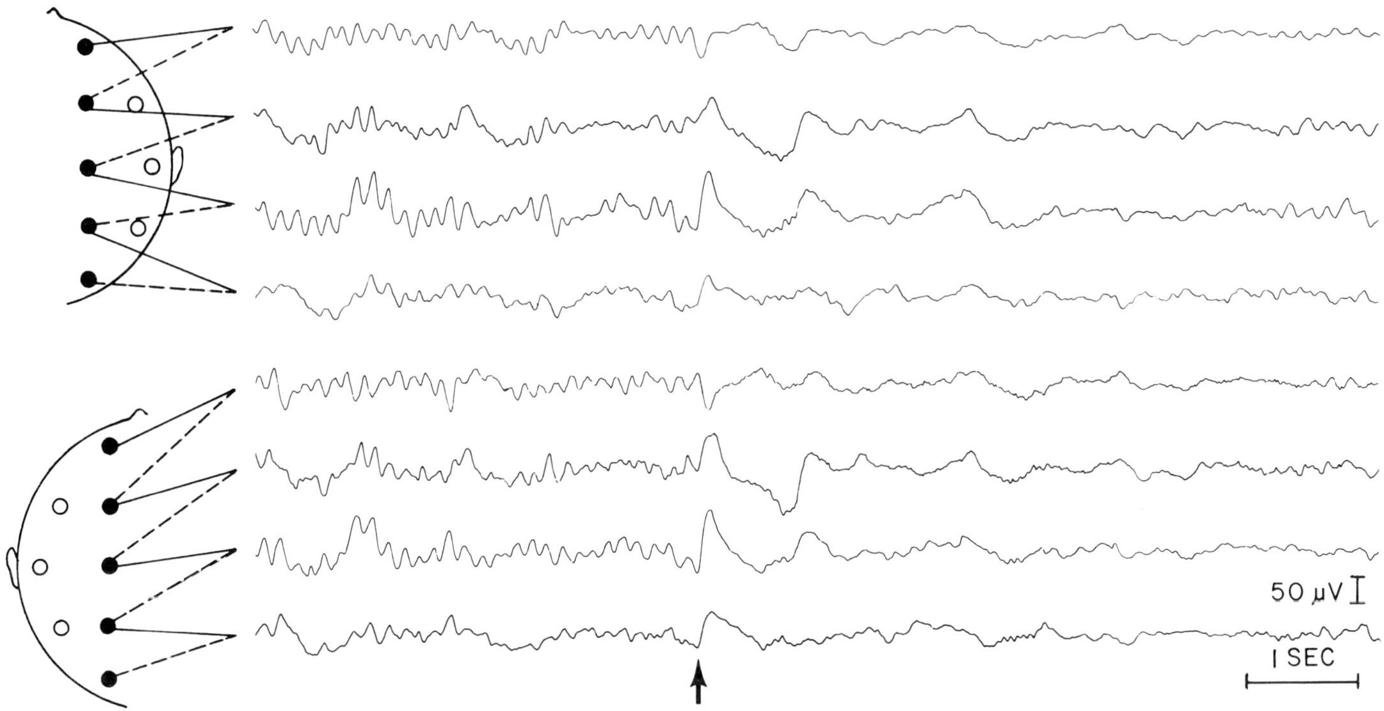


Fig. 25.2. Pattern of alpha frequency coma in a patient with a presumed pontine lesion. Sinusoidal 7 Hz waves, superimposed on delta waves, are seen in a wide distribution in the left part of the figure. Pinching of the left arm (arrow) blocks the sinusoidal waves promptly for several seconds. This 25-year-old woman sustained a severe head injury in a motorcycle accident 3 days before this recording and was in coma since then with pupillary and other signs suggestive of a pontine contusion.

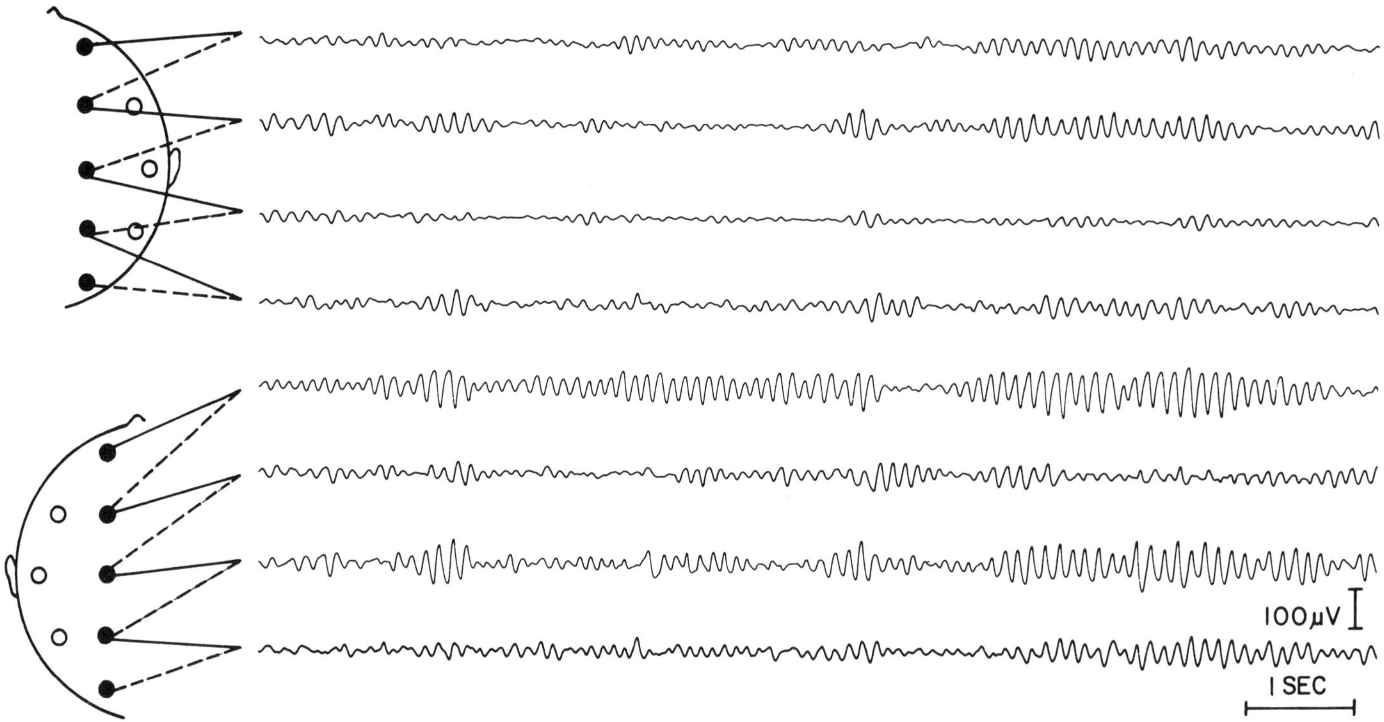


Fig. 25.3. Pattern of alpha frequency coma in a patient with widespread cerebral damage after cardiac arrest. Sinusoidal 8 Hz waves appear in a wide and asymmetrical distribution. They did not react to loud noises or noxious stimuli. This 27-year-old man was in postanoxic coma for 2 days after a cardiac arrest. A followup EEG 9 days later showed generalized slow waves of very low amplitude. The patient then was unresponsive and in a decerebrate posture and had roving vertical eye movements. He died 3 weeks later without regaining consciousness.

A similar pattern can be seen as a result of electrical injuries and of intoxication with sedative drugs even in the absence of respiratory depression. The prognosis in these cases is better.

**25.3.2** *Ictal alpha or beta activity* in a unilateral or focal and shifting distribution may be the only manifestation of intermittent seizures or status epilepticus in newborns; this condition is often due to diffuse or localized cortical damage resulting from perinatal injury or developmental defects (18.2.3). The rhythmical waves seen in a temporal, temporofrontal or wide distribution in one or both hemispheres of patients having partial complex seizures (17.1.3) occasionally fall into the alpha or beta frequency range even though they are usually slower.

### 25.4 ABNORMAL TIMING AND INCIDENCE OF SLEEP PATTERNS

**25.4.1** *Sleep activity in comatose patients* is occasionally superimposed on the slow waves or the alpha activity which characterize coma due to various structural lesions or toxic and metabolic encephalopathies. Sleep activity seems inappropriate in these patients insofar as they do not exhibit cycles of wakefulness and sleep. However, the appearance of sleep activity in such patients indicates a better prognosis than does the absence of sleep activity.

**25.4.2** *Paradoxical slow wave response to alerting stimuli* consists of a transient increase or appearance of generalized slow waves on a background of slow waves of lower amplitude or of alpha activity in patients with reduced alertness most often due to head injuries (Fig. 25.4). Although different from the normal response to alerting, this response indicates a better prognosis than does the absence of a response to alerting stimuli.

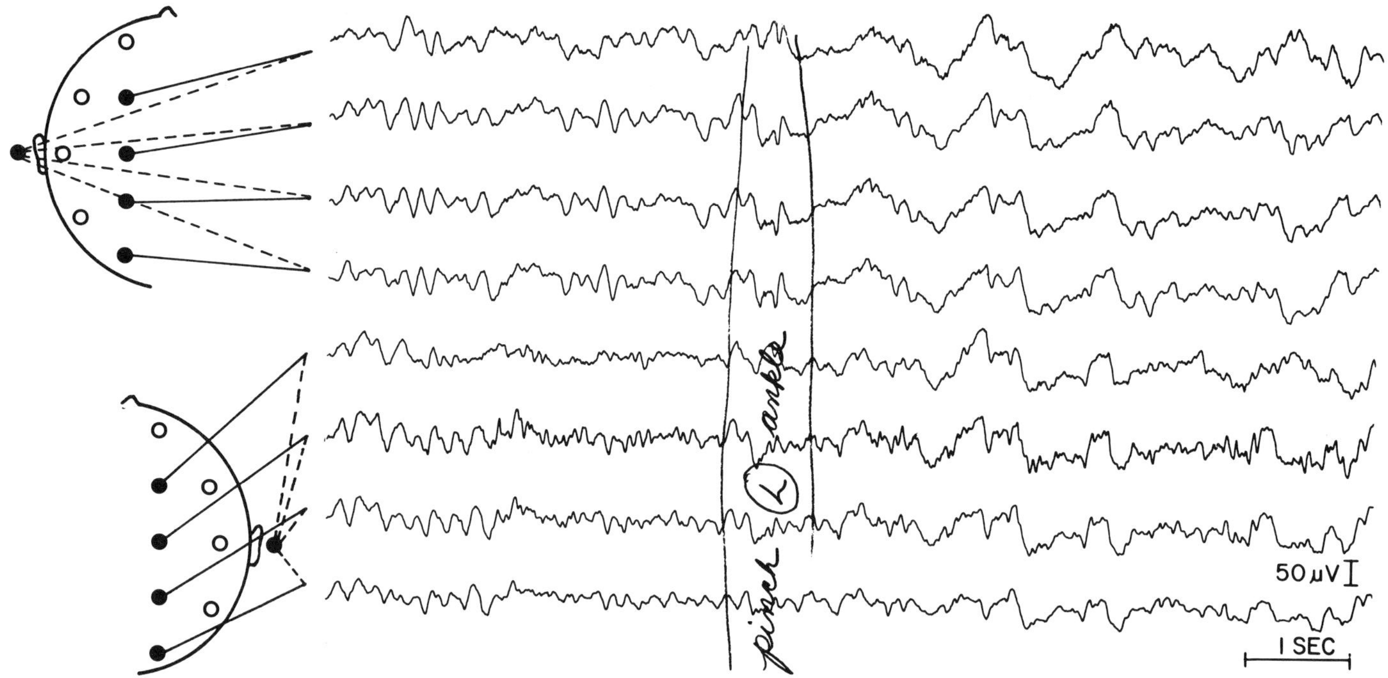


Fig. 25.4. Paradoxical slow wave response to alerting stimuli in an obtunded patient. Rhythmical 4–5 Hz waves at rest are replaced by generalized delta waves after pinching of the left ankle. This 70-year-old woman had repeated subarachnoid hemorrhages from an aneurysm on the left posterior communicating artery 2–3 weeks before this recording and began to recover from coma at the time of the recording.

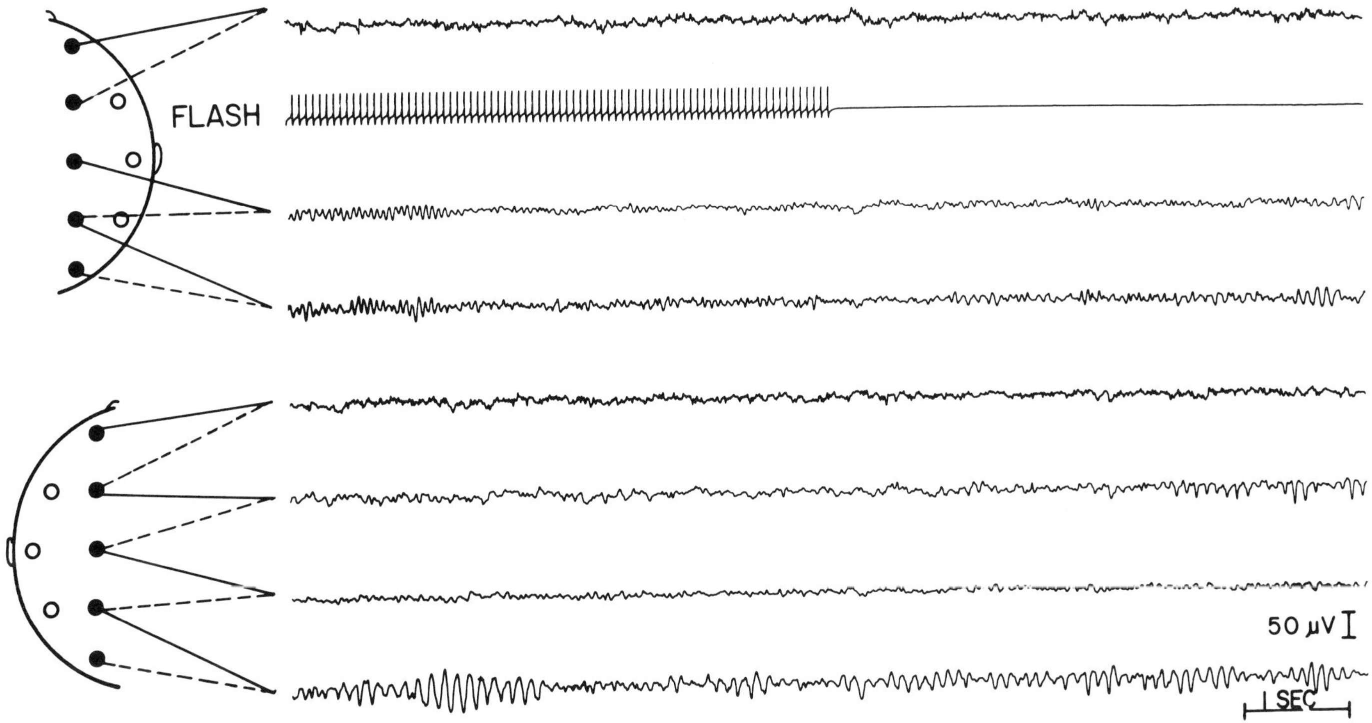


Fig. 25.5. Significant asymmetry of photic driving. Stimulation with repetitive flashes, monitored in channel 2, elicits moderate driving in the right parietal and occipital areas; there is no response on the left where alpha waves continue. This is a part of a recording also used in Fig. 25.1 to illustrate unilateral failure of alpha blocking on eye opening.

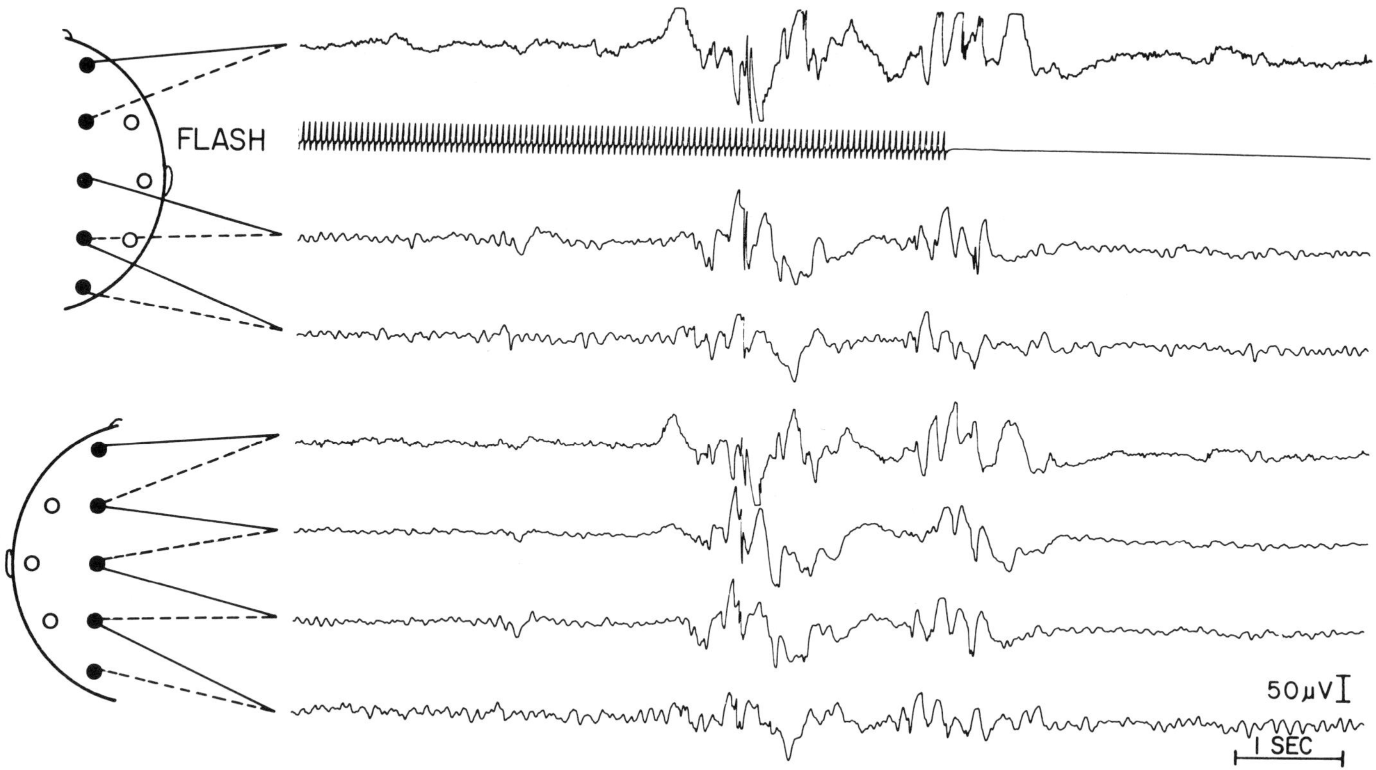


Fig. 25.6. Photoconvulsive response. Repetitive flash stimulation, monitored in channel 2, elicits no driving; rather, a paroxysm of irregular spikes, sharp and slow waves appears suddenly and in a wide distribution. The generalized epileptiform activity outlasts the end of photic stimulation. Similar paroxysms were elicited repeatedly with similar stimuli in other parts of the same recording. This 23-year-old woman had a generalized tonic-clonic seizure one day before the EEG recording. The seizure began while the patient looked at a television screen showing horizontal bars which turned over vertically.

**25.4.3** *Sleep onset REM periods (SOREMPs) and short latency to sleep onset* of less than 5 minutes occur in patients with narcolepsy, and Kleine-Levin syndrome (12.4.2; 12.4.3).

**25.4.4** *Reduction of REM sleep* can occur as the result of diseases causing structural damage, for instance mongolism, and Pelizaeus-Merzbacher disease, and as an effect of various drugs, for instance alcohol, barbiturates, tricyclic antidepressants and various other neuroleptic drugs.

**25.4.5** *Disordered sleep cycles* occur in sleep apnea, progressive supranuclear palsy and children with episodic sleep disturbances (12.4.4).

## 25.5 ABNORMAL PHOTIC RESPONSES

**25.5.1** *Abnormal amplitude of photic responses:*

(1) *Asymmetry* of the photic response may suggest an abnormality (23.7.3) the nature and location of which is best determined by correlation with other focal abnormalities (Fig. 25.5).

(2) *Abnormally high amplitude of a photic response,* recognizable only by comparison with a control record from the same subject (14.3.3), may be seen with hyperthyroidism, hyperparathyroidism, pseudohyperparathyroidism and renal encephalopathy.

**25.5.2** *Photoconvulsive or photoparoxysmal responses* consist of spikes, spike-and-slow-wave complexes and multiple spike-and-slow wave complexes of regular or irregular configuration and repetition (Fig. 25.6). They usually occur only at certain stimulus rates, most often in the range of 8–15 Hz. They often start not at the beginning of a stimulus train but appear during continued stimulation. Photic driving may precede the paroxysm (14.3). Paroxysms may develop from photic driving in the occipital regions and spread to the entire head, but they more often start abruptly and without transition from the posterior driving and have a wide and symmetrical distribution and bisynchronous timing from the start. In contrast to normal occipital driving, the rate of the paroxysmal discharges is usually unrelated to the stimulus frequency, and the discharges are often sustained, at least briefly, after the end of stimulation.

Photoparoxysmal responses are generally more likely to occur when the eyes are closed during stimulation than when they are open; the period immediately after eye closure seems most susceptible. During stimulation with the eyes open, flashes of colored or patterned light may be more effective in eliciting paroxysmal discharges. Some subjects with photoparoxysmal responses have epileptiform discharges in other parts of the EEG; these discharges are usually generalized and similar to those seen during photic stimulation. If the spontaneous discharges are frequent, it may be difficult to decide whether or not discharges during photic stimulation are triggered by photic stimulation. Triggering is more likely if repeated stimulation elicits paroxysmal responses consistently.

The ability to trigger paroxysmal discharges can be used to assess their clinical significance. While in many patients with photoparoxysmal discharges it would be possible to induce a generalized seizure by prolonged stimulation, this is obviously not desirable and the technician should limit photic stimulation to the safe minimum of eliciting brief, unquestionable photoparoxysmal responses. During such brief paroxysms, only a few patients show obvious clinical accompaniments, usually in the form of twitching movement. Other patients may show associated movements only on close inspection. For instance, 3 Hz spike-and-wave discharges may be associated with slight fluttering of the eyelids at 3 Hz. An arrest of motor function may go unnoticed by the technician but can be documented by having a patient count aloud

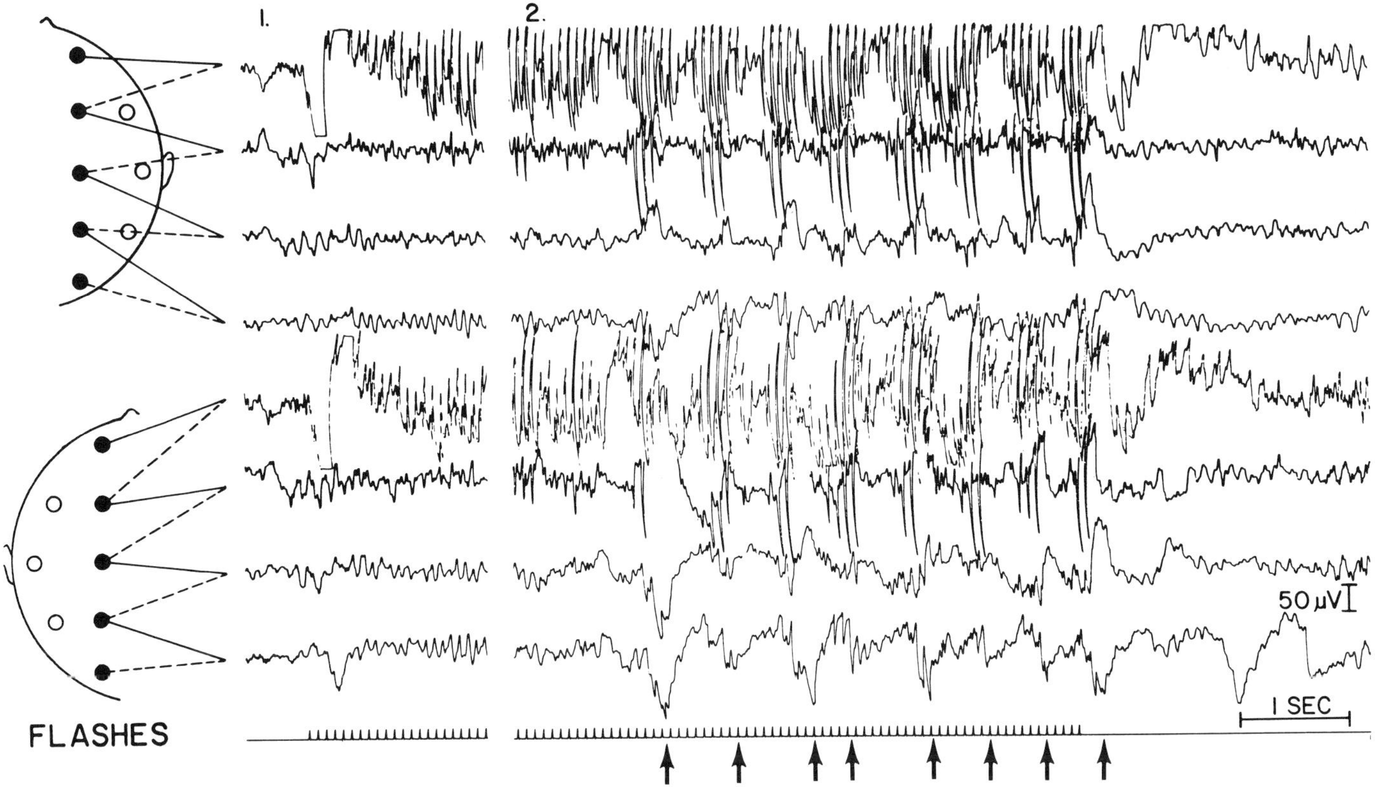


Fig. 25.7. Photomyoclonic response. 1. Stimulation with repetitive flashes at 13 Hz, monitored at the bottom, causes muscle artifact in the frontal regions at the rate of the flashes. The posterior head regions show the beginning of photic driving. 2. Five seconds after part 1, the muscle artifact is spreading to the posterior head regions and repetitive movement artifacts at 1–2 Hz (arros) develop, corresponding with jerking of the head and neck. Muscle and movement artifacts end promptly at the end of the flash stimuli. This 37-year-old woman has a history of syncope, headaches and high blood pressure; the neurological examination was normal.

beginning before stimulation with flashes which elicit photoparoxysmal responses. The patient may stop counting during the paroxysm and thus reveal a clinical correlate of the epileptiform activity. A loss of awareness can be demonstrated by giving a test word during a paroxysm and later asking the patient to recall the word (5.1).

Photoparoxysmal responses are definitely abnormal. Many patients with photoparoxysmal responses have a history of seizures, nearly always of primary generalized seizures; these cases are sometimes labelled 'photosensitive epilepsy'. However, photoparoxysmal responses can occur in other conditions, particularly in the hyperexcitable phase during the first few days after withdrawal from the chronic use of alcohol, barbiturates and other drugs which depress the central nervous system. In these instances, a patient may or may not have seizures during the withdrawal phase or a convulsive disorder independent of the withdrawal. Like other epileptiform activity, photoconvulsive responses occasionally are seen in persons who have no seizures. In very few cases does photic stimulation induce a generalized seizure in apparently normal subjects.

**25.5.3** *Photomyoclonic responses* must be distinguished from photoconvulsive responses. Photomyoclonic responses are muscle contractions which are triggered by bright flashes in a few susceptible individuals (14.3.2). The contractions usually involve the eyelids but may extend to involve muscles of the head, neck and body and lead to rhythmical twitches. The EEG shows these responses in the form of muscle and movement artifacts but contains no epileptiform activity (Fig. 25.7). Photomyoclonic responses are described here to distinguish them clearly from the abnormal photoconvulsive responses.

Photomyoclonic responses appear only when the eyes are closed. They are most prominent at flash rates of 8–20 Hz. Muscle artifacts, strictly tied to the preceding flash, appear usually first in the frontal electrodes. The response often increases in amplitude and spreads in distribution during continued stimulation at the same frequency; muscle and movement artifacts may obscure the recording from most or all electrodes on the head. In contrast to photoconvulsive responses, photomyoclonic responses begin in the frontal areas; like normal photic driving, photomyoclonic responses correspond exactly with the stimulus frequency and end promptly with the end of stimulation.

## 25.6 IMMATURE PATTERNS

*Immature patterns* are those found at an age when these patterns normally have disappeared. Immature patterns are probably slightly more common among patients with psychiatric afflictions such as behavior disorders, hysteria and reactive depression. However, too many normal persons have immature EEGs without immature personality features to permit equating EEG immaturity with emotional or other developmental immaturity.

## REFERENCES


Bancaud, J., Hacaen, H. and Lairy, G.C. (1955) Modifications de la réactivité EEG, troubles des fonctions symboliques et troubles confusionnels dans les lésions hémisphériques localisées. Electroenceph. clin. Neurophysiol. 7: 179–192.

Benoit, O., Goldenberg-Leygonie, F., Lacombe, J. and Marc, M.E. (1978) Sommeil de l'enfant presentant des manifestations episodiques du sommeil: Comparaison avec l'enfant normal. Electroenceph. clin. Neurophysiol. 44: 502–512.

Cadilhac, J. (1976) Section V. EEG in thyroid dysfunction. In: Rémond, A. (Ed.), Handbook of Electroenceph. clin. Neurophysiol., Vol. 15C, Elsevier, Amsterdam, pp. 70–76.

Carroll, W.M. and Mastaglia, F.L. (1979) Alpha and beta coma in drug intoxication uncomplicated by cerebral hypoxia. Electroenceph. clin. Neurophysiol. 46: 95–105.

Chatrian, G.E. and Perez-Borja, C. (1964) Depth electrographic observations in two cases of photo-

oculoclonic responses. Electroenceph. clin. Neurophysiol. 17: 71–75.
Chatrian, G.E. (1975) Section V. Electrographic and behavioral signs of sleep in comatose states. In: Rémond, A. (Ed.), Handbook of Electroenceph. clin. Neurophysiol., Vol. 12, Elsevier, Amsterdam, pp. 63–77.
Chokroverty, S. (1975) 'Alpha-like' rhythms in electroencephalograms in coma after cardiac arrest. Neurology 25: 655–663.
Fukuyama, Y. and Hayashi, M. (1979) Sleep electroencephalograms and sleep stages in hypoparathyroidism. Eur. Neurol. 18: 38–48.
Glass, J.D. (1977) Alpha blocking: Absence in visuobehavioral deprivation. Science 198: 58–60.
Gross, R.A., Spehlmann, R. and Daniels, J.C. (1978) Sleep disturbances in progressive supranuclear palsy. Electroenceph. clin. Neurophysiol. 45: 16–25.
Harner, R.N. (1975) EEG evaluation of the patient with dementia. In: Benson, D.F. and Blumer, D. (Eds.), Psychiatric Aspects of Neurological Disease. Grune and Stratton, New York, pp. 63–82.
Jeavons, P.M. and Harding, G.F.A. (1975) Photosensitive epilepsy: A review of the literature and a study of 460 patients. Clin. Dev. Med. 56: 1–121.
Knauss, T.A. and Carlson, C.B. (1978) Neonatal paroxysmal monorhythmic alpha activity. Arch. Neurol. 35: 104–107.
Laffont, F., Autret, A., Minz, M., Beillevaire, T., Gilbert, A., Cathala, H.P. and Castaigne, P. (1979) Étude polygraphique du sommeil dans 9 cas de maladie de Steele-Richardson. Rev. Neurol. 135: 127–142.
Meier-Ewert, K. and Broughton, R.J. (1967) Photomyoclonic response of epileptic and non-epileptic subjects during wakefulness, sleep and arousal. Electroenceph. clin. Neurophysiol. 23: 142–151.
Newmark, M.E. and Penry, J.K. (1979) Photosensitivity and Epilepsy: A Review. Raven Press, New York.
Reilly, E.L. and Peters, J.F. (1973) Relationship of some varieties of electroencephalographic photosensitivity to clinical convulsive disorders. Neurology 23: 1050–1057.
Schwartz, M.S. and Scott, D.F. (1978) Pathological stimulus-related slow wave arousal responses in the EEG. Acta Neurol. Scand. 57: 300–304.
Sørenson, K., Thomassen, A. and Wernberg, M. (1978) Prognostic significance of alpha frequency EEG rhythm in coma after cardiac arrest. J. Neurol. Neurosurg. Psychiat. 41: 840–842.
Westmoreland, B.F., Klass, D.W., Sharbrough, F.W. and Reagan, T.J. (1975) Alpha-coma. Electroencephalographic, clinical, pathologic, and etiologic correlations. Arch. Neurol. 32: 713–718.
Zander Olsen, P., Støier, M., Siersbaek-Nielsen, K., Mølholm Hansen, J., Schiøler, M. and Kristensen, M. (1972) Electroencephalographic findings in hyperthyroidism. Electroenceph. clin. Neurophysiol. 32: 171–177.

# 26 The EEG report

SUMMARY

The EEG report should give:

(26.1) *A description* of the essential features of normal and abnormal activity observed under the various conditions of recording, namely resting wakefulness, hyperventilation, photic stimulation and sleep;

(26.2) *An EEG diagnosis* listing the types of significant findings;

(26.3) *A clinical interpretation* of the EEG diagnosis in the light of the patient's clinical problems and the referring physician's queries.

EXAMPLE

The following is the report on the EEG of a 15-year-old boy referred because of four attacks of dizziness during the preceding three months; the referring physician wishes to investigate the possibility of a convulsive disorder.

*Report: The resting record* showed a background which was well developed for the age of this patient and well organized. Sinusoidal alpha rhythm of 10–11 Hz and of moderate amplitude appeared intermittently in a wide and essentially symmetrical distribution with a maximum in the posterior head regions. Beta rhythm of low amplitude was superimposed widely, mainly in the frontal regions. A mu rhythm of 9–10 Hz and of moderate, symmetrical amplitude occurred intermittently and independently in both central areas. Theta waves of 5–7 Hz and of an amplitude hardly exceeding that of the background were seen sporadically and diffusely, slightly more prominent in the temporal regions.

*Hyperventilation* was performed well and induced bilaterally synchronous slow waves but no abnormalities even though the patient complained of feeling dizzy and faint in a manner similar to that experienced during his recent attacks.

*Photic stimulation* elicited slight symmetrical driving in the occipital regions.

*Sleep* was induced with chloral hydrate and was associated with normal electrographic patterns. No epileptiform activity appeared during 10 minutes of sleep.

*Impression:* The EEG during wakefulness and sleep was normal for the age of this patient.

*Interpretation:* The absence of epileptiform activity does not exclude the diagnosis of a convulsive disorder as a possible cause of this patient's attacks because a significant portion of patients with such disorders have no epileptiform activity in their first recording. However, hyperventilation reproduced the dizziness which this patient experiences during his attacks. The absence of epileptiform activity in the EEG at that time strongly suggests that his dizziness is not a seizure manifestation.

## 26.1 DESCRIPTION OF THE RECORD

The report should describe the essential normal and abnormal patterns appearing under the various recording conditions so that a person with some knowledge of EEG can envisage the findings on which diagnosis and interpretation are based. Sufficient detail should be given to enable the reader of a later EEG to estimate whether the major features of the two recordings are similar or different. The report should not be exhaustive in describing normal detail but should include those rare or unusual features in the record which may have clinical significance. As far as possible, the report should use the terms defined in the glossary of the International Federation of Societies for EEG and Clinical Neurophysiology (9). Judgements like 'good' and 'poor' should be used only sparingly and only to characterize the overall composition of a record, but not to rate individual rhythms: Persons not familiar with the EEG cannot know that 'poor' driving has no different clinical significance than has 'good' or even 'excellent' driving.

Patterns should be described by indicating the frequency, amplitude and distribution of the component waves. Wave shape, rhythmicity, symmetry, synchrony, persistence, reactivity and periodicity may be important for the description of abnormal patterns. Because the frequency of a rhythm often varies, it is usually indicated in terms of a frequency range or band of a few hertz in width rather than in terms of a single frequency. In most instances, it is not sufficient to use only the wide bands of delta, theta, alpha and beta frequency to describe the frequencies of waves in a record; the frequency of alpha and beta rhythms and of theta and delta waves observed in a recording should be specified in narrower bands in every case. Amplitude may be reported in absolute or relative measurements. Absolute units must be used in the diagnosis of electrocerebral silence which requires a certification that no electrocerebral activity of over 2 $\mu$V is present. Even if activity of very low amplitude is found in these cases, the amplitude may be specified to indicate the severity of the abnormality and to give the basis for an exact comparison with subsequent recordings. In most other instances, it is sufficient to characterize amplitude as low, medium or high.

To avoid omitting important features in the report, one should adhere to a standard sequence of reporting. Here I will describe the format which I have used for many years.

**26.1.1** *The opening statement* should describe the general level of consciousness of the patient. In particular, it should mention behavioral abnormalities such as somnolence, coma, lack of cooperation, or persistent movement and muscle artifacts. All these factors could render the record technically unsatisfactory or reduce the length of the readable EEG to a sample shorter than the minimum required for reliable interpretation (5.1). The opening statement should indicate any unusual recording conditions, for instance recordings made at the bedside or in an intensive care unit, or the use of special recording techniques such as naso-pharyngeal electrodes or other special monitors.

The general appearance of the background activity should be stated. For adults, the report may open by saying 'The background of the resting record was well organized'. For a child, the opening may say 'The background of the resting record was well developed for the age of this patient and moderately well organized'. For old persons, it may say 'The background was poorly organized even considering the advanced age of this patient'. The waking record may show no normal background activity and be grossly and continuously abnormal, an observation which the opening statement should mention.

**26.1.2** *The resting record:*

(1) *Description of normal background. Alpha, beta, mu and other rhythms and patterns,* if present, are described in terms of their frequency range, relative amplitude and distribution. Wave shape, rhythmicity, symmetry, distribution, persistence and reactivity should be mentioned if they are abnormal. Excessive beta rhythm and unilateral blocking of alpha rhythm must be reported.

(2) *Description of abnormal patterns. Epileptiform activity* is characterized by its shape, amplitude, repetition rate, persistence, distribution, synchrony, symmetry, relationship between focal and generalized discharges and any other feature of possible clinical significance including the association with behavioral seizure manifestations.

*Slow waves* are described in terms of frequency, amplitude, shape, rhythmicity, regularity, persistence, distribution, symmetry, synchrony and any other parameter of clinical importance. If more than one type of slow wave is present, the specifications for each type must be given. Abnormal generalized asynchronous slow waves must be distinguished by amplitude, frequency, distribution and persistence from the range of asynchronous slow waves normally seen at the age of the patient.

*Asymmetries* and generalized changes of amplitude are usually noted when describing the normal background.

*Deviations from normal* must be described by indicating the specific features which make a pattern abnormal, for instance the appearance of alpha activity which has a frontal maximum, lacks reactivity and is associated with coma.

**26.1.3** *Hyperventilation. Normal responses* can be described in one short sentence, for instance 'Hyperventilation produced no change' or 'Hyperventilation produced buildup of bilaterally synchronous slow waves'. The performance of the patient may be mentioned. Symptoms induced by hyperventilation should be reported, particularly if the symptoms resemble episodic symptoms for which the patient is examined. Changes in the patient's behavior, such as jerking movements or loss of responsiveness must be reported.

*Abnormal responses* such as an asymmetrical buildup, enhancement of abnormalities of the resting record and induction of new abnormalities must be described in detail.

**26.1.4** *Photic stimulation.* *Normal responses* can be described briefly by stating 'Photic stimulation elicited no responses' or 'Photic stimulation elicited symmetrical occipital driving'.

*Abnormal responses* such as significant asymmetries and photoconvulsive responses must be described.

**26.1.5** *Sleep.* *Normal sleep* activity can be described by stating 'Sleep was associated with normal EEG patterns'. The report should indicate if sleep occurred spontaneously or was induced with a sedative. If no epileptiform activity appeared, the length and depth of sleep may be of importance. The report may state 'Sleep was induced with chloral hydrate and was associated with normal patterns during about 20 minutes of recording during light sleep'. An exact specification of sleep stages is usually not necessary.

*Abnormalities during sleep* should be described in detail. Most important is the appearance of epileptiform activity. Other abnormalities of clinical significance include persistence of abnormal patterns seen in the waking record, abnormal sleep patterns and sleep onset REM periods. Patterns of doubtful clinical significance such as 6 Hz spike-and-slow-wave, 14 and 6 Hz positive bursts, small sharp spikes and rhythmical midtemporal discharges may be mentioned, but their unknown significance must be stressed either in the report or in the interpretation to avoid confusion with clinically significant EEG abnormalities.

The diagnostically important features of the EEG should be summarized under a separate heading.

**26.2.1** *The diagnosis of a normal EEG* should state whether it was based on a waking record only or whether a sleep recording was also obtained: 'The EEG during wakefulness and sleep was normal'. Reports of patients younger or older than 20–60 years of age may indicate that the EEG was normal by age-dependent standards: 'The EEG during wakefulness and sleep was normal for the age of this patient'.

**26.2.2** *Abnormal findings* are categorized qualitatively and quantitatively as described in the preceding chapters. Only the major, diagnostically important features of abnormalities described in the report are repeated. Focal epileptiform activity is described by shape, distribution, incidence and clinical accompaniments, for example: 'The EEG showed intermittent sharp waves in the left anterior temporal area during sleep'; 'The EEG showed three episodes of seizure discharges in the right central and temporal areas, associated with rhythmical twitching of the left arm'.

*Generalized epileptiform activity* is characterized by its pattern, incidence and clinical associations: 'The EEG showed bursts of generalized 3 Hz spike-and-wave complexes during hyperventilation associated with loss of responsiveness'.

*Special patterns* should be mentioned by their name, especially if the name was given in the report: 'This record shows hypsarrhythmia' or 'This EEG shows periodic lateralizing epileptiform discharges over the left posterior head'.

*Focal slow waves* are described by distribution and degree: 'This record shows moderate focal slow waves in the right frontal area'.

*Generalized asynchronous slow waves* are described by distribution and degree: 'This record shows marked generalized asynchronous slow waves with a maximum in both temporal areas'.

*Bisynchronous slow waves* are described by distribution and degree: 'This record shows moderate bisynchronous slow waves with a maximum in both frontal areas'.

*Asymmetries* are described by distribution and degree; if it is doubtful whether the amplitude on one side is decreased or that on the other side is increased, this should be indicated: 'The EEG during wakefulness and sleep showed a mild asymmetry of amplitude over the frontal areas, consisting of an apparent reduction of amplitude on the right side'.

*Generalized changes of amplitude* should be described by degree: 'The EEG showed activity of very low amplitude' (i.e. less than 10 $\mu$V), or 'The EEG of this comatose patient on artificial respiration was made in the Intensive Care Unit with standards recommended by the American EEG Society. It shows no electrocerebral activity over 2 $\mu$V'.

*Deviations from normal patterns* are briefly summarized by their characteristic abnormality: 'The EEG showed failure of alpha rhythm to block over the left posterior head region on eye opening'.

## 26.3 CLINICAL INTERPRETATION

**26.3.1** *Normal records* generally do not need an interpretation. Exceptions should be made in cases of apparent discrepancies between the EEG and the clinical condition of the patient. This is especially true if the patient has clinical abnormalities during the recording as in the example of a report given above. Other interpretations of normal reports may be of interest to some, but not all recipients of EEG reports; the EEG reader should try to tailor his reports to the needs of the referring physician. Thus, in the case of a patient with dementia, the interpretation may add that 'a normal EEG may be seen in mild or even moderately advanced cases of presenile and senile dementia'. In the case of a person suspected of having seizures, the interpretation may be that 'many patients with epilepsy show no epileptiform activity in their first EEG, even if it includes a sleep recording'.

**26.3.2** *Abnormal findings* must be interpreted. Without interpretation, the report of an abnormal EEG finding is as meaningless as an X-ray report that lists opacities and translucencies but does not say whether they indicate a fracture. To interpret an abnormal EEG, the reader should take into consideration each abnormal pattern and mentally scan its general pathological and specific clinical correlates as outlined in the preceding chapters and tables. To arrive at a meaningful interpretation, he must compare the many possible clinical correlates of the EEG patterns with the clinical presentation of the case and must select the diagnoses most likely to satisfy both (15.3). Clearly, the interpretation will improve with the amount of clinical information given to the EEG reader and with the reader's ability to match the abnormal patterns with the clinical presentation.

**26.3.3** *Recommendations for further diagnostic work* may be appropriate in some cases. Repeat EEG recordings may help to answer questions whether focal slow waves are postictal, i.e. whether they disappear after several days without seizures. The failure to obtain a sleep recording in a patient suspected of having partial complex seizures may lead to the suggestion to have the patient return sedated. A patient with a suspected seizure disorder who shows no epileptiform activity in his first EEG including a sleep recording may show epileptiform discharges in a second or third EEG recording. Repeat recordings may better evaluate the condition of patients with acute and transient changes resulting from head injuries, cardio-respiratory arrest or drug effects. The presence of muscle artifact preventing the interpretation of an EEG of a patient with suspected cerebral death may lead to the proposal to use neuromuscular blocking agents during the recording. All-night sleep recordings may be indicated for patients with possible diagnoses of narcolepsy, sleep apnea and other disturbances of wakefulness and sleep. Unexplained focal slow waves may prompt the recommendation of further diagnostic studies.

## REFERENCES

Schneider, J. (1977) Section IV. The EEG report. In: Rémond, A. (Ed.), Handbook of Electroenceph. clin. Neurophysiol., Vol. 11A, Elsevier, Amsterdam, pp. 97–109.

# Appendix

## LIST OF MAJOR MANUFACTURERS OF EEG MACHINES

This list is incomplete and does not mean to indicate that the equipment of the manufacturers listed is better than other equipment.

**Alvar Electronic**
6 bis, rue du progrès
F 93511 Montreuil Cedex
France

**Beckman Instruments, Inc.**
3900 N. River Road
Schiller Park
Illinois 60176
U.S.A.

**DISA Elektronik A/S**
DK-2740 Skovlunde
Denmark

**Fritz Schwarzer GmbH**
Bärmanstr. 38
D-8000 Munich
West Germany

**Grass Instrument Co.**
101 Old Colony Ave.
Quincy
Massachusetts
U.S.A.

**Medelec Limited**
Manor Way
Woking
Surrey
England

**Nihon Kohden Kogyo Co. Ltd.**
31-4, Nishiochiai 1-chome
Shinjuku-ku
Tokyo 161
Japan

**O.T.E. Biomedica**
P.O. Box 400
50100 Florence
Italy

**San-ei Instrument Co. Ltd.**
1-57, Tenjin-cho
Kodaira City
Tokyo 187
Japan

**Siemens-Elema AB**
Medicinsk Teknik
Solna
Sweden

# Index

Numbers in the index refer to pages; italicized numbers distinguish major from minor items.


Abnormal EEG, definition, 235–236
Abscess
  *see* Brain abscess
Absence, *254–256*, 291
  atypical, *254–255*, 314
  status, *255*, 291
Abundance, 156
Action potential, 10–11
Activation procedures, 219–229
Active reference electrode, 67–68
Active sleep, 163
Activité moyenne, 165
Acute intermittent porphyria, 305, 353, 390, 434
Acute stroke
  *see* Stroke, acute
Acute subdural hematoma, 356, *393*, 406
Addison's disease, 305, 390, 434
Adversive seizure, 251
Agyria, 278, 305
Air embolism, 354, *373*, 426
Akinetic seizures, 257
Alcohol, intoxication, *370*, 434, 445
  withdrawal, 306, *370*, 448
Alerting response, 15, *421*
All-night sleep recording, 95–96, 207–208
Alpha frequency, definition, 151
  coma pattern, 438–441
  ictal, *330*, 435, *441*
Alpha rhythm. description, 183–189
  asymmetry, abnormal, 410–411
    normal, 186
  frequency, decrease, 434–435
    increase, 435–437
    normal, 185
  normal development, adults, 183–189
    children, 177
    old people, 213–214
  paradoxical, 187
Alpha variant, fast, *189*, 432
  slow, 178, *187*
Alternating current (A.C.) amplifier, 55
Alternating current, impedance measurement, 27
  *see also* Interference
Alternating montages, 73
Alternating seizures, 258
Alzheimer's disease *see* Senile dementia
Amaurotic familial idiocy, 369
American EEG Society, guidelines in EEG
  minimum technical standards, general, 85–92
    pediatric EEG, 92–95
    suspected cerebral death, 96–100
  standard montages, 73–75
  telephone transmission, 101–102
Amplifier, 41–48
Amplitude, measurement, 152
  result of impedance of tissue, 16
    of interelectrode distance, 68, 418
Amplitude, abnormality, 239–240
  asymmetry, 397–412
  increase and decrease, 415–429
Anesthesia, barbiturates, 325, *371*
Aneurysm, cerebral, 355
  *see also* Subarachnoid hemorrhage
Anoxia, 9, 353, 369, 390, 403, *423*, 425, 434
Anoxic encephalopathy
  *see* Postanoxic encephalopathy
Anterior–posterior bipolar montages, 72
Anxiety, 427, 428
Aphasic seizures, 251
Arousal, 15, *421*
Arrhythmical waves, 151, 341
Artifacts, 17–18, *105–117*
  blink, 105
  cardiac pacemaker, 111, 115
  chewing, *110*, 112
  coughing, 112
  dental restoration, 113
  electrocardiogram, 110–112
  electrode, 115–117
  eye movement, 105–109
  glossokinetic, 112–113
  heart beat, 110–111
  hiccoughing, 112
  interference, 113–115
  intravenous drip, 115
  lid flutter, 107

movement, 110
muscle, 109–110
palatal myoclonus, 113
paper stop, 61
perspiration, 112
pulse wave, 112
rapid eye movement, 105–107
rejection, 46–47
60 Hz, 29, 46, 57, *113–115*
sobbing, 113
sucking, 110,112
swallowing, 112
tongue movement, 112–113
tremor, 110, 367
Ascending reticular activating system, 15
Asymmetry, 152–153
abnormal, 239–240, 397–412
alpha rhythm, 186, 410–411
beta and mu rhythms, 411
photic response, 411–412
sleep activity, 412
Asychronous, 155
Atonic seizure, 257
Atropine, 370
Attention, 15
Atypical absence, 314
Auditory evoked potential, 134–135
Auditory seizures, 251
Aura, 257
Autocorrelation, 125–128
Automatism, 253
Average evoked potential, 128–136
Average reference electrode, 40, *68–69*

Balanced amplifier, 43
Balanced noncephalic reference electrode, 111
Barbiturate, effect, 325, *371*, 423–425, 428, 434, 445
withdrawal, 306, *371*, 448
Basilar artery, insufficiency, 425–426
migraine, 279, *306*, 355, 392
Bemegride, 228–229
Benign epilepsy of childhood with rolandic spikes, 281
Benign epileptiform transients of sleep (BETS), 338
Benign intracranial hypertension, 394
Benzodiazepines, 428
Beta activity, ictal, 298, 311, *330*, 411, 441
Beta frequency, 151
Beta rhythm, asymmetry, 411
excessive, 418, 420, *428–429*
normal development, adults, 189–191
children, 178
old persons, 214
Bias potential, 30
Bilateral massive epileptic myoclonus, 256
Bilaterally synchronous, definition, 17, *155*
slow waves, 379–395
Binswanger's disease, 327
Bipolar montage, 65–67, 73–75
Bisynchronous
*see* Bilaterally synchronous
Blindness, 338, *437*
Blink artifact, 105
Block montage, 72–73
Blocking of amplifiers, 30
Blood sugar, 221
*see also* Hypoglycemia
Brain abscess, 281, 321, *357*, 409, 411
Brain death
*see* Cerebral death
Brain stem auditory evoked potential, 134–135
Brain stem stroke, 354, *373*, 392, 438
Brain stem tumor, 356, *393–394*, 435
Brain surgery, 279, 280, 356, 393, *406–407*, 412
Brain tumor, infratentorial, 356, *393–394*, 435
multiple metastases, 356, *374*
supratentorial, *280*, 321, 327, *356*, 374, 394, 409, 411, 412, 435
Burr holes, 33–34, *406–407*
Burst-suppression pattern, 325

Calibration, description of procedure, 40–41
filter effects, 53, 56
recommendations, electrocerebral silence, 98
general recording, 87–88
sensitivity testing, 48
Capacitor input coupling, 55
Carbon monoxide poisoning, 353, *371–372*, 390
Cardiac pacemaker artifact, 111, 115
Carotid endarterectomy, *354*, 405
Cell membrane potential, 7–13
Central beta rhythm, 330
Centrencephalic, definition, 17
seizures, 303
Cerebellar fits, 330, *426*
Cerebral abscess
*see* Brain abscess
concussion
*see* Head injury
contusion, *356*, 406
*see also* Head injury
death, diagnosis, 425
minimum recording standards, 96–100
*see also* Electrocerebral silence
infarct
*see* Stroke
palsy, 368
*see also* Perinatal cerebral damage
tumor
*see* Brain tumor

Channel, definition, 37
Channels, number of recording
all-night sleep recording, 96
electrocerebral silence 97
general recordings, 86
infants and small children, 93
magnetic tape, 122
Chewing artifact, *110*, 112
Chorea
*see* Huntington's, Sydenham's chorea
Chronic subdural hematoma
*see* Subdural hematoma, chronic
Classification of seizures, 248–249, 250–258
Clip electrode, 24
Clonic seizures, *256*, 258, *294*, 314
CNS depressant drugs, 325, *370–372*, 423–425
Closed circuit TV monitoring, 120
Coherence function, 125
Collodion technique, 23
Common mode, *43*, 47
Complex, definition, 147–148
Compressed spectral array, 125
Computer analysis of EEG, 122–128
Computer averaging, 128–136
Computer, general purpose, special purpose, 123
Conceptional age, 95, 159
Concussion
*see* Head injury
Conduction, neuronal potentials, 11
*see also* Volume conduction
Contingent negative variation, 136
Contraversive seizures, 251
Contusion, *356*, 406
*see also* Head injury
Convulsant drugs, 228–229
Convulsions, definition, 246
*see also* Seizures
Coronal montages
*see* Montages, bipolar, transverse
Correlation analysis, 125–128
Cortical epilepsy, 303–304
Cortico-reticular seizures, 304
Coughing artifact, 112
Cranial defect, 356, *406–407*, 411
Cross-correlation, 125
Ctenoids, 337
Cup electrode, 23
Curvilinear distortion, 58–59

Death
*see* Cerebral death
DDT, 305
Decerebrate attacks, 330, 426
Decibels, 48
Déjà vu, entendu, vécu, 252
Delirium tremens, 370
Delta brushes 161
Delta frequency, 151
Dementia
*see* Senile dementia
Denervation supersensitivity, 277
Dental restoration artifact, 113
Depolarization, 10–11
Depression, endogenous, 435
Depth EEG (DEEG), 17
Depth electrodes, 26
Derivations,
*see* Montages
Descriptors, *147–157*, 452–453
Desynchronization, 15, 421
Deviations from normal patterns, 240, 431–449
Dialysis encephalopathy, 305, 390, 391
Diazepam, 428
Differential amplification, 43
Diffuse, definition, 153
Diffuse, cortical epilepsy, 303
Diphasic, definition, 147
Dipole, 71
Direct current (D.C.) amplifier, 55
Direct current, resistance measurement, 27
Disc electrode, 23
Discontinous pattern, 159–161
Discrimination, *43–47*, 115
Double grounding, 39
Down's syndrome, 368, 445
Dreamy state, 252
Drop attack, epileptic, 257
Drowsiness patterns, adults, 203
children and adolescents, 178
infants, 173
newborns, 165
old persons, 217
Drug intoxication, 325, *370–372*
Dyssynergia cerebellaris myoclonica, *304*, 389

Ear electrode, 73–75
Early posttraumatic seizures, 279–280
EEG diagnosis, 456–457
generator, 7–13
machines, manufacturers, 461
report, 451–459
Electrical field plotting, 69–71, 128
Electrocardiogram (ECG) artifact, 110–111
Electrocerebral silence or inactivity, 84
barbiturate intoxication, 423–425
cerebral death, 425
hypothermia, 423
low amplitude, 420
montages, 75
prognosis, 372–373

recording standards, 96–100
reporting, 452–453
Electroconvulsive therapy (ECT), 374
Electrocorticogram (ECoG), 16, 26, 280
Electrode, 21–34
application, 23–24
artifact, 115–117
average reference, 40, 68–69
ear, 73–75
clip, 24
cup, 23–24
depth, 26
disc, 23–24
electrocorticographic, 26
ground, 33, 38–39, 47, 85–86
impedance, measurement, *27–29*, 38, 88
recommended, general recording, 86
electrocerebral silence, 97
lead wire, 23
mandibular, 73–75
material, 26
nasopharyngeal, 25
needle, *24*, 85, 97
nonpolarizable, 30
paste, 23–24
placement, electrocerebral silence, 97
general recordings, 85–86
infants, 93
International 10-20 System, 30–34
polarization, 29–30
popping, 116
reference, 67, 73–75
active, 67–68
average, 40, *68–69*
balanced noncephalic, 111
resistance, *27*, 30
shape, 21–26
sphenoidal 25
tympanic 25
Electrodecremental seizure, 298, 311, 314, 325, *329–330*, 409, 426
Electrographic ictal epileptiform activity, 265
Electrographic status epilepticus, 269–270
Electrolyte imbalance, 301, 302, 369, *389–391*, 395
Electromagnetic interference, 113–115
Electromyogram (EMG), 79
Electrostatic interference, 113–115
Electrotonic conduction, 11, 17, 346, 407
Embolism
*see* Stroke, Air embolism, Fat embolism
Encephalitis, 281, 321, 325, *375*, 395, 409, 426–427, 435
*see also* Herpes simplex encephalitis
Epidural hematoma, 356, 393, 406
Epilepsia partialis continua, *247*, 321, 329, 357
Epilepsy, 246
*see also* Convulsions
Idiopathic epilepsy
Lafora's inclusion body epilepsy
Photosensitive epilepsy
Posttraumatic epilepsy
Rolandic epilepsy
Seizures
Status epilepticus
Symptomatic epilepsy
Epileptic drop attack, 257
Epileptic neuronal aggregate, 275
Epileptiform activity, definition, 149–150
focal, 261–283, 309–338
generalized, 285–307, 309–338
ictal, interictal, 149–150
Etat lacunaire, 354, 373, 434
Evoked potential, 128–136
auditory brain stem, 134–135
cortical *versus* brain stem, 130
somatosensory, 135
spinal, 135–136
visual, 130–133
diffuse flash, 133, 225
pattern reversal, 131–133
Excitatory postsynaptic potential, 10
Eye movement artifact, 90–92

Facial myokymia, 110
Familial dysautonomia, 305, 368
Far field evoked potential, 130
Fast alpha variant, *189*, 432
Fast waves, definition, 152
Fat embolism, 323, 354, *373*
Febrile seizures, 306
Fever
*see* Hyperthermia
Field plotting, *69–71*, 128
Filters, function, 49–57
high frequency, 55–57
low frequency, 49–55
recommended setting, electrocerebral silence, 98
general recordings, 87
infants and small children, 94
Flash response, 133, 223–225
Flat EEG, 84
*see also* Electrocerebral silence
Low amplitude
Low voltage EEG
Floating input, 47
Flurazepam, 429
Focal distribution, definition, 154
Focal epileptiform activity, 261–283
ictal, 262–265, 267–268

electrographic or subclinical, 265
interictal, 262–265, 265–267
special epileptiform patterns, 309–338
Focal motor seizures, 250
Focal seizures, 250
*see also* Partial seizures
Focal slow waves, 341–358
localizing value, 346
old persons, 215
time course, 345–346
14 and 6 Hz positive bursts, 179, *337*
Frequency, 151–152
Frequency modulation (FM), 121
Frontal intermittent rhythmical delta activity (FIRDA), 381–386

Gain, 48
Generalized, definition, 153
Generalized asynchronous slow waves, 359–376
Generalized epileptiform activity, 285–307
Generalized seizures, ictal patterns, 291–298, 311, 314, 317, 323, 327–330
interictal patterns, 289–291, 311, 314, 323
special epileptiform patterns, 309–338
*see also* Absence
Akinetic seizures
Atonic seizures
Bilateral massive epileptic myoclonus
Clonic seizures
Infantile spasms
Tonic-clonic seizures
Tonic seizures
Generator of the EEG, 7–13
Gestational age, 95, 159
Glossokinetic artifact, 112–113
Grand mal seizures
*see* Tonic-clonic seizures
Grid 1, grid 2, 43
Ground electrode, 33, 38–39, 47, 85–86
Grounded input, 40
Guidelines in EEG, 85

Haloperidol, 305, 371
Headache, 373
Head injury, 279–280, 325, 355–356, *373–374,* 393, 406, 411, 426, 434–435
Heart beat artifact, 110–111
Heart beat monitoring, 78, 93, 99
Hematoma
*see* Epidural hematoma
Stroke
Subarachnoid hematoma
Subdural hematoma
Subgaleal hematoma
Hemiconvulsions, hemiplegia and epilepsy (HHE) syndrome, 283
Hemispherectomy, 356, *407–409*
Hepatic encephalopathy, 305, 327, 369, 371, 390, 423, 428, 429, 434
Heredity in epilepsy, 304
Herpes simplex enephalitis, 283, 325–327, 357
Hiccoughing artifact, 112
High amplitude, 152, 418
High frequency filter, 55–57
Holoprosencephaly, 278, 305, 353, 368, 404
Huntington's chorea, 367, *422*
Hydrocephalus, 278, 352, *368*, 389
Hypercalcemia, 327, 353, 390, 434, 445
Hypernatremia, 327
Hyperosmolar coma, 353
Hyperosmolar nonketotic hyperglycemia, 278, 305, 390
Hyperparathyroidism, 353, 390, 434, 445
Hyperpolarization, 10
Hypersynchrony, 275
Hyperthermia, 306, 375, 395, *423*, 435, 437
Hyperthyroidism, 370, 390, 428, *435–437*, 445
Hyperventilation, 88, 91, *219–222*
Hypnagogic hypersynchrony, 173
Hypocalcemia, 305, 390, 423, 427, 429, 434
Hypoglycemia, 221, 305, 311, 353, 369, 390, 403, 434, 438
Hypokalemia, 390
Hyponatremia, 305, 327, 390
Hypoparathyroidism, 305, 390, 423, 427, 429, 434
Hypothermia, 325, *423*
Hypothyroidism, 370, *423*, 426, 427, 429, 434
Hypoxia
*see* Anoxia
Hypsarrhythmia, 311

Ictal alpha frequency waves, *330*, 435, 441
Ictal beta activity, 298, 311, *330*, 411, 441
Ictal decrease of amplitude
*see* Electrodecremental seizure
Ictal epileptiform activity, 148–149
focal, 262–268
generalized, 286, 291–298
Ictal fast activity, 294, 311, 330
Ictal slow waves, focal, 329, 357
generalized, 329, 374
Idiopathic epilepsy, 299, *307*
Imbalance of input impedance, 46–47
Immature patterns, 449
Impedance, electrode
*see* Electrode impedance
Impedance meter, *27–29*, 38
Impedance causing asymmetry, 404
Increased amplitude, 302, 418

Increased intracranial pressure, 387
Independent, definition, 155–156
Independent multifocal spikes, 317
Index of activity, 156
Infantile hemiplegia, 368
Infantile spasms, 256, 311, 329
Infants, montages, 75
  recording standards, 92–95
Infarct, cerebral
  *see* Stroke
Infratentorial brain tumors, 356, *393–394*, 435
INH treatment, 305
Inhibitory motor seizures, 251
Inhibitory postsynaptic potential, 10
In phase, 154
Input board, 38–39
Input, closed, 40
  differential, 43
  floating, 47
  grounded, 40
  leakage current, 38–39
  selector switches, 39–40
  short-circuited, 40
  single-ended, 46–47
Input 1, input 2, 43, 65
Interelectrode distance, effect on amplitude, 68, 418
  electrocerebral silence, 97–98
  heart beat artifact, 110–111
Interference, 29, 46, 57, *113–115*
Interictal asymmetry, 409
Interictal epileptiform activity, 149–150
  focal, 261–283, 309–338
  generalized, 285–307, 309–338
Interictal slow waves, focal, 357
  generalized, 374, 394
International classification of seizures, 247–258
International 10-20 System, 30–34
Intoxication, alcohol, 370
  drugs, 305, 371–372
Intracerebral hemorrhage, spontaneous
  *see* Stroke
  traumatic, 356, 406
Intravenous drip artifact, 115
Irregular, definition, 147
Isoelectric EEG, 84
  *see also* Electrocerebral silence
    Low amplitude
    Low voltage EEG
Isopotential lines, 69–71

Jacksonian seizures, 251
Jakob-Creutzfeldt disease, 23, 277–278, 304, *323*, 327, 352, 367, 422
Jamais vu, entendu, vécu, 252

Kappa rhythm, 194
K complex, 175, 203
Kindling, 277
Kleine–Levin syndrome, 395, 445
Korsakoff's psychosis, 370
Krabbe's disease, 369, 391

Labelling of EEG record, 82–92, 95
Lacunar state, 354, 373, 434
Lafora's inclusion body epilepsy, 304
Lambda waves, 193
Late traumatic epilepsy, 280
Lateralized, definition, 153
Lead poisoning, 305, 372
Lead wire, electrodes, 23
Leakage current at input, 38–39
Leber's hereditary optic atrophy, 368, 389
Leigh's disease, 368
Length of recording, electrocerebral silence, 100
  general recordings, 88
  infants, 94
Lennox–Gastaut syndrome, 314
Lid flutter artifact, 107
Linear EEG, 84
  *see also* Electrocerebral silence
    Low amplitude
    Low voltage EEG
Lithium intoxication, 327, 372, 434
Longitudinal bipolar montages, 73–75
Low amplitude, 152, 418
Low frequency filter, 49–55
Low pressure hydrocephalus, 352, 367–368
Low voltage EEG, 195, 419, 427

Magnetic tape recording, 121–122
Mandibular electrode, 73–75
Marihuana, 434
Master selector switch, 39–40
Master sensitivity switch, 48
Membrane potential, 9
Meningitis, 281, 321, 357, 375, 395, 426–427, 435
Mercury poisoning, 305, 372
Metachromatic leukodystrophy, 369, 391, 429
Metal cup and disc electrodes, 23–24
Metastatic brain tumors, multiple, 356, *374*
Metrizamide, 353, 370
Midbrain reticular formation, 15
Microcephaly, 368, 422
Microgyria, 278, 305
Migraine, *355*, 373, *406*, 411, 412
Minimum technical standards, 83–102
  general recordings, 85–92
  infants and small children, 92–95
  sleep recordings, all-night, 95–96

suspected cerebral death, 96–100
telephone transmission, 101–102
Mirror focus, 265–267, 277, 280
Mongolian idiocy, 368, 445
Monitoring extracerebral activity, 75–79
electrocerebral silence, 99–100
eye movements, 76–78
all-night sleep, 95, 208
newborns, 93
sleep, 205–207
heart beat, 78, 93, 99
movement, 79, 99
muscle activity, 75, 95, 208
respiration, 78–79, 93, 96, 209
Monophasic, definition, 147
Monopolar, definition, 47
*see also* Montages, referential
Monorhythmic frontal delta (MFD), 386
Montages, 72–75
alternating, 73
bipolar, longitudinal and transverse, 65–67, 73–75
block, 72–73
electrocerebral silence, 75
recommended, general recording, 86
infants, 93
suspected cerebral death, 97–98
infants, 75
labelling, 92
monopolar
*see* referential
referential, 67–68, 73–75
Movement-activated myoclonus, 330
Movement, artifact, 110
monitoring, 79
Moyamoya disease, 393
Multichannel recordings, 63–71
Multifocal spikes, 317
Multiple metastases, 356, *374*
Multiple sclerosis, 353, *368*, 389, 405, 422
Multiple sleep latency test, 209
Multiple spike
*see* Polyspike
Multiple spike-and-slow-wave
*see* Polyspike-and-slow-wave
Multiple strokes, *354*, 373, 434, 438
*see also* Lacunar state
Mu rhythm, adults, 191–192
children, 178
paradoxical, 192
Muscle activity monitoring, 79, 95, 208
Muscle artifact, 109–110
Musicogenic epilepsy, 228
Myoclonic jerks, 256, 323, 325, 327, 329, 330
Myoclonus epilepsy, 304, 327
Myotonic dystrophy, 368, 389, 434

Narcolepsy, 209, 445
Nasopharyngeal electrode, 25
Needle electrode, *24*, 85, 97
Negative polarity, *43*, 65
Neurotransmitter, 10
Nonketotic hyperosmolar hyperglycemia, 253, 278, 305, 390
Nonpolarizable electrode, 30
Non-REM sleep, 174–175, 203–205, 207–208
Normal EEG, definition, 143–146
Normal pressure hydrocephalus, 352, 367–368
Number of recording channels
*see* Channels, number of recording

Occipital spikes of blind persons, 338
Ohmmeter, 27
Old strokes, 279, 345
Olfactory seizures, 251
Optic neuritis, 131, 278, 353
Organic solvents, poisoning, 305, 372
Oscillograph, 57
Oscilloscope display, 119–120
Out of phase, 154

Pacemaker hypotheses, bisynchronous slow waves, 388–389
epilepsy, 303
rhythmical activity of thalamus, 13–15
Pachygyria, 278
Palatal myoclonus artifact, 113
Paper speed, 61, 88
Paper stop artifact, 61
Paper transport, 61–62
Paradoxical alpha rhythm, 187
mu rhythm, 192
sleep, 205
slow wave respons to alerting, 441
Parkinson's disease, 110, *367*, 389
Paroxysm, definition, 150
Paroxysmal depolarizing shift, 275
Partial seizures, ictal patterns, 267–268, 327–330, 441
interictal patterns, 265–267, 317
with complex symptoms
*see also* Automatism
Déjà vu
Dreamy state
Jamai vu
Psychomotor seizures
Psychosensory seizures
with elementary symptoms
*see also* Adversive seizures
Aphasic seizures
Auditory seizures

Contraversive seizures
Focal motor seizures
Gustatory seizures
Inhibitory motor seizures
Jacksonian seizures
Olfactory seizures
Phonatory seizures
Postural seizures
Somatosensory seizures
Versive seizures
Vertiginous seizures
Visual seizures
Pattern reversal evoked potential, 131–133
Pattern sensitivity, 227
Pattern shift evoked potential, 131–133
Pelizaeus-Merzbacher's disease, 369, 445
Pen alignment, 59–61
Pen, writing, 58–61
Penicillin intoxication, 327
Pentylene tetrazol, 228–229
Perinatal cerebral damage, *272*, 309, 311, 314, 317, 330, 353, 404, 441
Periodic complexes, 317–327
definition, 151
generalized complexes of SSPE, 323–325
generalized sharp waves of Jakob-Creutzfeldt disease, 323
lateralizing epileptiform discharges (PLEDs), 321
slow waves, 329
temporal sharp waves of herpes simplex encephalitis, 325–327
Pernicious anemia, 353, 390, 391, 434
Perspiration artifact, 112
Persistence, definition, 156
Pesticide intoxication, 305
Petit mal
*see* Absence
Petit mal pattern
*see* 3 Hz spike-and-wave pattern
Petit mal variant pattern
*see* Slow spike-and-wave pattern
Phase, definition, 154
reversal, 65, 154
Phenothiazine, 305, 371, 429, 434
Phenylketonuria, 311, 369, 429
Phonatory seizures, 251
Photic driving, *225*, 411–412, 445
Photic stimulation, 88–89, 94, 223–226
Photoconvulsive response, 226, 370, 371, *445–448*
Photometrazol test, 229
Photomyoclonic response, 226, *448–449*
Photosensitive epilepsy, 88–89, 448
Pick's disease, 367
Poisons
*see* Intoxication
Polarity, electrical, *43*, 65
Polarization of electrodes, 29–30
Polymorphic delta waves
*see* Arrhythmical waves
Polyphasic wave, definition, 147
Polyspike-and-slow-wave, definition, 149
ictal, 294
interictal, 289
Polyspike, definition, 149
interictal, 291
Pontine lesions, 373, 438
Porencephaly, 278, 353, 404, 411
Porphyria, 305, 353, 390, 434
Positive occipital sharp transients of sleep (POSTs), 179, *201–202*
Positive polarity, *43*, 65
Postanoxic encephalopathy, 306, 323, 325, 327, 330, *372–373*, 392, 405, 425, 434, 438
Postanoxic myoclonus, 323, 330, 411
Postictal decrease of alpha rhythm frequency, 435
Postictal decrease of amplitude, 409
Postictal slow waves, focal, 357
generalized, 374, 395
Postoperative focal seizures, 279–280
Postsynaptic potentials, 9–10
Posttraumatic epilepsy, 280
Posttraumatic seizures, early, 279–280
Postural seizures, 251
Potential, action, 10–11
bias, 30
membrane, 9
postsynaptic, 9–10
resting, 9
Power spectrum, 123–125
Presenile dementia,
*see* Senile dementia
Primary generalized seizures
*see* Generalized seizures
Primary subcortical seizures, 303
Progressive multifocal leukoencephalopathy, 358, 375, 409, 427
Progressive supranuclear palsy, *367*, 389, 429, 445
Progressive traumatic encephalopathy, 356, *374*, 393, 434–435
Projected rhythms, 17
slow waves, 386
Prominence, definition, 156
Pseudo-epileptogenic patterns, 331–338
Pseudohypoparathyroidism, 390, 423, 427
Pseudotumor cerebri, 394
Psychomotor seizures, 253
varant pattern

*see* Rhythmical midtemporal discharges
Psychosensory seizures, 253
Psychotropic drugs, 370, 371, 434, 445
Pulse wave artifact, 112
Pyramidal neurons, 11
Pyridoxine deficiency, 305, 311

Quiet sleep, 163

Rage, 253
Ramsey-Hunt syndrome, *304*, 389
Random, 156
Rapid eye movement (REM)
*see* Artifact, rapid eye movement
Monitoring, eye movement
REM sleep
Rauwolfia derivatives, 305, 371
Reactivity, definition, 156–157
test in electrocerebral silence, 99
Reading epilepsy, 228
Recording channel
*see* Channel
Recording techniques
*see* Minimum technical standards
Recording strategy of montages, 63–79
Reference electrode
*see* Electrode, reference
Referential montage, 67–68, 73–75
Reflex epilepsy, 227–229, 247, 269, 298
Regular, definition, 147
Rejection ratio, 45
REM sleep, normal patterns, adults, 205–207
children, 179
infants, 174
old persons, 217
*see also* Active sleep
reduction, 445
sleep cycles, 208
Renal encephalopathy
*see* Uremic encephalopathy
Resistance, electrode, *27*, 30
Respiration monitoring, 78–79, 93, 96, 209
Respiratory arrest, 425
Resting potential, 9
Reticular activating system, 15
Retrobulbar neuritis, 131, 278, 353
Reye's syndrome, 325, 337
Rhythmes à distance, 17, 386
Rhythmical, definition, 150
midtemporal discharges (RMTD), 337–338
Rhythmicity, 13–15
Riley-Day syndrome, 305, 368
Ripples of prematurity, 161
Rolandic epilepsy, 281

Scalp edema, 406
Schilder's disease, 353, *368*
Schizophrenia, *376*, 395, 435
Secondary bilateral synchrony, 303
Secondary generalization, 272–274, 303
Secondary generalized seizures, 254
Sedation for sleep recordings, 89, 94
Seitelberger's disease, 368
Seizures, centrencephalic, 303
classification, 247–258
definition, 245–246
generalized
*see* Generalized seizures
partial
*see* Partial seizures
pattern, definition, 149
unclassified, 258
unilateral, 258
Selector switch, input, 39–40
Senile dementia, 277, 352, *366*, 389, 422, 434
Sensitivity, definition, 48
recommended, electrocerebral silence 98
general recordings, 86–87
infants, 94
Sensitivity switch, amplifier, 48
Sharp transient, definition, 149
Sharp-and-slow-wave, definition, 149
ictal and interictal, 291–294, 314
Sharp wave, definition, 149
*see also* Epileptiform activity
Shielding of recording room, 115
*see also* 60 Hz artifact
Short latency to sleep onset, 209, 445
Shorted input, 40
Signal averaging, 128–129
Simultaneous, definition, 155
Single-ended recording, 46–47
Sinusoidal, definition, 147
6 Hz spike-and-slow-wave pattern, 291, *331*
60 Hz artifact, 29, 46, 57, *113–115*
filter, 57
Skull defect, 356, *406–407*, 411
Sleep, activation of epileptiform activity, 222–223
active, 163
all-night recording, 95–96
*see also* Sleep cycles
apnea, 209, 445
cycles, 207–208
disordered, 445
deprivation, 223
onset latency, 209, 445
onset REM periods (SOREMP), 209,445
patterns, asymmetry, 412
coma, 441
normal adult, 201–208

children and adolescents, 178–179
infants, 174–175
newborns, 165–170
old persons, 217
prematures, 161–163
quiet, 163
rapid eye movement
*see* REM sleep
slow eye movements, 203
spindles, 175, 202
stages, 174–175, 203–207
Slow alpha variant, 178, *187*
Slow eye movements of sleep, 203
Slow spike-and-wave pattern, definition, 149, 291
ictal and interictal patterns, 291–294, *311–314*, 329
Slow wave, definition, 152
abnormality, 238–239, 341–395
Small sharp spikes (sss), 338
Sobbing artifact, 113
Sphenoidal electrodes, 25
Sodium pump, 9
Somatosensory evoked potential, 135
Somatosensory seizures, 251
Spectral analysis, 123–125
Spike-and-wave, definition, 149
ictal and interictal patterns, 289, 291
Spike, definition, 148–149
*see also* Epileptiform activity
Spinal evoked potential, 135–136
Spindles, definition, 151
*see also* Sleep spindles
Sporadic, definition, 156
Standards, minimum technical
*see* Minimum technical standards
Startle myoclonus, 323
seizures, 227–228
Status epilepticus, absences, 255, 291
definition, 246–247
neonatal and infantile, 330, 441
partial, 269, 357
subclinical or electrographic, 270
Status lacunaris, 354, 373, 434
Stereotaxic operations, 280, 393
Stimulation, activation procedures, 223–229
coma, electrocerebral silence, 99, 441
evoked potentials, 128–136
photic, 88–89, 94, 223–226
Stokes-Adams attacks, 372, 425
Stroke, brain stem, 354, *373*, 392, 438
cerebral, *353*, 392, 405, 410–411, 412, 434
acute, *279*, 306, 321, 325, 327, 345
multiple,
*see* Multiple strokes
old, 279, 345–346
Sturge-Weber syndrome, *278*, 305, 311, *404–405*, 409, 412
Subacute sclerosing panencephalitis (SSPE), 314, *323–325*, 329, 375
Subarachnoid hemorrhage, *355*, 393, 406, 434
Subclinical ictal epileptiform activity, 150, 265
Subclinical status epilepticus, 269–270
Subcortical epilepsy, 303
Subdural hematoma, acute, 356, *393*, 406
chronic, 279, 321, 327, *355*, 371, 373, 392, *405–406*, 410, 425, 434
Subgaleal hematoma, 406
Sucking artifact, 110, 112
Suppression-burst pattern, 325
Supratentorial brain tumor
*see* Brain tumor, supratentorial
Swallowing artifact, 112
Sydenham's chorea, 283, *375*, 395
Sylvian seizures, 281
Symptomatic epilepsy, 245, 271–272
Synaptic potentials, 9–10
transmitter, 10
Synchronization, 13–15, 388–389
Synchronous, defintion, 155
Syncope, 372, 392, *425*

Telemetry, 120
Telephone transmission of EEG, 101–102
Television seizures, 227
Temporal lobectomy, 229
Temporal lobe seizures
*see* Partial seizures with complex symptoms
Temporal slow waves of old persons, 215
10 Hz spike discharge, 294, 314
10-20 System, International, 30–34
Terminology, 147–157, 452–453
Thalamic pacemaker, 13–15
Theta frequency, 151
Thiamine deficiency
*see* Leigh's disease, Wernicke's encephalopathy
3 Hz rhythmical slow waves, 329, 394
3 Hz spike-and-wave pattern, 289, 291
Thrombophlebitis of the cerebral venous sinuses, 281–283, 409
Thrombosis
*see* Stroke
Time constant, 53–55
Time marker, 61
Todd's paralysis, 246
Tongue movement artifact, 112–113
Tonic seizures, *256*, 258, *294*, 311, 314, 325, 329, 330
Tonic-clonic seizures, *257*, 258, *294*, 314
Tracé alternant, 165

Tranquilizer, 428
Transient, definition, 147–148
Transient global amnesia, 279, *354*
Transient ischemic attack, brain stem, 372, 392, 434
  cerebral, 354, 405, 434
Transverse bipolar montages, 73–75
Traumatic seizures, 279–280
Tremor artifact, 110, 367
Tricyclic antidepressants, 305, *371*, 429, 445
Triphasic, definition, 147
  waves, 327
Trouble shooting, 115–117
Tuberous sclerosis, *278*, 311, 353, *368*, 389
Tumors
  *see* Brain tumors
Tympanic electrodes, 25

Unclassified seizures, 258
Unilateral epileptiform activity, 274
Unilateral seizures, 258
Unipolar
  *see* Monopolar
Unverricht-Lundborg's myoclonus epilepsy, *304*, 327
Uremic encephalopathy, 305, 327, 369, 390, 405, 423, 429, 434, 445

Vascular malformation, 355
Ventricular shunt, 280
Versive seizures, 251
Vertebro-basilar insufficiency, 425–426
  *see also* Transient ischemic attack, brain stem
Vertex sharp transient (V wave), *175*, 193–194, *202*
Violence in seizures, 253
Visual evoked potential,
  *see* Evoked potential, visual
Visual seizures, 251
Vitamin $B_{12}$ deficiency, 353, 390, *391*, 434
Volume conduction, 11–13, 17, 346, 406–409
V wave (vertex sharp transient), *175*, 193–194, 202

Wave, definition, 147
  form, 147–150
Wavelength, 151
Wernicke's encephalopathy, 325, *370,* 390, 391, 434
West syndrome, 311
Wicket rhythm
  *see* mu rhythm
Wicket spikes, 338
Widespread, definition, 153
Wilson's disease, 353, *369*, 390, 391
Withdrawal, from alcohol, 306, *370*, 448
  from barbiturates, 306, *371*, 448
Writing unit, 57–62